T0226852

Aging and Endocrinology

Editor

ANNE R. CAPPOLA

ENDOCRINOLOGY AND METABOLISM CLINICS OF NORTH AMERICA

www.endo.theclinics.com

Consulting Editor
DEREK LEROITH

June 2013 • Volume 42 • Number 2

ELSEVIER

1600 John F. Kennedy Boulevard • Suite 1800 • Philadelphia, Pennsylvania, 19103-2899

http://www.theclinics.com

ENDOCRINOLOGY AND METABOLISM CLINICS OF NORTH AMERICA Volume 42, Number 2 June 2013 ISSN 0889-8529, ISBN-13: 978-1-4557-7085-4

Editor: Pamela Hetherington

Endocrinology and Metabolism Clinics of North America (ISSN 0889-8529) is published quarterly by Elsevier Inc., 360 Park Avenue South, New York, NY 10010-1710. Months of issue are March, June, September, and December. Periodicals postage paid at New York, NY and additional mailing offices. Subscription prices are USD 313.00 per year for US individuals, USD 557.00 per year for US institutions, USD 159.00 per year for US students and residents, USD 393.00 per year for Canadian individuals, USD 681.00 per year for Canadian institutions, USD 456.00 per year for international individuals, USD 681.00 per year for international institutions, and USD 234.00 per year for international and Canadian and foreign students/residents. To receive student/resident rate, orders must be accompanied by name of affiliated institution, date of term, and the signature of program/residency coordinator on institution letterhead. Orders will be billed at individual rate until proof of status is received. Foreign air speed delivery is included in all *Clinics* subscription prices. All prices are subject to change without notice. **POSTMASTER:** Send address changes to *Endocrinology and Metabolism Clinics of North America*, Elsevier Health Sciences Division, Subscription Customer Service, 3251 Riverport Lane, Maryland Heights, MO 63043. **Customer Service: Telephone: 1-800-654-2452** (U.S. and Canada); **1-314-447-8871** (outside U.S. and Canada). **Fax: 1-314-447-8029. E-mail: journalscustomerservice-usa@elsevier.com** (for print support); **journalsonlinesupport-usa@elsevier.com** (for online support).

Reprints. For copies of 100 or more, of articles in this publication, please contact the Commercial Rights Department, Elsevier Inc., 360 Park Avenue South, New York, NY 10010-1710; phone: (+1) 212-633-3813; fax: (+1) 212-462-1935; e-mail: reprints@elsevier.com.

Endocrinology and Metabolism Clinics of North America is covered in *MEDLINE/PubMed (Index Medicus), EMBASE/Excerpta Medica, Current Contents/Clinical Medicine, Current Contents/Life Sciences, Science Citation Index, ISI/BIOMED, BIOSIS,* and *Chemical Abstracts*.

Printed and bound by CPI Group (UK) Ltd, Croydon, CR0 4YY

Transferred to digital print 2012

Contributors

CONSULTING EDITOR

DEREK LEROITH, MD, PhD
Director of Research, Division of Endocrinology, Metabolism, and Bone Diseases, Department of Medicine, Mount Sinai School of Medicine, New York, New York

EDITOR

ANNE R. CAPPOLA, MD, ScM
Associate Professor of Medicine, Division of Endocrinology, Diabetes, and Metabolism, Smilow Center for Translational Research, Perelman School of Medicine, University of Pennsylvania, Philadelphia, Pennsylvania

AUTHORS

ELIZABETH BARRETT-CONNOR, MD
Distinguished Professor, Department of Family and Preventive Medicine, University of California, San Diego, La Jolla, California

SHEHZAD BASARIA, MD
Associate Professor of Medicine, Medical Director, Men's Health, Aging and Metabolism, Brigham and Women's Hospital, Harvard Medical School, Boston, Massachusetts

ANNE CAUFRIEZ, MD, PhD
Associate Professor of Endocrinology and Faculty of Medicine, Laboratory of Physiology, Physiopathology, and CHU Saint-Pierre, Université Libre de Bruxelles, Brussels, Belgium

GEORGES COPINSCHI, MD, PhD
Professor Emeritus of Endocrinology and Faculty of Medicine, Laboratory of Physiology and Physiopathology, Université Libre de Bruxelles, Brussels, Belgium

LAURA E. COWEN, MD
Endocrinology Fellow, Division of Endocrinology and Metabolism, Georgetown University Medical Center, Washington, DC

CAROLYN J. CRANDALL, MD, MS
Professor of Medicine, Department of Medicine, David Geffen School of Medicine, University of California at Los Angeles, Los Angeles, California

DIMA L. DIAB, MD
Assistant Professor of Clinical Medicine, Division of Endocrinology/Metabolism, Department of Internal Medicine, Cincinnati VA Medical Center, Bone Health and Osteoporosis Center, University of Cincinnati, Cincinnati, Ohio

JOSEPHINE M. EGAN, MD
National Institute on Aging/National Institutes of Health, Baltimore, Maryland

J. CHRISTOPHER GALLAGHER, MD, MRCP
Professor of Medicine and Endocrinology, Endocrine Department, Creighton University Medical School, Omaha, Nebraska

STEVEN P. HODAK, MD
Medical Director, Center for Diabetes and Endocrinology, University of Pittsburgh Medical Center, Pittsburgh, Pennsylvania

RITA RASTOGI KALYANI, MD, MHS
Division of Endocrinology and Metabolism, Department of Medicine, Johns Hopkins University School of Medicine, The Johns Hopkins University, Baltimore, Maryland

THEODORE K. MALMSTROM, PhD
Assistant Professor, Division of Geriatric Medicine; Department of Neurology and Psychiatry, Saint Louis University School of Medicine, St Louis, Missouri

ALVIN M. MATSUMOTO, MD
Associate Director and Director, Geriatric Research, Education and Clinical Center and Clinical Research Unit, VA Puget Sound Health Care System; Professor and Acting Head, Division of Gerontology and Geriatric Medicine, Department of Medicine, University of Washington School of Medicine, Seattle, Washington

JOHN E. MORLEY, MB, BCh
Dammert Professor of Medicine and Director, Division of Geriatric Medicine, Saint Louis University School of Medicine, St Louis, Missouri

RALF NASS, MD
Research Assistant Professor, Division of Endocrinology and Metabolism, University of Virginia, Charlottesville, Virginia

ROBIN P. PEETERS, MD, PhD
Thyroid Division, Department of Internal Medicine, Erasmus Medical Center, Rotterdam, The Netherlands

FERDINAND ROELFSEMA, MD, PhD
Professor, Department of Endocrinology and Metabolic Diseases, Leiden University Medical Center, Leiden, The Netherlands

ANIMESH SHARMA, MBBS
Pediatric Endocrinology Fellow, Endocrine Research Unit, Mayo School of Graduate Medical Education, Center for Translational Science Activities, Mayo Clinic, Rochester, Minnesota

JOHANNES D. VELDHUIS, MD
Professor and Clinical Investigator, Endocrine Research Unit, Mayo School of Graduate Medical Education, Center for Translational Science Activities, Mayo Clinic, Rochester, Minnesota

JOSEPH G. VERBALIS, MD
Professor of Medicine and Chief, Division of Endocrinology and Metabolism, Georgetown University Medical Center, Washington, DC

THEO J. VISSER, PhD
Thyroid Division, Department of Internal Medicine, Erasmus Medical Center, Rotterdam, The Netherlands

W. EDWARD VISSER, MD, PhD
Thyroid Division, Department of Internal Medicine, Erasmus Medical Center, Rotterdam, The Netherlands

NELSON B. WATTS, MD
Director, Mercy Health Osteoporosis and Bone Health Services, Cincinnati, Ohio

Contents

Foreword **xiii**

Derek LeRoith

Preface **xvii**

Anne R. Cappola

Growth Hormone Axis and Aging **187**

Ralf Nass

Growth hormone (GH) and/or ghrelin mimetics represent potential treatment and/or prevention options for musculoskeletal impairment associated with aging. Use of improvement in muscle function as an outcome in studies of GH and ghrelin mimetics is complicated by the lack of a standardized definition for clinically meaningful efficacy of this end point. Based on preliminary study results, the use of ghrelin mimetics may be more suitable for use in this age group than GH itself. There are still several unanswered questions related to the use of ghrelin mimetics in the elderly, which prevents recommendation for its use at the current time.

Age-Dependent and Gender-Dependent Regulation of Hypothalamic-Adrenocorticotropic-Adrenal Axis **201**

Johannes D. Veldhuis, Animesh Sharma, and Ferdinand Roelfsema

Tightly regulated output of glucocorticoids is critical to maintaining immune competence, the structure of neurons, muscle, and bone, blood pressure, glucose homeostasis, work capacity, and vitality in the human and experimental animal. Age, sex steroids, gender, stress, body composition, and disease govern glucocorticoid availability through incompletely understood mechanisms. According to an ensemble concept of neuroendocrine regulation, successful stress adaptations require repeated incremental signaling adjustments among hypothalamic corticotropin-releasing hormone and arginine vasopressin, pituitary adrenocorticotropic hormone, and adrenal corticosteroids. Signals are transduced via (positive) feedforward and (negative) feedback effects. Age and gonadal steroids strongly modulate stress-adaptive glucocorticoid secretion by such interlinked pathways.

Endogenous Sex Steroid Levels and Cardiovascular Disease in Relation to the Menopause: A Systematic Review **227**

Carolyn J. Crandall and Elizabeth Barrett-Connor

Heart disease remains a major cause of death among women in the United States. This article focuses on physiologic endogenous estrogen levels with a systematic review of literature related to endogenous sex steroid levels and coronary artery disease (CAD) among postmenopausal women with natural or surgical menopause. There is adequate reason to seek

restriction, which is currently experienced by a substantial and rapidly growing proportion of children and young adults, might contribute to accelerate the senescence of endocrine and metabolic function. The mechanisms of sleep-hormonal interactions, and therefore the endocrino-metabolic consequences of age-related sleep alterations, which markedly differ from one hormone to another, are reviewed in this article.

Frailty, Sarcopenia, and Hormones **391**

John E. Morley and Theodore K. Malmstrom

Frailty is now a definable clinical syndrome with a simple screening test. Age-related changes in hormones play a major role in the development of frailty by reducing muscle mass and strength (sarcopenia). Selective Androgen Receptor Molecules and ghrelin agonists are being developed to treat sarcopenia. The role of Activin Type IIB soluble receptors and Follistatin-like 3 mimetics is less certain because of side effects. Exercise (resistance and aerobic), vitamin D and protein supplementation, and reduction of polypharmacy are keys to the treatment of frailty.

Index **407**

ENDOCRINOLOGY AND METABOLISM CLINICS OF NORTH AMERICA

FORTHCOMING ISSUES

September 2013
Endocrinology and Neuropsychiatric Disorders
Eliza Geer, MD, *Editor*

December 2013
Acute and Chronic Diabetic Complications
Leonid Poretsky, MD and Emilia Liao, MD, *Editors*

March 2014
Associated Diabetic Complications
Leonid Poretsky, MD and Emilia Liao, MD, *Editors*

RELATED INTEREST

Endocrinology Clinics, Volume 42, Issue 1 (March 2013)
Neuroendocrine Control of Metabolism
Christoph Buettner, *Editor*

Foreword

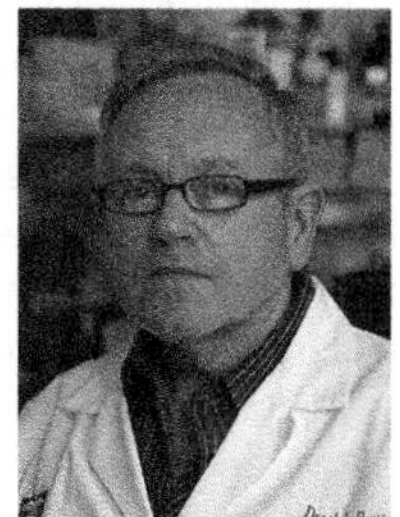

Derek LeRoith, MD, PhD
Consulting Editor

Worldwide, the proportion of older individuals is increasing possibly due to improvements in lifestyle and advances in medicine. As hormonal homeostasis is a fundamental aspect of normal physiology, the concept of "Endocrinology in the Aging Process" is a timely contribution to our *Endocrinology and Metabolism Clinics of North America* series and Dr Anne Cappola has compiled a number of very relevant topics.

During the aging process there is often a parallel between lower circulating GH levels and loss of muscle mass. The reduced GH levels maybe related to alterations in Ghrelin, a hormone secreted from the stomach that stimulates GH secretion via the GHS receptor. As described by Dr Nass, a number of studies have demonstrated the efficacy of GH replacement or the use of Ghrelin mimetics. However, many questions remain to be answered, including the dose, the expected outcomes on muscle mass and quality of life, and the potential side effects of these agents.

Drs Veldhuis, Sharma, and Roelfsema discuss the importance of the adrenal cortex in maintaining adequate production of glucocorticoids for many varied functions of the body and how the hypothalamic-pituitary-adrenal axis is controlled and affected by aging. Furthermore, there are distinct gender differences in the levels of cortisol secretion, the response to ACTH, effects of sex hormones, and other factors that seemingly explain these differences. Some experimental evidence suggests a decrease in brain glucocorticoid receptors that may affect the feedback of peripheral corticosteroids on the hypothalamic-pituitary axis. Finally, diurnal variation in activity of this axis may also be affected and contribute to the reduced response of the axis to stress.

There is continuing controversy regarding the role of sex steroids and coronary heart disease (CHD) in women, whether it relates to the postmenopausal increase in CHD or to the benefits or harmful effects of hormone replacement therapy commonly used in postmenopausal women. Drs Crandell and Barrett-Connor discuss the epidemiologic studies and clinical trials that have attempted to address these issues. Although it seems that postmenopausal increases in CHD are both a real and a major cause of death in women, prevention of this effect with hormone replacement therapy remains to be determined. More recent evidence also points to levels of androgens and sex hormone-binding globulin as playing a role and the relationship of the metabolic syndrome and diabetes is another factor to be considered.

Endocrinol Metab Clin N Am 42 (2013) xiii–xv
http://dx.doi.org/10.1016/j.ecl.2013.03.001
0889-8529/13/$ – see front matter © 2013 Published by Elsevier Inc.
endo.theclinics.com

The aging man may present with a number of features suggestive of impaired reproductive function, namely, erectile dysfunction. Although late-onset hypogonadism secondary to failure of the pituitary-gonadal axis may be the underlying factor, this has only been found in about 2% of aging men. Thus numerous other causes seem to be involved, in particular, obesity or other comorbidities. As Dr Basaria describes, there is often a desire to use testosterone replacement therapy for fatigue, sexual dysfunction, psychologic symptoms, and physical dysfunction; however, the value of such therapy in the absence of lower testosterone levels remains uncertain.

As a corollary to the previous article on hypogonadism in the aging man, Dr Matsumoto in his article discusses in more depth the importance of both the correct diagnosis and the careful monitoring of outcomes if testosterone therapy is to be used. Androgen replacement therapy should only be used for symptoms that are accompanied with low testosterone levels; its efficacy, including any potential side effects, should be monitored carefully and reevaluated constantly.

Drs Visser, Visser, and Peeters describe the physiologic changes in thyroid function in aging, specifically age-related alterations in thyroid function tests. If overt hypothyroidism or hyperthyroidism is diagnosed, then therapy is indicated. On the other hand, subclinical hypothyroidism and hyperthyroidism may be evident and treated accordingly; namely, hyperthyroidism should be treated once the low thyroid stimulating hormone (TSH) due to nonthyroidal illness has been excluded. In the case of subclinical hypothyroidism, "watchful waiting" maybe the more appropriate approach, and special consideration should be given to consider a TSH level of up to 10 mU/L as being normal.

Osteoporosis is a common component of the aging process in both women and men. Osteoporosis increases the risk for fractures that are particularly devastating in elderly people due to the immobilization that often occurs. The use of DEXA technology to evaluate the degree of bone mineral density and the potential for fractures is widely used for diagnostic purposes as well as to evaluate response to therapy. As Dr Diab discusses, vitamin and calcium supplementation is important for preventing osteoporosis and there are numerous therapeutic agents now available for the treatment of low bone mineral density; decisions on which is appropriate for the individual patient should be judicious.

Vitamin deficiency, which is very common in elderly people, can be diagnosed by simply measuring 25 OH vitamin D levels. In addition, there is a decrease in 1,25 OH vitamin D production in the aging population. Thus, as described by Dr Gallagher, the end result is increased osteoporosis and an increased risk for fracture. Standard therapy comprises 800 IU daily that will increase 25 OH vitamin D levels and prevent fractures and should be considered in all elderly people after measuring serum levels, especially elderly people who are institutionalized.

Drs Kalyani and Egan describe the deterioration in insulin action and β-cell function that is commonly seen with aging. These changes explain the greater incidence of type 2 diabetes in older individuals. However, they suggest that any abnormality in glucose homeostasis is generally due to a genetic predisposition. Regarding antidiabetic medications and glycemic goals, it behooves the health care provider to be more judicious in choices to avoid side effects and complications that are more evident in this population.

Disorders of the hypothalamic-neurohypophyseal-renal axis related to water balance and osmolality are common in elderly people and, as described by Drs Cowen, Hodak, and Verbalis, may affect cognition, gait stability, morbidity, and even mortality in this population. Studies have demonstrated that abnormalities may originate at all levels and careful evaluation is critical in dealing with these changes to allow for appropriate therapy, as thirst perception, for example, maybe decreased and not reflect changes in plasma volume, AVP secretion, and kidney responses to fluid alterations.

Drs Copinschi and Caufriez describe the normal physiology related to sleep-wake cycles, circadian rhythms, and the endocrine system. It is becoming well recognized that this system is critical for normal hormonal function and alterations may affect a variety of hypothalamic-pituitary-endocrine organ systems. They describe how sleep deprivation in young individuals alters normal endocrine physiology and how similarly sleep derangements that are common in the elderly population may explain a number of endocrine disorders, including deteriorations glucose homeostasis. Given this important control mechanism, it is not surprising that this is a rapidly burgeoning area of research.

The list of hormonal changes that occur in the aging process and that maybe causative in the events related to sarcopenia and frailty are described in the article by Drs Morley and Malstrom. Thesehormonal agents range from GH, androgens, vitamin D, and protein supplements. Many studies have demonstrated that replacement therapy with some of these hormonal agents have proven efficacy, although side effects may occur. The authors correctly suggest that cocktails may be developed that use low doses of various therapeutic agents in combination and complement the nutrition and exercise programs that should be a major component of the prevention or therapeutic regimens.

I thank Dr Cappola and all the authors for their outstanding contributions.

Derek LeRoith, MD, PhD
Division of Endocrinology, Metabolism, and Bone Diseases
Department of Medicine
Mount Sinai School of Medicine
One Gustave L. Levy Place
Box 1055, Altran 4-36
New York, NY 10029, USA

E-mail address:
derek.leroith@mssm.edu

Preface

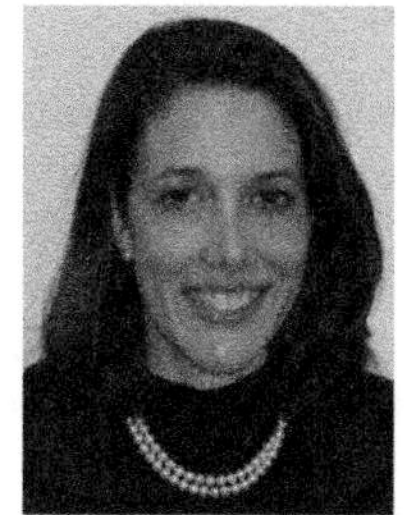

Anne R. Cappola, MD, ScM
Editor

As larger numbers of individuals live into their 80s and 90s, it is becoming increasingly important to understand the underlying hormonal alterations with age and the clinical impact of these changes. In this issue of *Endocrinology and Metabolism Clinics of North America*, we examine the hormonal underpinnings of human aging on an axis-by-axis basis. The authors have done a masterful job of summarizing the existing literature, and I thank them for their wonderful contributions. Several cross-axis themes are apparent in this work.

When comparing healthy younger and older people, major physiologic changes in hormones are apparent. These include decreases in growth hormone and sex steroid secretion in parallel with increased secretion of cortisol and abnormal glucose metabolism. These hormonal alterations are largely considered to represent age-related changes rather than true endocrine disease. In addition, confounding influences affect secretion of each of these hormones, with obesity and sleep playing major, potentially bidirectional, roles.

The overlap in symptoms between these age-related hormonal alterations and the phenotype of aging is unmistakable and has been raised in each article in this issue. In turn, this association and the question of its causality have led to hormonal intervention trials. Studies of replacement of growth hormone, growth hormone secretagogues, estrogen, and testosterone have largely been conducted in the healthy older population, with disappointing results in terms of effects on muscle function and cardiovascular risk. Even quantifying what constitutes vitamin D deficiency in the elderly—a population in whom intake, skin conversion, and activation are all known to be impaired—is an area of controversy, as is the appropriate dose of vitamin D supplementation to provide.

The question then becomes the optimal target population for hormonal replacement therapy. Should it be healthy elderly, or those with illness or disability? Those with illness or disability arguably have the most to gain from hormonal interventions, but are also more likely to incur adverse events and complications from polypharmacy. The goals should be not just gains in muscle mass, for example, but improved mobility and quality of life. Unanswered questions abound, including the age at which to start replacement, the degree of change to define hormonal deficiency, and whether

Endocrinol Metab Clin N Am 42 (2013) xvii–xviii
http://dx.doi.org/10.1016/j.ecl.2013.04.001

therapy should be ongoing for chronic effects or for acute recovery needs. The delivery method of available replacement therapies cannot mimic the underlying hormonal milieu of youth and the line between physiologic and pharmacologic replacement is easily blurred.

These issues become even more complex when the interplay among hormonal axes is introduced, as with effects of estrogen on the adrenal axis, and when patterns are not strictly overabundance or underabundance, such as is seen with less orderly cortisol secretion patterns with age. Whether hormones should be administered in low doses together as a hormonal cocktail and in conjunction with known beneficial nonpharmacologic interventions such as exercise and appropriate nutrition is a looming unknown.

In contrast to changes considered to be associated inevitably with aging, there are the increases in endocrine disease found with age, such as subclinical hypothyroidism and hyperthyroidism, hyponatremia and hypernatremia, diabetes mellitus, and osteoporosis. Once identified, each of these disorders is amenable to treatment, but who should be screened for these disorders, the threshold for treatment, and the therapeutic goals are evolving and becoming more refined over time. Diagnosis of thyroid dysfunction can be challenging in the older person due to the presence of nonclassical symptoms, and there is increasing recognition that thyroid function testing ranges that define disease may need to be shifted in older people. Recommendations for individualization of target hemoglobin A1c levels in older patients depend on the underlying health of the patient and balancing risk of complications with risk of hypoglycemia. Focus is shifting toward treatment of the entire geriatric syndrome leading to fracture, including attention to nonskeletal risk factors such as fall prevention in addition to osteoporosis drug therapy.

This issue provides a comprehensive, thoughtful examination of the state of knowledge of the endocrinology of aging. May future studies provide breakthroughs in enhancing the lives of older people through a better understanding of hormonal regulation and the development of effective hormone-based therapies.

Anne R. Cappola, MD, ScM
Division of Endocrinology, Diabetes, and Metabolism
Perelman School of Medicine
University of Pennsylvania
Smilow Center for Translational Research
12th Floor, 3400 Civic Center Blvd, Building 421
Philadelphia, PA 19104-5160, USA

E-mail address:
acappola@med.upenn.edu

Growth Hormone Axis and Aging

Ralf Nass, MD

KEYWORDS

- Growth hormone • Ghrelin mimetic • Aging

KEY POINTS

- Growth hormone (GH) and/or ghrelin mimetics represent potential treatment and/or prevention options for musculoskeletal impairment associated with aging.
- Use of improvement in muscle function as an outcome in studies of GH and ghrelin mimetics is complicated by the lack of a standardized definition for clinically meaningful efficacy of this end point.
- Based on preliminary study results, the use of ghrelin mimetics may be more suitable for use in this age group than GH itself.
- There are still several unanswered questions related to the use of ghrelin mimetics in the elderly, which prevents recommendation for its use at the current time.

INTRODUCTION

The physiology of aging is one of the least-well understood phases of human life, and at the same time the current demographic changes occurring worldwide suggest that more insight into the underlying mechanism of the aging process is mandatory. The worldwide population aged older than 65 years is projected to increase from about 249 million in 2000 to an estimated 690 million in 2030.[1] In 2050, individuals aged 60 years and older will represent 25% of the world's population. It is expected that by 2050 there will be more than 4.5 million hip fractures annually[2]; complications resulting from falls are the sixth leading cause for death in people older than 65 years.[3] The Third National Health and Nutrition Examination Survey (NHANES III) data show that 23% of people 80 years and older are unable to prepare their own meals and 17% are unable to walk.

From an endocrine point of view, the question arises as to what extent the aging phenotype can be explained by the age-dependent decline of one of the well-described hormone axes and whether the replacement of such hormones would prevent or even reverse some of the age-specific changes. This article focuses on growth hormone (GH) and ghrelin and it addresses the question of whether there is a potential role for GH and/or GH secretagogues (GHS), also known as ghrelin

Division of Endocrinology and Metabolism, University of Virginia, 450 Ray C. Hunt Drive, Room 1412C, Charlottesville, VA 22903, USA
E-mail address: rmn9a@virginia.edu

Endocrinol Metab Clin N Am 42 (2013) 187–199
http://dx.doi.org/10.1016/j.ecl.2013.02.001 endo.theclinics.com
0889-8529/13/$ – see front matter

mimetics, as an intervention in the elderly to prevent/reverse some of the aspects of the phenotype of aging.

REGULATION OF GH RELEASE: ROLE OF GHRELIN?

GH secretion is pulsatile and is thought to be controlled by the 2 neurohormones, GH-releasing hormone (GHRH) and somatostatin.[4,5] Current data suggest that besides GHRH and somatostatin, other factors play a role in the regulation of GH release from the pituitary.[6] The most reproducible GH pulse is observed shortly after sleep onset.[7] Several studies observed that the nocturnal rise in GH is not abolished by an infusion of the somatostatin analog octreotide,[8–10] which indirectly supports the hypothesis that a factor that antagonizes the effects of somatostatin might be involved in the regulation of GH. Patients with inactivating mutations of the GHRH receptor have rhythmic GH secretion, which supports a role for an additional GH-releasing factor besides GHRH in the regulation of GH.[11] Animal studies also support the involvement of an additional factor in the regulation of GH secretion.[12] Portal blood measurements of GHRH and somatostatin in rodents showed that although most GH pulses were closely related to GHRH pulses, about 30% of GH pulses were completely dissociated.[13] Data from several animal studies implicate the hormone ghrelin, which is produced in the stomach, as a major factor affecting GH release from the pituitary. Experiments on transgenic rats that have decreased expression of the ghrelin receptor (GHS receptor [GHSR]) in the arcuate nucleus of the hypothalamus, and decreased GHRH containing neurons, support an interaction of the GHRH and ghrelin systems at the hypothalamic level.[14]

Clinical studies show conflicting results: (1) a relationship between GH and circulating ghrelin,[15] (2) no relationship,[16] or (3) a relationship under certain conditions, such as fasting or the time of day.[17] Koutkia and colleagues[15] studied ghrelin pulsatility with cross-approximate entropy analysis and found that there is significant regularity in cosecretion between ghrelin levels and GH in the fasted state during the night. Similarly, Misra and colleagues,[18] using deconvolution analysis for GH and total ghrelin in healthy adolescents and adolescents with anorexia, found that fasting ghrelin is an independent predictor of basal GH secretion and GH secretory burst frequency. Data published by Espelund and colleagues,[19] Norrelund and colleagues,[20] and Avram and colleagues[16] did not find a correlation between GH and circulating ghrelin levels. One limitation of most published studies is the measurement of total ghrelin, which does not distinguish between acyl-ghrelin and desacyl-ghrelin. In addition, the negative studies may have collected samples too infrequently or of too short duration to detect correlations. Studies from our group examining 8 healthy young men[21] showed a significant correlation between the amplitudes of GH secretory events and the average acyl-ghrelin concentration in the 60-minute interval during and before the GH pulse. Based on the similar diurnal rhythm, the results suggest that during fed conditions, acyl-ghrelin acts as a positive modifier of GH release (**Fig. 1**).

Several studies have confirmed that ghrelin acts through the GHSR to stimulate GH release. MK-677 is an orally active, long-acting GHS that acts as a ghrelin mimetic at the ghrelin receptor. Long-term administration of MK-677 in older adults[22] increased GH pulse amplitude and the preexisting pulsatile GH profile was preserved. Pantel and colleagues[23] showed that in humans, a missense mutation that impairs the constitutive activity of the GHSR is associated with short stature. Similarly, GHSR-null mice have lower insulinlike growth factor-I (IGF-I) levels when compared with wild-type animals[24] and ghrelin null mice tend to have lower IGF-I concentrations when compared with the control animals.[25] The unexpectedly modest changes found in

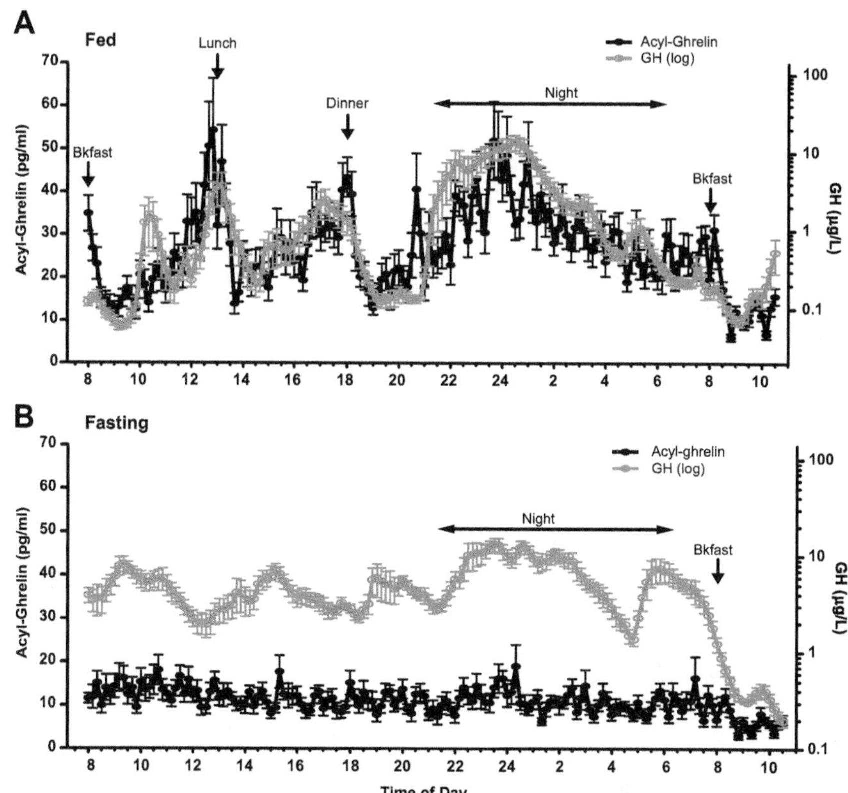

Fig. 1. Mean (± SEM) plasma acyl-ghrelin (pg/mL) and serum GH levels (µg/L, shown on log scale); n = 8 young men. (*A*) Fed admission. (*B*) Fasted admission. (*From* Nass R, Farhy LS, Liu J, et al. Evidence for acyl-ghrelin modulation of growth hormone release in the fed state. J Clin Endocrinol Metab 2008;93:1988–94; with permission. Copyright 2008, The Endocrine Society.)

these knockout models could be because of physiologic compensations, such as constitutive activity of the receptor and the presence of a complex redundant system. Conversely, application of a GHS receptor antagonist results in a decrease in GH pulse amplitude in rodents.[26]

CHANGES IN BODY COMPOSITION IN THE ELDERLY

Circulating GH levels show a significant decline with aging. In elderly subjects, the 24-hour integrated GH concentration is equal to levels observed in young patients with GH deficiency. Several investigators have described a reduction in GH secretory parameters from 15% to 70% in men and women older than 60.[27,28] The age-dependent decrease in GH levels is paralleled by changes in body composition similar to those seen with GH deficiency. There is a change in the distribution of fat mass in the elderly, with an increase in total body fat by about 9% to 18% in men and 12% to 13% in women.[29,30] This age-dependent increase in body fat is associated with an excess of intra-abdominal fat,[31–33] rather than subcutaneous abdominal fat.[29,34–36] In addition, a reduction of subcutaneous fat in the upper leg region has been described with aging.[37] Peak bone mass is usually reached by the third decade of life, followed by a significant gradual decline in bone mineral density (BMD),[30,38–40] which is associated with an increased incidence of fractures. Several studies show an age-dependent decrease in lean body mass (fat-free mass).[29,41,42] Janssen and colleagues[43] report that the decrease of skeletal muscle mass starts in the third decade when expressed as relative muscle mass. This is not the case when reporting absolute muscle mass, which remains stable until the age of 45 years and starts to decline afterward. Thus, the relative decrease in muscle mass before age 45 is mainly the result of an increase in body fat. This finding is in accordance with studies showing that muscle fiber cross-sectional area (ie, contractile muscle), body cell mass, and strength do not change substantially until approximately age 45.[44–49] These findings suggest that interventions targeting age-dependent changes in body composition should be started earlier than age 60 years, which is the lower age limit of most of the GH studies to date.

When reaching the eighth decade, men have lost about 7 kg of absolute muscle mass and women about 3.8 kg of muscle mass.[43] The age-related decrease in lower extremity strength is in the order of 20% to 40% in the seventh and eighth decades and exceeds 50% in the ninth decade.[50]

FUNCTIONAL IMPLICATIONS OF LOSS OF MUSCLE MASS

Several studies suggest that the age-dependent loss of muscle mass and function is linked to physical frailty and decreased capacity of independent living. Sarcopenia is recognized as one component of the multisystemic decline leading to frailty.[51–58] Janssen and colleagues[59] studied the relationship between sarcopenia and functional impairment in 4504 adults aged 60 years and older using NHANES III data. Skeletal muscle mass was estimated using bioelectrical impedance and expressed as the skeletal muscle mass index (SMI) (skeletal muscle mass/body mass × 100) and compared with young adults. The likelihood of functional impairment and physical disability was 2 times greater in older men and 3 times greater in older women with class II sarcopenia (defined as SMI of 2 SD below young adults). Interestingly, class I sarcopenia (defined as SMI within −1 to −2 SD of young adults), when adjusted for age, race, health behaviors, and comorbidity, was no longer associated with an increased likelihood of functional impairment and disability. This study suggests that modest reductions in skeletal muscle mass with aging do not cause functional impairment and disability; however, when skeletal muscle mass relative to body weight is 30% below the mean of young adults, there is an increased risk of functional impairment and disability.

EFFECTS OF GH THERAPY IN THE ELDERLY

The expectation that GH treatment will have beneficial effects in the elderly is based on the observation that there is an age-dependent decline in GH and IGF-I levels,[28] and the study results in patients with adulthood-onset or childhood-onset GH deficiency, which show that GH treatment increases lean body mass in patients with adulthood as well as childhood-onset GH deficiency. Several studies also show that the alterations in body composition with aging are similar to those observed in adult GH deficiency.[27,29,30,34]

There have been a number of small studies of GH administration in older adults, in study populations ranging from healthy to frail. The first 2 publications, both in 1990, set the field in motion. The first showed that treatment of healthy older adults, aged 60 years and older, for 1 week using different doses of GH could produce a dose-dependent increase in IGF-I.[60] In the second, Rudman and coworkers[61] showed that 6 months of treatment with a high dose of GH (0.03 mg/kg per week subcutaneously given 3 times per week) increased lean body mass and spinal bone density and decreased fat mass in men older than 60 years with low pretreatment IGF-I levels. It should be noted that the GH dose used in this study was a pharmacologic dose, significantly higher than the current recommendation for the GH starting dose for GH-deficient adults. Similar results were found by Papadakis and colleagues,[62] who studied 52 men 70 years and older using the same GH dose. After 6 months of GH treatment, fat mass decreased by 13.1% and lean body mass increased by 4.3%; however, these changes did not improve functional ability in this study population. Positive effects on body composition were also found in a 10-week study in 18 healthy elderly men when strength training was combined with GH treatment (0.02 mg/kg per day).[63] In postmenopausal women, the combination of exercise, diet, and GH resulted in an enhanced loss of truncal fat rather than peripheral fat, when compared with placebo.[64] Treatment (0.02 mg/kg body weight subcutaneously given 3 times per week) resulted in a decrease in visceral fat (compared with baseline)[65] in men 65 years or older; however, no change was found when compared with placebo. In a study of elderly malnourished patients,[66] 3 weeks of GH treatment increased midarm muscle circumference. In a 12-week study with a small number of participants (n = 17), treatment with GH of healthy older men increased lean body mass by 3.2 kg.[67]

A meta-analysis of 31 studies of GH administration in healthy older adults showed that despite a significant increase in IGF-I, an average reduction of fat mass by 2.08 kg, and an average increase in lean body mass by 2.13 kg, there were no beneficial effects on function or strength.[68] Whether there are subpopulations of nonhealthy elderly people who may benefit from GH therapy remains undefined, however.

GHS AS A POTENTIAL THERAPEUTIC IN THE ELDERLY

Data from our group show that mean 24-hour acyl-ghrelin levels are lower in a group of adults aged 60 years and older when compared with a group of young adults aged 30 years and younger; both groups had a similar body mass index.[69] The results from several other groups support an age-dependent decline of ghrelin.[70] Aging is also associated with a decrease in circulating GH levels, with the decline starting in the second decade and with a half-life of 7 years.[71] The pituitary ghrelin receptor content does not decline with aging[72] and the secretory response of the pituitary to ghrelin and GH secretagogues is sustained in the elderly.[73]

Ghrelin or ghrelin mimetics have been shown to enhance the preexisting pulsatile GH release[74] and several short-term studies demonstrate a GH increasing effect in the elderly. Chapman and colleagues[75] showed, in a 4-week double-blind placebo-controlled study, that once-daily oral MK-677, given to healthy older adults, enhances pulsatile GH release and IGF-I concentrations reaching levels seen in young adults.

In a multicenter, randomized, double-blind placebo-controlled 18-month study in 292 postmenopausal women, MK-677, given in combination with alendronate, increased BMD at the femoral neck versus alendronate alone; however, at the lumbar spine, total hip, or total body, MK-677 did not improve BMD more than alendronate alone.[76] The investigators concluded that although MK-677 in combination with alendronate has significant positive effects on bone formation at the femoral neck, the lack of enhancement at other sites made it a less attractive choice when compared with alendronate alone.[76] Bach and colleagues[77] showed that MK-677, when given to patients with hip fracture after hip surgery in a group of patients aged 65 years and older, resulted in a greater improvement relative to placebo in 3 of 4 lower-extremity functional performance measures. A 2-year study using an orally active ghrelin mimetic in healthy older adults was published in 2008.[22] This study found that 1-year treatment with MK-677 resulted in an increase in fat-free mass by 1.1 kg and that the effect was maintained through the second year. No significant increase in total body fat was found; however, there was a significant increase in subcutaneous limb fat (**Fig. 2**). The changes in muscle mass did not result in measurable changes in muscle strength or function. This study included mainly physically fit, active, healthy older adults. This may explain the apparent discrepancy between the increase in muscle mass and lack of detectable change in function and strength, whereas in a similar study examining frail subjects, functional improvements were detectable.[77] Similar changes in body composition were found with the pyrazoline-piperidine ghrelin mimetic capromorelin. Studies showed that this ghrelin mimetic was able to increase lean body mass by 1.4 kg in a group of older adults with mild functional limitation. The results also showed an improvement in tandem walk and stair climb. However, the study used different dosing groups, which had to be pooled to demonstrate significance.[78] Overall, these data suggest a potential role for ghrelin or ghrelin mimetics in the treatment of the anorexia/sarcopenia of aging.

POTENTIAL RISKS OF GH REPLACEMENT IN THE ELDERLY

One of the main concerns about GH treatment, as well as using a ghrelin mimetic in the elderly, is the risk of developing cancer or cancer progression. GH/IGF-I has antiapoptotic effects, leading to proliferation of almost all tissues. This might be especially a concern in the older population with an increased number of genetically damaged cells. However, long-term data in children and adults treated with GH for 27,000 patient-years have shown no increased overall occurrence of de novo neoplasia or an increased rate of regrowth of primary pituitary tumors.[79,80] A review of the current data suggests that GH replacement therapy in GH-deficient adults is safe and does not lead to tumor formation.[81,82] However, these are patients who are GH-deficient and receive GH as a replacement therapy to restore age-appropriate levels, whereas in the healthy elderly it is being given to restore "youthful" levels. Previous studies

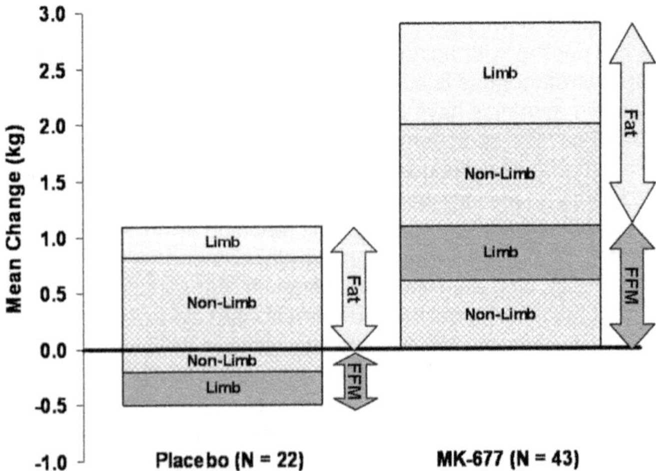

Fig. 2. Mean changes in fat and fat-free mass (FFM) at 12 months treatment with MK-677 or placebo in healthy older adults. Limb = appendicular lean soft tissue and appendicular fat; nonlimb = total minus limb.

suggested that increased IGF-I levels are associated with increased cancer risk. A published study from Amsterdam with 1273 older persons, who were followed over an 11.6-year period, showed no association with fatal and nonfatal cancer.[83] Data by Roddam and colleagues[84] suggested that IGF-I levels are related to an increase in prostate cancer, whereas more recent data by Holly,[85] in 111,000 men, showed that IGF-I is not related to PSA-detected prostate cancer. The overall number of studies in older individuals, as well as the total number of volunteers tested, is too low to estimate cancer risk from GH or ghrelin mimetic administration.

Another of the safety concerns about using GH and ghrelin mimetics includes the potential deterioration of insulin sensitivity and ultimately the development of diabetes mellitus in the elderly, especially with impaired glucose tolerance. Only 2 cases of reversible diabetes were reported from a combined series of 400 treated GH-deficient adults[86] and insulin sensitivity may even normalize with GH treatment as shown in a 1-year study.[87] After 7 years of GH treatment in GH-deficient adults, no change in insulin sensitivity was found.[88] In the meta-analysis of healthy older adults, those treated with GH were more likely to experience onset of diabetes mellitus and impaired fasting glucose, although the number of studies that assessed this outcome was small.[68] In our study with healthy older adults treated for 1 year with the ghrelin mimetic MK-677, HBA1c and fasting glucose levels increased significantly; however, this change was small when expressed in absolute terms, and the fasting glucose levels remained in the normal range. Similar effects on glucose metabolism were reported by Bach and colleagues[77] after 6 months of treatment with MK-677 in healthy older adults after hip fracture. Similar changes in glucose and insulin were described by White and colleagues[78] with the ghrelin mimetic Capromorelin. Svensson and colleagues[89] did not find an increase in fasting glucose or insulin concentrations after 8 weeks of treatment with MK-677; however, the glucose tolerance test showed an impairment of glucose homeostasis. The synthetic ghrelin mimetic SUN 11031, administered to patients with chronic obstructive pulmonary disease with cachexia for 3 months, did not result in changes in fasting or post oral glucose tolerance test glucose or HBA1c.[90] Additional side effects from GH administration include soft tissue edema, arthralgias, carpal tunnel syndrome, and gynecomastia.[68] Other points to consider when discussing the use of GH treatment in the elderly are the data showing that GH-knockout rodents live longer when compared with their GH intact controls.[91,92] Whether these findings in rodents maintained under laboratory conditions can be applied to humans is questionable.[93] Besson and colleagues[94] showed that patients with isolated childhood-onset GH deficiency caused by a GH-1 gene deletion who were untreated during childhood and adulthood have a reduction in life span when compared with controls.

SUMMARY

Overall, the use of GH or GHS represents potential treatment and/or prevention options for musculoskeletal impairment associated with aging; however, there are still a considerable number of unanswered questions related to the use of GH in the elderly that prevent recommendations for use. These include the age, degree of relative GH deficiency, and functional status of the treatment group, as well as long-term safety concerns. Improved muscle function and/or a decrease in the age-dependent muscle loss in the elderly should result in more independent living and improved quality of life in this population group. However, use of improvement in muscle function as an outcome in studies of GH and ghrelin mimetics is complicated by the lack of a standardized definition for clinically meaningful efficacy of this end point. Based on preliminary study results, the use of ghrelin mimetics may be more suitable for use in this age group than GH itself. Future well-controlled studies of adequate duration are required to answer these questions.

REFERENCES

1. CDC. Public health and aging: trends in aging—United States and Worldwide. JAMA 2003;289:1371–3.
2. Gullberg B, Johnell O, Kanis JA. World-wide projections for hip fracture. Osteoporos Int 1997;7:407–13.
3. Tinetti ME, Baker DI, McAvay G, et al. A multifactorial intervention to reduce the risk of falling among elderly people living in the community. N Engl J Med 1994;331(13):821–7.
4. Hartman ML, Faria AC, Vance ML, et al. Temporal structure of in vivo growth hormone secretory events in humans. Am J Physiol 1991;260(1 Pt 1):E101–10.
5. Thorner MO, Chapman IM, Gaylinn BD, et al. Growth hormone-releasing hormone and growth hormone-releasing peptide as therapeutic agents to enhance growth hormone secretion in disease and aging. Recent Prog Horm Res 1997;52:215–44 [discussion: 244–6].
6. Wagner C, Caplan SR, Tannenbaum GS. Interactions of ghrelin signaling pathways with the GH neuroendocrine axis: a new and experimentally tested model. J Mol Endocrinol 2009;43(3):105–19.
7. Van Cauter E, Plat L, Copinschi G. Interrelations between sleep and the somatotropic axis. Sleep 1998;21(6):553–66.
8. Vance ML, Kaiser DL, Evans WS, et al. Pulsatile growth hormone secretion in normal man during a continuous 24-hour infusion of human growth hormone releasing factor (1-40). Evidence for intermittent somatostatin secretion. J Clin Invest 1985;75(5):1584–90.
9. Webb CB, Vance ML, Thorner MO, et al. Plasma growth hormone responses to constant infusions of human pancreatic growth hormone releasing factor. Intermittent secretion or response attenuation. J Clin Invest 1984;74(1):96–103.
10. Dimaraki EV, Jaffe CA, Demott-Friberg R, et al. Generation of growth hormone pulsatility in women: evidence against somatostatin withdrawal as pulse initiator. Am J Physiol Endocrinol Metab 2001;280(3):E489–95.
11. Maheshwari HG, Pezzoli SS, Rahim A, et al. Pulsatile growth hormone secretion persists in genetic growth hormone-releasing hormone resistance. Am J Physiol Endocrinol Metab 2002;282(4):E943–51.
12. Muller EE, Locatelli V, Cocchi D. Neuroendocrine control of growth hormone secretion. Physiol Rev 1999;79(2):511–607.
13. Frohman LA, Downs TR, Clarke IJ, et al. Measurement of growth hormone-releasing hormone and somatostatin in hypothalamic-portal plasma of unanesthetized sheep. Spontaneous secretion and response to insulin-induced hypoglycemia. J Clin Invest 1990;86(1):17–24.
14. Mano-Otagiri A, Nemoto T, Sekino A, et al. Growth hormone-releasing hormone (GHRH) neurons in the arcuate nucleus (Arc) of the hypothalamus are decreased in transgenic rats whose expression of ghrelin receptor is attenuated: Evidence that ghrelin receptor is involved in the up-regulation of GHRH expression in the arc. Endocrinology 2006;147(9):4093–103.
15. Koutkia P, Canavan B, Breu J, et al. Nocturnal ghrelin pulsatility and response to growth hormone secretagogues in healthy men. Am J Physiol Endocrinol Metab 2004;287(3):E506–12.

16. Avram AM, Jaffe CA, Symons KV, et al. Endogenous circulating ghrelin does not mediate growth hormone rhythmicity or response to fasting. J Clin Endocrinol Metab 2005;90(5):2982–7.
17. Muller AF, Lamberts SW, Janssen JA, et al. Ghrelin drives GH secretion during fasting in man. Eur J Endocrinol 2002;146(2):203–7.
18. Misra M, Miller KK, Kuo K, et al. Secretory dynamics of ghrelin in adolescent girls with anorexia nervosa and healthy adolescents. Am J Physiol Endocrinol Metab 2005;289(2):E347–56.
19. Espelund U, Hansen TK, Hojlund K, et al. Fasting unmasks a strong inverse association between ghrelin and cortisol in serum: studies in obese and normal-weight subjects. J Clin Endocrinol Metab 2005;90(2):741–6.
20. Norrelund H, Hansen TK, Orskov H, et al. Ghrelin immunoreactivity in human plasma is suppressed by somatostatin. Clin Endocrinol (Oxf) 2002;57(4):539–46.
21. Nass R, Farhy LS, Liu J, et al. Evidence for acyl-ghrelin modulation of growth hormone release in the fed state. J Clin Endocrinol Metab 2008;93(5):1988–94.
22. Nass R, Pezzoli SS, Oliveri MC, et al. Effects of an oral ghrelin mimetic on body composition and clinical outcomes in healthy older adults: a randomized trial. Ann Intern Med 2008;149(9):601–11.
23. Pantel J, Legendre M, Cabrol S, et al. Loss of constitutive activity of the growth hormone secretagogue receptor in familial short stature. J Clin Invest 2006; 116(3):760–8.
24. Sun Y, Wang P, Zheng H, et al. Ghrelin stimulation of growth hormone release and appetite is mediated through the growth hormone secretagogue receptor. Proc Natl Acad Sci U S A 2004;101(13):4679–84.
25. Sun Y, Ahmed S, Smith RG. Deletion of ghrelin impairs neither growth nor appetite. Mol Cell Biol 2003;23(22):7973–81.
26. Zizzari P, Halem H, Taylor J, et al. Endogenous ghrelin regulates episodic growth hormone (GH) secretion by amplifying GH Pulse amplitude: evidence from antagonism of the GH secretagogue-R1a receptor. Endocrinology 2005;146(9):3836–42.
27. Finkelstein JW, Roffwarg HP, Boyar RM, et al. Age-related change in the twenty-four-hour spontaneous secretion of growth hormone. J Clin Endocrinol Metab 1972;35(5):665–70.
28. Zadik Z, Chalew SA, McCarter RJ Jr, et al. The influence of age on the 24-hour integrated concentration of growth hormone in normal individuals. J Clin Endocrinol Metab 1985;60(3):513–6.
29. Novack L. Aging, total body potassium, fat-free mass, and cell mass in males and females between ages 18 and 85 years. J Gerontol 1972;27:438–43.
30. Rudman D. Growth hormone, body composition, and aging. J Am Geriatr Soc 1985;33(11):800–7.
31. Haarbo J, Marslew U, Gotfredsen A, et al. Postmenopausal hormone replacement therapy prevents central distribution of body fat after menopause. Metabolism 1991;40(12):1323–6.
32. Ashwell M, Cole TJ, Dixon AK. Obesity: new insight into the anthropometric classification of fat distribution shown by computed tomography. Br Med J (Clin Res Ed) 1985;290(6483):1692–4.
33. DeNino WF, Tchernof A, Dionne IJ, et al. Contribution of abdominal adiposity to age-related differences in insulin sensitivity and plasma lipids in healthy nonobese women. Diabetes Care 2001;24(5):925–32.
34. Clasey JL, Weltman A, Patrie J, et al. Abdominal visceral fat and fasting insulin are important predictors of 24-hour GH release independent of age, gender, and other physiological factors. J Clin Endocrinol Metab 2001;86(8):3845–52.

35. Enzi G, Gasparo M, Biondetti P, et al. Subcutaneous and visceral fat distribution according to sex, age and overweight, evaluated by computed tomography. Am J Clin Nutr 1986;44:739–46.
36. Shimokata H, Tobin J, Muller D, et al. Studies in the distribution of body fat. I. Effects of age, sex, and obesity. J Gerontol 1989;44:67–73.
37. Borkan GA, Hults DE, Gerzof SG, et al. Age changes in body composition revealed by computed tomography. J Gerontol 1983;38(6):673–7.
38. Marcus R. Skeletal aging—understanding the functional and structural basis of osteoporosis. Trends Endocrinol Metab 1991;2:53–8.
39. Hannan M, Felson D, Anderson J. Bone mineral density in elderly men and women: results from the Framingham Osteoporosis Study. J Bone Miner Res 1992;7:547–53.
40. Stiegler C, Leb G. One year of replacement therapy in adults with growth hormone deficiency. Endocrinol Metab 1994;1(Suppl A):37–42.
41. Forbes G, Reina J. Adult lean body mass declines with age: some longitudinal observations. Metabolism 1970;19:653–63.
42. Thompson JL, Butterfield GE, Marcus R, et al. The effects of recombinant human insulin-like growth factor-I and growth hormone on body composition in elderly women. J Clin Endocrinol Metab 1995;80(6):1845–52.
43. Janssen I, Heymsfield SB, Wang ZM, et al. Skeletal muscle mass and distribution in 468 men and women aged 18-88 yr. J Appl Physiol 2000;89(1):81–8.
44. Tseng BS, Marsh DR, Hamilton MT, et al. Strength and aerobic training attenuate muscle wasting and improve resistance to the development of disability with aging. J Gerontol A Biol Sci Med Sci 1995;50(Spec No):113–9.
45. Bemben MG, Massey BH, Bemben DA, et al. Isometric muscle force production as a function of age in healthy 20- to 74-yr-old men. Med Sci Sports Exerc 1991; 23(11):1302–10.
46. Clement FJ. Longitudinal and cross-sectional assessments of age changes in physical strength as related to sex, social class, and mental ability. J Gerontol 1974;29(4):423–9.
47. Hurley BF. Age, gender, and muscular strength. J Gerontol A Biol Sci Med Sci 1995;50(Spec No):41–4.
48. Kehayias JJ, Fiatarone MA, Zhuang H, et al. Total body potassium and body fat: relevance to aging. Am J Clin Nutr 1997;66(4):904–10.
49. Lexell J, Downham D, Sjostrom M. Distribution of different fibre types in human skeletal muscles. Fibre type arrangement in m. vastus lateralis from three groups of healthy men between 15 and 83 years. J Neurol Sci 1986;72(2–3):211–22.
50. Doherty TJ. Invited review: aging and sarcopenia. J Appl Physiol 2003;95(4): 1717–27.
51. Walston J, Hadley EC, Ferrucci L, et al. Research agenda for frailty in older adults: toward a better understanding of physiology and etiology: summary from the American Geriatrics Society/National Institute on Aging Research Conference on Frailty in Older Adults. J Am Geriatr Soc 2006;54(6):991–1001.
52. Brown WF. A method for estimating the number of motor units in thenar muscles and the changes in motor unit count with ageing. J Neurol Neurosurg Psychiatry 1972;35(6):845–52.
53. Young VR. Amino acids and proteins in relation to the nutrition of elderly people. Age Ageing 1990;19(4):S10–24.
54. Roubenoff R, Harris TB, Abad LW, et al. Monocyte cytokine production in an elderly population: effect of age and inflammation. J Gerontol A Biol Sci Med Sci 1998;53(1):M20–6.

55. Argiles JM, Busquets S, Felipe A, et al. Molecular mechanisms involved in muscle wasting in cancer and ageing: cachexia versus sarcopenia. Int J Biochem Cell Biol 2005;37(5):1084–104.
56. Delbono O. Molecular mechanisms and therapeutics of the deficit in specific force in ageing skeletal muscle. Biogerontology 2002;3(5):265–70.
57. Gamper N, Fillon S, Huber SM, et al. IGF-1 up-regulates K+ channels via PI3-kinase, PDK1 and SGK1. Pflugers Arch 2002;443(4):625–34.
58. Labrie F, Belanger A, Luu-The V, et al. DHEA and the intracrine formation of androgens and estrogens in peripheral target tissues: its role during aging. Steroids 1998;63(5–6):322–8.
59. Janssen I, Heymsfield SB, Ross R. Low relative skeletal muscle mass (sarcopenia) in older persons is associated with functional impairment and physical disability. J Am Geriatr Soc 2002;50(5):889–96.
60. Marcus R, Butterfield G, Holloway L, et al. Effects of short term administration of recombinant human growth hormone to elderly people. J Clin Endocrinol Metab 1990;70:519–27.
61. Rudman D, Feller A, Nagraj H, et al. Effects of human growth hormone in men over 60 years old. N Engl J Med 1990;323:1–6.
62. Papadakis MA, Grady D, Black D, et al. Growth hormone replacement in healthy older men improves body composition but not functional ability [see comments]. Ann Intern Med 1996;124(8):708–16.
63. Taaffe DR, Pruitt L, Reim J, et al. Effect of recombinant human growth hormone on the muscle strength response to resistance exercise in elderly men. J Clin Endocrinol Metab 1994;79(5):1361–6.
64. Taaffe DR, Thompson JL, Butterfield GE, et al. Recombinant human growth hormone, but not insulin-like growth factor-I, enhances central fat loss in postmenopausal women undergoing a diet and exercise program. Horm Metab Res 2001;33(3):156–62.
65. Muenzer T, Harman S, Hees P, et al. Effects of GH and/or sex steroid administration on abdominal subcutaneous and visceral fat in healthy aged women and men. J Clin Endocrinol Metab 2001;86:3604–10.
66. Kaiser FE, Silver AJ, Morley JE. The effect of recombinant human growth hormone on malnourished older individuals. J Am Geriatr Soc 1991;39(3):235–40.
67. Lange KH, Isaksson F, Rasmussen MH, et al. GH administration and discontinuation in healthy elderly men: effects on body composition, GH-related serum markers, resting heart rate and resting oxygen uptake. Clin Endocrinol (Oxf) 2001;55(1):77–86.
68. Liu H, Bravata DM, Olkin I, et al. Systematic review: the safety and efficacy of growth hormone in the healthy elderly. Ann Intern Med 2007;146(2):104–15.
69. Nass R, Liu J, Pezzoli SS, et al. 24-h mean acyl-ghrelin levels are decreased in older adults. 4th International Congress of the GRS and the IGF Society. Genova, September 19, 2008.
70. Rigamonti AE, Pincelli AI, Corra B, et al. Plasma ghrelin concentrations in elderly subjects: comparison with anorexic and obese patients. J Endocrinol 2002; 175(1):R1–5.
71. Nass R, Johannsson G, Christiansen JS, et al. The aging population—is there a role for endocrine interventions? Growth Horm IGF Res 2009;19(2):89–100.
72. Sun Y, Garcia JM, Smith RG. Ghrelin and growth hormone secretagogue receptor expression in mice during aging. Endocrinology 2007;148(3):1323–9.
73. Broglio F, Benso A, Castiglioni C, et al. The endocrine response to ghrelin as a function of gender in humans in young and elderly subjects. J Clin Endocrinol Metab 2003;88(4):1537–42.

74. Smith RG. Development of growth hormone secretagogues. Endocr Rev 2005; 26(3):346–60.
75. Chapman IM, Hartman ML, Pezzoli SS, et al. Effect of aging on the sensitivity of growth hormone secretion to insulin-like growth factor-I negative feedback. J Clin Endocrinol Metab 1997;82(9):2996–3004.
76. Murphy MG, Weiss S, McClung M, et al. Effect of alendronate and MK-677 (a growth hormone secretagogue), individually and in combination, on markers of bone turnover and bone mineral density in postmenopausal osteoporotic women. J Clin Endocrinol Metab 2001;86(3):1116–25.
77. Bach MA, Rockwood K, Zetterberg C, et al. The effects of MK-0677, an oral growth hormone secretagogue, in patients with hip fracture. J Am Geriatr Soc 2004;52(4):516–23.
78. White HK, Petrie CD, Landschulz W, et al. Effects of an oral growth hormone secretagogue in older adults. J Clin Endocrinol Metab 2009;94(4):1198–206.
79. Monson JP. Long-term experience with GH replacement therapy: efficacy and safety. Eur J Endocrinol 2003;148(Suppl 2):S9–14.
80. Jenkins PJ, Mukherjee A, Shalet SM. Does growth hormone cause cancer? Clin Endocrinol (Oxf) 2006;64(2):115–21.
81. Orme SM, McNally RJ, Cartwright RA, et al. Mortality and cancer incidence in acromegaly: a retrospective cohort study. United Kingdom Acromegaly Study Group. J Clin Endocrinol Metab 1998;83(8):2730–4.
82. Growth Hormone Research Society. Consensus: critical evaluation of the safety of recombinant human growth hormone administration: statement from the Growth Hormone Research Society. J Clin Endocrinol Metab 2001;86:1868–70.
83. van Bunderen CC, van Nieuwpoort IC, van Schoor NM, et al. The association of serum insulin-like growth factor-I with mortality, cardiovascular disease, and cancer in the elderly: a population-based study. J Clin Endocrinol Metab 2010; 95(10):4616–24.
84. Roddam AW, Allen NE, Appleby P, et al. Insulin-like growth factors, their binding proteins, and prostate cancer risk: analysis of individual patient data from 12 prospective studies. Ann Intern Med 2008;149(7):461–71 W83–8.
85. Holly J. Insulin-like growth factors (IGFs) and IGF binding proteins in PSA-detected prostate cancer: a population-based case control study. 5th International Congress of the GRS and IGF-I Society. New York, October 4, 2010.
86. Chipman JJ, Attanasio AF, Birkett MA, et al. The safety profile of GH replacement therapy in adults. Clin Endocrinol (Oxf) 1997;46(4):473–81.
87. Hwu CM, Kwok CF, Lai TY, et al. Growth hormone (GH) replacement reduces total body fat and normalizes insulin sensitivity in GH-deficient adults: a report of one-year clinical experience. J Clin Endocrinol Metab 1997;82(10):3285–92.
88. Svensson J, Fowelin J, Landin K, et al. Effects of seven years of GH-replacement therapy on insulin sensitivity in GH-deficient adults. J Clin Endocrinol Metab 2002;87(5):2121–7.
89. Svensson J, Lonn L, Jansson JO, et al. Two-month treatment of obese subjects with the oral growth hormone (GH) secretagogue MK-677 increases GH secretion, fat-free mass, and energy expenditure. J Clin Endocrinol Metab 1998; 83(2):362–9.
90. Gertner J. SUN 11031 (synthetic human ghrelin) improves lean body mass and function in advanced COPD cachexia in a placebo controlled trial. 5th International Congress of the GRS and IGF-I Society. New York, October 4, 2010.
91. Bartke A. Long-lived Klotho mice: new insights into the roles of IGF-1 and insulin in aging. Trends Endocrinol Metab 2006;17(2):33–5.

92. Berryman DE, Christiansen JS, Johannsson G, et al. Role of the GH/IGF-1 axis in lifespan and healthspan: lessons from animal models. Growth Horm IGF Res 2008;18(6):455–71.
93. Nass R, Thorner MO. Life extension versus improving quality of life. Best Pract Res Clin Endocrinol Metab 2004;18(3):381–91.
94. Besson A, Salemi S, Gallati S, et al. Reduced longevity in untreated patients with isolated growth hormone deficiency. J Clin Endocrinol Metab 2003;88(8):3664–7.

Age-Dependent and Gender-Dependent Regulation of Hypothalamic-Adrenocorticotropic-Adrenal Axis

Johannes D. Veldhuis, MD[a,*], Animesh Sharma, MBBS[a],
Ferdinand Roelfsema, MD, PhD[b]

KEYWORDS

• ACTH • Human • Aging • Cortisol • Feedback

KEY POINTS

- Aging increases adrenocorticotropic hormone (ACTH)/cortisol responses to corticotropin-releasing hormone (CRH) (especially in women) and to vasopressin/CRH (especially in men).
- Estrogen treatment reduces hyperresponsiveness in postmenopausal women.
- Age decreases glucocorticoid feedback (inhibition), leading to slow ACTH recovery after stress.
- There is no age effect on corticosteroid-binding globulin.
- Cortisol responses to hypoglycemia (insulin tolerance test) are preserved in aging.
- How body composition interacts with age in hypothalamic-corticotropic-adrenal regulation is not known.

Disclosure Statement: The authors have nothing to disclose.
Supported in part via R01 DK073148 and DK050456 (Metabolic Studies Core of the Minnesota Obesity Center) from the National Institutes of Health (Bethesda, MD). The content is solely the responsibility of the authors and does not necessarily represent the official views of the National Institutes of Health. The project described was supported by the National Center for Research Resources and the National Center for Advancing Translational Sciences, National Institutes of Health, through Grant Number 1UL1 RR024150-01.
[a] Endocrine Research Unit, Mayo School of Graduate Medical Education, Center for Translational Science Activities, Mayo Clinic, 200 First Street SW, Rochester, MN 55905, USA; [b] Department of Endocrinology and Metabolic Diseases, Leiden University Medical Center, Albinusdreef 2, Leiden 2333ZA, The Netherlands
* Corresponding author.
E-mail address: veldhuis.johannes@mayo.edu

Endocrinol Metab Clin N Am 42 (2013) 201–225
http://dx.doi.org/10.1016/j.ecl.2013.02.002 **endo.theclinics.com**
0889-8529/13/$ – see front matter

OVERVIEW OF REGULATED GLUCOCORTICOID PRODUCTION

Clinical observations indicate that diverse disorders disrupt hypothalamic-corticotropic-adrenal (HPA) homeostasis. Prominent examples include depression, mania, dementia, posttraumatic stress disorder, chronic fatigue syndrome, alcoholism, visceral adiposity, diabetes mellitus, polycystic ovarian disease, acute illness, systemic disease, and multiorgan failure.[1–19] Age, gender, and sex steroids are salient physiologic factors that determine the magnitude and duration of stress-adaptive cortisol production, albeit via mechanisms that are essentially unknown in the human.[20–34]

Understanding the regulation of normal HPA outflow is significant, because chronically increased glucocorticoid concentrations correlate with metabolic features of syndrome X (visceral adiposity, insulin resistance, low high-density lipoprotein levels, high blood pressure, increased triglyceride levels), physical frailty (reduced bone and muscle mass, decreased aerobic capacity), immune suppression, hypogonadism, growth hormone (GH), and insulinlike growth factor 1 deficiency and impaired memory and spatial cognition (**Fig. 1**).[15,35–44] Aging itself is associated with similar changes (**Box 1**). Accordingly, there is an ongoing scientific need to elucidate the basic mechanisms that govern cortisol homeostasis in the aging human.[22,26,27,32,45–51] Inferable effects of aging on HPA function may be confounded by multiple factors, including gender, stress, and genetics (**Box 2**).

DIURNAL ADRENOCORTICOTROPIC HORMONE AND CORTISOL RHYTHMS

In principle, age could modulate mean hormone concentrations, secretion rates, elimination kinetics, pulse size (amplitude) or number (frequency), pattern regularity, or circadian (approximately 24-hour) rhythms. Nycthemeral (night-day) cortisol rhythms are consistently altered in aging individuals (**Box 3**). Most clinical studies report a phase-advanced acrophase (clock time of maximal adrenocorticotropic hormone (ACTH) or cortisol concentrations within the 24-hour day), eg, 06:30 AM (older) vis-à-vis 09:00 AM (young). Concomitantly, there is an increased circadian nadir (lowest 24-hour concentration) in the late evening and through midnight.[52–54] The higher nadir blunts the overall 24-hour increase in cortisol levels. Possible relevance of these findings is that certain target-tissue effects of cortisol, such as reduced lymphocyte subtype populations, share in the phase shift.[55,56]

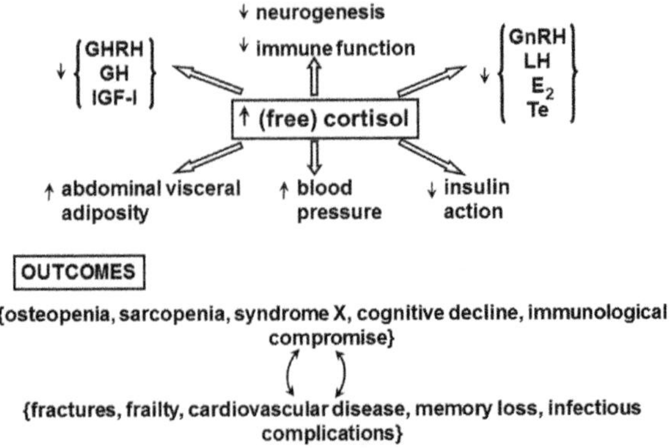

Fig. 1. Putative clinical sequelae of excessive HPA axis activation. An increase in (free) cortisol availability is associated with adverse outcomes in diverse body systems.

Box 1
Similar changes occur in aging as in HPA hyperactivity

↓ physical performance if ↑ evening cortisol

↓ walking speed

↓ bone-mineral density in postmenopausal women

↑ functional disabilities

↓ immune responses

↑ syndrome X (visceral adiposity, ↑ blood pressure, ↓ insulin action)

↓ cognitive function ↓ memory

↑ depression

↑ blood pressure

↓ lean muscle mass

↑ insulin resistance ↓ glucose tolerance

Abbreviations: ↑, increase; ↓, decrease.

Sleep disruption (reduced deep sleep or early awakening) occurs in many older people.[57–59] The degree to which these alterations reflect or cause aging-associated changes in functional disability, anxiety, depression, social support, caloric intake, and lifestyle modifications is not clear.[60–65] However, structural alterations in the hippocampus, suprachiasmatic nuclei, hypothalamus, adrenal gland, and possibly the

Box 2
Confounding factors in HPA evaluation with age

- Gender differences[90]
- Sex-steroid milieu[184]
- Cumulative glucocorticoid exposure[185]
- Dementia or depression[186]
- Genetic polymorphisms in HPA genes[187]
- Inflammation, obesity, weight loss, medication use, illness[130,188]
- Type of stress (psychosocial, physical, metabolic, cognitive)[189]
- Onset versus recovery of stress response[190]
- Structural brain changes[191]
- Cigarette smoking[63]
- Impaired sleep[192]
- Socioeconomic insecurity[63]
- Ethnicity, psychological traits[193]
- ↑, ↓ or unchanged serum total cortisol (ages 19–89 years)[125,130,194–198]
- ↓ urinary free cortisol in centenarians[65]
- ↓ circannual free cortisol rhythm[197]

Box 3
Circadian cortisol changes with age

- Late-day and evening increases in cortisol levels[54,63,125,199]
- Earlier morning cortisol maximum (phase advance)[68,125,195,200,201]
- Lower circadian amplitude (24-hour decrement for peak minus nadir)[54]
- More irregular (less orderly) cortisol secretion patterns[200]

autonomic nervous system can accompany aging in animals (**Box 4**).[66–68] A confounding unresolved issue is the extent to which memory or cognitive decline in older adults results from (is caused by) versus elicits (causes) increased cortisol secretion in the late day.[69–71] Available data do not exclude bidirectional effects.[72–74]

HPA ALTERATIONS IN AGED ANIMALS

Significant functional changes occur in the HPA axis of aged laboratory animals (**Box 5**). A consistent adaptation is reduction in brain corticosteroid receptors, type I (MR) and type II (GR).[75] Both mRNA and protein levels of MR and GR decline in the aged male Fischer rat. This model shows increased hypothalamopituitary portal venous CRH, consistent with a functional decrement in corticosteroid negative feedback. However, species and strain differences limit the consistency of laboratory animal models.

EXPERIMENTAL INSIGHTS INTO AND CLINICAL INFERENCES REGARDING SEX-STEROID REGULATION OF GLUCOCORTICOID AVAILABILITY

Experimental Insights

Sex steroids direct key regulatory mechanisms within the HPA axis of several mammalian species (ie, rat,[76–84] mouse,[85] sheep,[86,87] monkey[88,89] and human[46,90–92]). How gonadal steroids regulate ACTH and cortisol secretion is well articulated in the young adult rat, as highlighted in **Fig. 2**. Sex differences in HPA regulation in the rodent arise from both neuronal imprinting during early development and distinct actions of estradiol (E_2) and testosterone (Te) in adulthood.[93–97] In the young adult animal, exposure

Box 4
Age modifies selective components of HPA axis in animals and humans

Component of Axis	Age Effect
Hippocampus	↓ GR and ↓ MR
Suprachiasmatic nucleus (circadian)	↓ VIP (older men only)[202]
Hypothalamus (paraventricular nucleus)	↑ CRH ↑ AVP[a,203]
Pituitary gland	No change in ACTH
Adrenal gland zona reticularis	↓ DHEA[a,204,205]
Autonomic nervous system	↓ NE outflow[a]
Plasma cortisol-binding globulin	No change[a,130]
Monocytes	↓ GR (both sexes)[206]

Abbreviations: AVP, arginine vasopressin (ADH); DHEA, dehydroepiandrosterone; GR, glucocorticoid receptor; MR, mineralocorticoid receptor; NE, norepinephrine; VIP, vasoactive intestinal polypeptide.

[a] Human data.

Box 5
Aged animals: HPA alterations

↓ hippocampal MR and GR in Fischer-344 rat[207]

↑ portal venous CRH (Fischer)[208]

↓ portal venous AVP (Fischer)[208]

↑ corticosterone (Long-Evans rat)[209,210]

↓ hippocampal MR but not GR[209]

↑ evening cortisol (female Rhesus monkey)[211]

↓ cortisol escape after dexamethasone (DEX)[211]

to E_2 typically potentiates stress-induced ACTH secretion by: (1) attenuating negative feedback in the hypothalamus, hippocampus, amygdala, and pituitary gland[98,99]; (2) inducing AVP, CRH, and CRH-R1 gene expression in the paraventricular nucleus (PVN)[77,93,100–103]; (3) enhancing adrenal responsiveness to ACTH[104–107]; (4) muting hippocampal and bed nucleus of the stria terminalis–directed inhibition of PVN neurons[108]; and (5) blunting homologous downregulation of limbic GR.[76] Conversely, Te and 5α-dihydrotestosterone (5α-DHT) generally exert opposing effects on the foregoing mechanisms, resulting in diminished stress-stimulated ACTH secretion (see **Fig. 2**).[6,81,84,109–114] What remains unclear is how aging per se modulates the sex-steroid effects.

The impact of gonadal steroids in the rat is not expressly dichotomous, because E_2 may augment certain actions of 5α-DHT, whereas 5α-DHT can impede other effects of E_2.[115–117] In addition, in some studies, low concentrations of estrogen diminish rather than amplify stress-induced ACTH and glucocorticoid secretion in the ovariprival state.[82,118,119]

Clinical Inferences

Certain HPA modulators and stressors affect ACTH and cortisol homeostasis, with strong age dependence and female or male predominance (**Box 6**).[21,22,46,120–122] Modulators in this category include CRH, AVP, DEX, somatostatin, social stress,

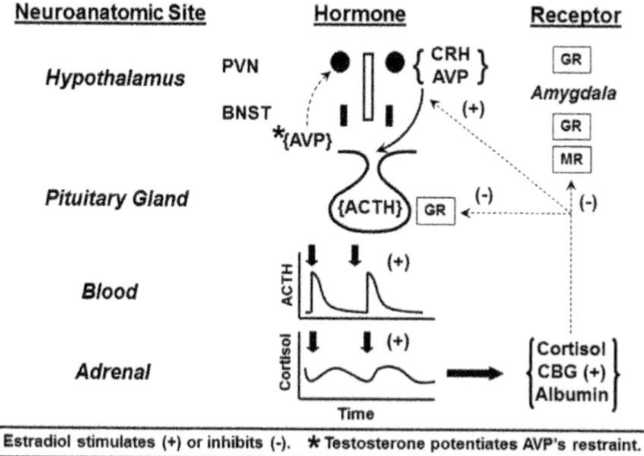

Fig. 2. Experimentally based schema of loci of sex-steroid (estradiol and testosterone) control of HPA axis outflow. The + and – signs denote stimulation and inhibition, respectively.

Box 6
Gender-related and age-related distinctions in human HPA responsiveness

↑ or unchanged plasma ACTH with age[212–214]

↑ stimulation of CRH of ACTH and cortisol secretion[a,48]

↑ AVP/CRH (combined) stimulation[a,46]

↓ glucocorticoid suppression of effect of basal ACTH and CRH[48,56,74,148,149,213,215]

↑ paradoxic ACTH/cortisol response to somatostatin[216]

↑ social stress effect[a,22]

↑ response to cognitive stress[a,217]

↑ stimulation by 5HT-1A agonist (ipsapirone)[a,218]

↑ response to hypothermic stress[218]

↑ effect of physostigmine[a,219]

↑ cortisol response to naltrexone (opiate blocker)[a,220]

↑ ACTH/cortisol response to MR blocker[221,222]

[a] More prominent age contrast in women than men.

cognitive stress, and pharmacologic probes. Most often, greater responses occur in aging, especially in women. The precise bases for age-associated gender selectively in these clinical settings is not established. Investigations in the human are limited in scope and discrepant in inference. Critical review shows the following fragmentary and disparate observations:

a. Daily cortisol secretion rates are higher in men,[123,124] greater in older women,[125] comparable in women and men,[126–130] and increased in young women in the luteal compared with follicular phase of the menstrual cycle[131,132];
b. Maximal ACTH-stimulated cortisol secretion is greater in women,[33,49,133] similar by gender,[126] accentuated by Te administration in women,[134] or unaffected by estrogen in men[31,34,135];
c. Maximal CRH-stimulated ACTH or cortisol secretion is equivalent in the 2 sexes,[26,27,46] higher in men,[136] greater in women,[32,42,48,136–139] not affected by E_2 in women,[140] augmented by E_2 in men[141] or suppressed by Te in men[142];
d. AVP-induced ACTH secretion is comparable in the 2 genders[47] or greater in women[48];
e. Synergy between CRH and AVP is greater in men than women or comparable by gender[46];
f. Stress-induced elevations in ACTH and cortisol concentrations are greater in men,[22,23,25,143–146] greater in women,[28,145,147] comparable by gender,[26,32] repressed by E_2 in women, and dependent on age[22,25,26,28,122,144] or independent of age[32];
g. Delayed (integral) glucocorticoid negative feedback is either muted in women[32,48,148] or accentuated in women[148,149] compared with men;
h. Rapid cortisol-mediated negative feedback has been studied in men,[149] but responses have not been compared in women and men; and
i. The metabolic clearance rate of cortisol is the same in the 2 sexes,[126,130] decreased in women[150] or increased in women.[91]

Box 7
Age-related changes in human HPA dynamics

1. Various stressors
   a. Depression
      i. ↑ cortisol with age in both sexes[196]
      ii. ↑ post-DEX/CRH cortisol with age[223]
   b. Memory impairment
      i. ↑ basal and post-DEX cortisol in older women with (vs without) memory impairment[69]
   c. Awakening
      i. ↑ salivary cortisol after meal[224]
      ii. ↓ salivary cortisol in older (vs young) adults especially women[60,224–227]
      iii. Salivary cortisol predicts:
         1. executive function positively in older adults[228]
         2. working memory positively in older men and declarative memory negatively (both sexes)[229]
   d. Hypoglycemia
      i. Normal cortisol response to ↓ glucose of 50 mg/dL with age[153]
   e. Speech task
      i. ↓ (salivary) cortisol response in older men only[230]
   f. Socioeconomic status
      i. ↓ (salivary) cortisol with age in socioeconomically matched women only[227]
   g. Sleep
      i. ↓ deep sleep and amplitude of 24-hour cortisol rhythm with age (men)[58,192]
   h. Abdominal visceral adiposity in older women
      i. ↓ estimated ACTH efficacy[231]
   i. Psychosocial stress
      i. ↓ ACTH increment after DEX/CRH in older (vs young) men[22]
   j. Mineralocorticoid agonist (9α-fludrocortisone)
      i. ↓ ACTH/cortisol suppression in older (vs young) men[232]
   k. Mineralocorticoid antagonist (spironolactone)
      i. ↑ cortisol more in older (than young) adults[222]
2. Adrenal feedback
   a. Hydrocortisone-imposed negative feedback (25-mg IV bolus)
      i. ↓ ACTH suppression in older men[149]
   b. DEX (0.25–3 mg orally)
      i. ↓ ACTH/cortisol suppression in:
         1. older volunteers[48,233,234]
         2. and in luteal-phase women[235]
3. Pharmacologic interventions
   a. ACTH infusion

i. No age effect on maximal cortisol response[234]

b. Naloxone infusion (stimulus to ACTH/cortisol)

i. No effect of age on cortisol response in men[236]

c. Selective serotonin reuptake inhibitor (citalopram)

i. ↑ ACTH secretion with age in men[237]

4. Sex-steroid interactions

a. Short-term (2-week–8-week) E_2 treatment

i. ↓ cortisol hyperresponsiveness after DEX/CRH in older women treated with estrogen[32,118,238]

ii. Progesterone potentiates cortisol release to exercise[239–241]

iii. E_2 has no effect (vs hypogonadism) on exercise response in young women[240]

The foregoing inconsistencies and the lack of precise data on body compositional effects preclude definitive inferences regarding putatively joint interactions among age, gender, sex steroids and body-fat distribution in regulating glucocorticoid availability in humans.

Glucocorticoid Negative Feedback Studies in the Human: Confounding by Gender and Age

Increased glucocorticoid concentrations and impaired suppression of ACTH and cortisol concentration by DEX tend to correlate with increased age and decreased cognitive function.[15,38,151,152] Although such observations could signify that aging increases mean cortisol levels and reduces glucocorticoid negative feedback, clinical data are controversial. For example, awakening morning salivary cortisol seems to decrease with age, especially in women (**Box 7**). In contrast, cortisol responses to glucose less than 50 mg/dL are preserved in aging.[153] In 1 study, feedback inhibition of ACTH and cortisol concentrations by graded doses of DEX did not differ in older and young men.[29] In other investigations, intravenous (IV) infusion of cortisol suppressed ACTH concentrations less in older than young men, and more in postmenopausal women than elderly men.[149,154,155] Analogously, DEX administration lowered cortisol concentrations more in 106 women than 203 men aged 66 to 78 years.[156] Assessments of rapid negative feedback have typically used pharmacologic doses of cortisol (5–50 mg IV) without evaluating age and gender effects.[149,157,158] Experimental data indicate that feedback effects and loci of inhibition differ between synthetic glucocorticoids and cortisol.[159] **Box 7** presents several other age (and gender) effects on human HPA dynamics, showing variously no effect, diminution, and accentuation of ACTH/cortisol responses to distinct stressors in aging humans. Age does not seem to alter responses to infusions of insulin, naloxone, or ACTH. Aging attenuates ACTH/cortisol responses to speech stress, low socioeconomic status, deep sleep, psychosocial stress, and MR stimulation with 9α-fludrocortisone, and potentiating HPA responses to an MR antagonist and a selective serotonin uptake inhibitor.

UNRESOLVED ISSUES

Delineating Relevant in Vivo Cortisol Feedback Signals

Free (protein-unbound), cortisol-binding globulin (CBG), and albumin-bound cortisol concentrations constitute respectively 6%, 80%, and 14% of total plasma cortisol

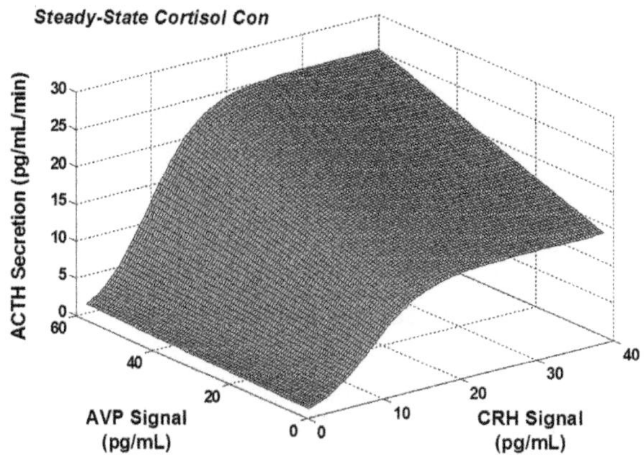

Fig. 3. Joint AVP and CRH drive of ACTH secretion under fixed cortisol concentration (*con*) estimated from hypothalamopituitary portal venous sampling in the horse.

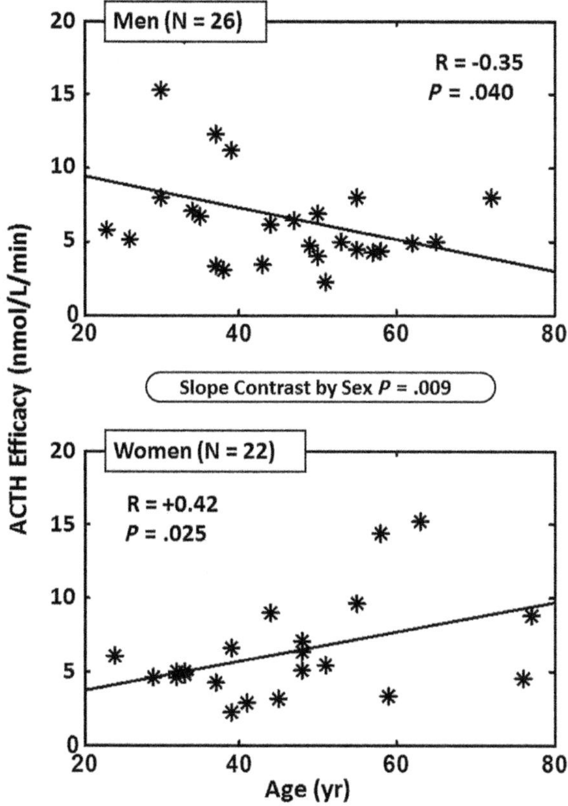

Fig. 4. Opposite impact of age (independent variable) on ACTH efficacy (asymptotically maximal ACTH-stimulated pulsatile cortisol secretory rate) in men (N = 26, *top*) and women (N = 22, *bottom*). Pearson's product-moment correlation coefficients are shown for the regressions. The *P* value in the ellipse denotes the gender difference in slopes. (*Adapted from* Keenan DM, Roelfsema F, Carroll BJ, et al. Sex defines the age dependence of endogenous ACTH-cortisol dose responsiveness. Am J Physiol Regul Integr Comp Physiol 2009;297(2):R515–23; with permission.)

in the human.[126,160] Indirect evidence points to greater biological relevance of free than total glucocorticoid concentration in mediating certain tissue-specific effects, such as hippocampal GR occupancy, negative feedback efficacy, stimulation of glycogen synthesis, fractional hepatic extraction, and uptake into cerebrospinal fluid.[161–164] Clinical studies are needed to quantify negative feedback control of CRH and AVP secretion and stimulation of ACTH secretion by each of free, CBG-bound, and albumin-bound cortisol in young and older women and men exposed to E_2, Te, and GR or MR antagonists.

Estimating Condition-Specific and Subject-Specific Kinetics of Cortisol and ACTH Elimination

In the human, the nominal half-life of total cortisol is 35 to 65 minutes.[126,127,165,166] Longer half-lives occur with higher CBG concentrations in estrogen-rich young women than Te-predominant men.[167,168] Model-based analyses of the fate of cortisol in plasma in middle-aged adults predict gender-independent half-lives of free cortisol diffusion of 1.8 minutes and of free and total cortisol elimination of 4.1 minutes and 48 minutes, respectively.[126] Such calculations also forecast higher free and albumin-bound cortisol concentrations in the morning than evening and thereby more rapid clearance, as observed clinically.[169] The half-life of human ACTH is reportedly 8 to 25 minutes by bioassay and immunoassay.[126,165,170,171] Rapid ACTH disappearance imposes a requirement for frequent blood sampling to monitor pulsatile secretion.[172–174]

Noninvasive Analyses of Multisignal Regulation of ACTH Secretion

New analytical procedures are needed to reconstruct feedforward and feedback dose-response properties using only paired measurements of linked hormones. The

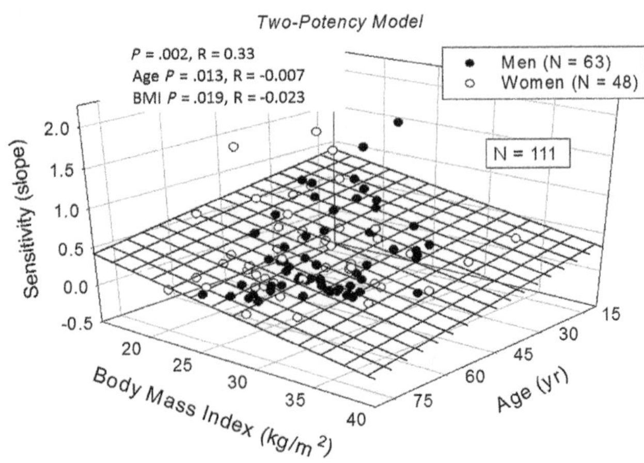

Fig. 5. Age and body mass image (BMI) jointly attenuate adrenal sensitivity (maximal slope of ACTH-cortisol dose-response function) in a cohort of 111 healthy adults (overall P = .0017). Sensitivity was negatively associated with both age (P = .014) and BMI (P = .019), indicating reduced adrenal cortisol secretory responsiveness per unit increase in ACTH concentrations. R values are the correlation coefficients. (*Adapted from* Veldhuis JD, Iranmanesh A, Roelfsema F, et al. Tripartite control of dynamic ACTH-cortisol dose-responsiveness by age, body mass index and gender in 111 healthy adults. J Clin Endocrinol Metab 2011;96(9):2874–81; with permission.)

Box 8
Other diurnal rhythms affected in aging

↓ melatonin secretion at night[194,213]

↓ core body temperature rhythm[242]

↓ DHEA-sulfate levels[201]

↓ CD4 T-helper cell rhythm[243]

↓ δ (slow-wave) [and rapid-eye-movement] sleep[57,59]

↓ salivary amylase on awakening[62]

↓ free Te peak and phase advance (earlier)[201]

↓ thyrotropin (centenarians)[65]

↓ interleukin 6, interleukin 1β concentrations[59,244]

objective is to obviate the previous long-standing necessity to inject agonists, antagonists, or marked molecules.[126,175,176] Implementation of 1 such methodology in 32 healthy adults ages 26 to 79 years permitted estimation of unstressed ACTH feedforward efficacy (maximal cortisol secretion), potency (one-half maximally effective concentration, [EC_{50}]) and adrenal sensitivity (absolute slope of effector-response relationship).[126] A computed EC_{50} (potency) of endogenous ACTH of 24 ± 3.3 ng/L was associated with a mean plasma ACTH concentration in the same cohort of 19 ± 6.2 ng/L. Empirical validation of the equation set was by frequent (5-minute), extended (4-hour–12-hour) direct sampling of hypothalamopituitary portal and internal-jugular blood to measure CRH, AVP, ACTH, and cortisol as well as gonadotropin-releasing hormone, luteinizing hormone, and Te concentration in the awake unrestrained horse and sheep.[175,176] Statistical verification was by direct mathematical proof of maximum-likelihood estimation of all parameter asymptotes.[176] An extension of this concept is to reconstruct the 3-parameter relationship among CRH concentration, AVP concentration, and ACTH secretion at a given steady-state cortisol concentration using data from pituitary portal vessels (**Fig. 3**).[177] Based on these methods, estimated ACTH efficacy decreases in men and increases in women with age (**Fig. 4**).[178] In addition, age and body mass index together determine adrenal sensitivity to endogenous ACTH (**Fig. 5**).

Other Diurnal Rhythms in Aging

Melatonin, core body temperature, DHEA, T-helper cells, slow-wave sleep, and other nycthemeral rhythms are also flattened with age (**Box 8**). The relationship between these and HPA changes is not known. GH secretagogues also drive ACTH/cortisol secretion, but the mechanism is not defined.[179]

SUMMARY

Age, gender, and sex steroids represent key modulators of physiologically incremental and pathologically overt adaptations in the ensemble regulation of CRH, AVP, ACTH, and cortisol output.[126,165,175,180,181] Challenges in this arena include development and application of new safe rational approaches to identify, prevent, and treat deficient or excessive cortisol production. Further clinical investigations should aid in clarifying mechanistic HPA changes in aging and comorbid states (eg, increased visceral adiposity), with the goal of obviating HPA-associated morbidity, mortality, disability, and impaired quality of life in aging women and men.[181–183]

ACKNOWLEDGMENTS

We thank Jill Smith for support with manuscript preparation.

REFERENCES

1. Mortola JF, Liu JH, Gillen JC, et al. Pulsatile rhythms of adrenocorticotropin (ACTH) and cortisol in women with endogenous depression: evidence for increased ACTH pulse frequency. J Clin Endocrinol Metab 1987;65:962–8.
2. Huizenga NA, Koper JW, De Lange P, et al. A polymorphism in the glucocorticoid receptor gene may be associated with an increased sensitivity to glucocorticoids *in vivo*. J Clin Endocrinol Metab 1998;83(1):144–51.
3. Joels M, de Kloet ER. Mineralocorticoid and glucocorticoid receptors in the brain. Implications for ion permeability and transmitter systems. Prog Neurobiol 1994;43(1):1–36.
4. Fries E, Hesse J, Hellhammer J, et al. A new view on hypocortisolism. Psychoneuroendocrinology 2005;30(10):1010–6.
5. Vamvakopoulos NC, Chrousos GP. Hormonal regulation of human corticotropin-releasing hormone gene expression: implications for the stress response and immune/inflammatory reaction. Endocr Rev 1994;15(4):409–20.
6. Spinedi E, Suescun MO, Hadid R, et al. Effects of gonadectomy and sex hormone therapy on the endotoxin-stimulated hypothalamo-pituitary-adrenal axis: evidence for a neuroendocrine-immunological sexual dimorphism. Endocrinology 1992;131(5):2430–6.
7. Cameron OG, Kronfol Z, Greden JF, et al. Hypothalamic-pituitary-adrenocortical activity in patients with diabetes mellitus. Arch Gen Psychiatry 1984;41(11):1090–5.
8. Karanth S, Linthorst AC, Stalla GK, et al. Hypothalamic-pituitary-adrenocortical axis changes in a transgenic mouse with impaired glucocorticoid receptor function. Endocrinology 1997;138(8):3476–85.
9. Invitti C, De Martin M, Delitala G, et al. Altered morning and nighttime pulsatile corticotropin and cortisol release in polycystic ovary syndrome. Metabolism 1998;47(2):143–8.
10. Makino S, Smith MA, Gold PW. Increased expression of corticotropin-releasing hormone and vasopressin messenger ribonucleic acid (mRNA) in the hypothalamic paraventricular nucleus during repeated stress: association with reduction in glucocorticoid receptor mRNA levels. Endocrinology 1995;136(8):3299–309.
11. Spinedi E, Salas M, Chisari A, et al. Sex differences in the hypothalamo-pituitary-adrenal axis response to inflammatory and neuroendocrine stressors. Evidence for a pituitary defect in the autoimmune disease-susceptible female Lewis rat. Neuroendocrinology 1994;60(6):609–17.
12. Rasmusson AM, Lipschitz DS, Wang S, et al. Increased pituitary and adrenal reactivity in premenopausal women with posttraumatic stress disorder. Biol Psychiatry 2001;50(12):965–77.
13. McCormick CM, Smythe JW, Sharma S, et al. Sex-specific effects of prenatal stress on hypothalamic-pituitary-adrenal responses to stress and brain glucocorticoid receptor density in adult rats. Brain Res Dev Brain Res 1995;84(1):55–61.

14. Hudson JI, Hudson MS, Rothschild AJ, et al. Abnormal results of dexamethasone suppression tests in nondepressed patients with diabetes mellitus. Arch Gen Psychiatry 1984;41(11):1086–9.
15. Fonda SJ, Bertrand R, O'Donnell A, et al. Age, hormones, and cognitive functioning among middle-aged and elderly men: cross-sectional evidence from the Massachusetts Male Aging Study. J Gerontol A Biol Sci Med Sci 2005; 60(3):385–90.
16. Pfohl B, Sherman B, Schlechte J, et al. Differences in plasma ACTH and cortisol between depressed patients and normal controls. Biol Psychiatry 1985;20(10): 1055–72.
17. Fliers E, Swaab DF, Pool CW, et al. The vasopressin and oxytocin neurons in the human supraoptic and paraventricular nucleus; changes with aging and in senile dementia. Brain Res 1985;342(1):45–53.
18. Gotthardt U, Schweiger U, Fahrenberg J, et al. Cortisol, ACTH, and cardiovascular response to a cognitive challenge paradigm in aging and depression. Am J Physiol 1995;268(4 Pt 2):R865–73.
19. Griffin MG, Resick PA, Yehuda R. Enhanced cortisol suppression following dexamethasone administration in domestic violence survivors. Am J Psychiatry 2005;162(6):1192–9.
20. Lundberg U. Stress hormones in health and illness: the roles of work and gender. Psychoneuroendocrinology 2005;30(10):1017–21.
21. Kessler RC, McGonagle KA, Zhao S, et al. Lifetime and 12-month prevalence of DSM-III-R psychiatric disorders in the United States. Results from the National Comorbidity Survey. Arch Gen Psychiatry 1994;51(1):8–19.
22. Kudielka BM, Buske-Kirschbaum A, Hellhammer DH, et al. HPA axis responses to laboratory psychosocial stress in healthy elderly adults, younger adults, and children: impact of age and gender. Psychoneuroendocrinology 2004;29(1):83–98.
23. Kudielka BM, Hellhammer J, Hellhammer DH, et al. Sex differences in endocrine and psychological responses to psychosocial stress in healthy elderly subjects and the impact of a 2-week dehydroepiandrosterone treatment. J Clin Endocrinol Metab 1998;83(5):1756–61.
24. Weiss JM, McEwen BS, Silva MT, et al. Pituitary-adrenal influences on fear responding. Science 1969;163(863):197–9.
25. Collins A, Frankenhaeuser M. Stress responses in male and female engineering students. J Human Stress 1978;4(2):43–8.
26. Kirschbaum C, Wust S, Hellhammer D. Consistent sex differences in cortisol responses to psychological stress. Psychosom Med 1992;54(6):648–57.
27. Ohashi M, Fujio N, Kato K, et al. Aging is without effect on the pituitary-adrenal axis in men. Gerontology 1986;32(6):335–9.
28. Traustadottir T, Bosch PR, Cantu T, et al. Hypothalamic-pituitary-adrenal axis response and recovery from high-intensity exercise in women: effects of aging and fitness. J Clin Endocrinol Metab 2004;89(7):3248–54.
29. Waltman C, Blackman MR, Chrousos GP, et al. Spontaneous and glucocorticoid-inhibited adrenocorticotropin hormone and cortisol secretion are similar in healthy young and old men. J Clin Endocrinol Metab 1991;73:495–502.
30. Heuser I, Yassouridis A, Holsboer F. The combined dexamethasone/CRH test: a refined laboratory test for psychiatric disorders. J Psychiatr Res 1994;28(4): 341–56.
31. Ohashi M, Kato K, Nawata H, et al. Adrenocortical responsiveness to graded ACTH infusions in normal young and elderly human subjects. Gerontology 1986;32(1):43–51.

32. Kudielka BM, Schmidt-Reinwald AK, Hellhammer DH, et al. Psychological and endocrine responses to psychosocial stress and dexamethasone/corticotropin-releasing hormone in healthy postmenopausal women and young controls: the impact of age and a two-week estradiol treatment. Neuroendocrinology 1999;70(6):422–30.
33. Parker CR Jr, Slayden SM, Azziz R, et al. Effects of aging on adrenal function in the human: responsiveness and sensitivity of adrenal androgens and cortisol to adrenocorticotropin in premenopausal and postmenopausal women. J Clin Endocrinol Metab 2000;85(1):48–54.
34. Vermeulen A, Deslypere JP, Schelfhout W, et al. Adrenocortical function in old age: response to acute adrenocorticotropin stimulation. J Clin Endocrinol Metab 1982;54(1):187–91.
35. Giustina A, Veldhuis JD. Pathophysiology of the neuroregulation of growth hormone secretion in experimental animals and the human. Endocr Rev 1998;19(6):717–97.
36. Montaron MF, Drapeau E, Dupret D, et al. Lifelong corticosterone level determines age-related decline in neurogenesis and memory. Neurobiol Aging 2006;27(4):645–54.
37. Bjorntorp P. Stress and cardiovascular disease. Acta Physiol Scand Suppl 1997;640:144–8.
38. Wright CE, Kunz-Ebrecht SR, Iliffe S, et al. Physiological correlates of cognitive functioning in an elderly population. Psychoneuroendocrinology 2005;30(9):826–38.
39. Rosmond R, Dallman MF, Bjorntorp P. Stress-related cortisol secretion in men: relationships with abdominal obesity and endocrine, metabolic and hemodynamic abnormalities. J Clin Endocrinol Metab 1998;83(6):1853–9.
40. Jacobson L. Hypothalamic-pituitary-adrenocortical axis regulation. Endocrinol Metab Clin North Am 2005;34(2):271–92.
41. de Kloet ER, Joels M, Holsboer F. Stress and the brain: from adaptation to disease. Nat Rev Neurosci 2005;6(6):463–75.
42. Burke HM, Davis MC, Otte C, et al. Depression and cortisol responses to psychological stress: a meta-analysis. Psychoneuroendocrinology 2005;30(9):846–56.
43. Watts LM, Manchem VP, Leedom TA, et al. Reduction of hepatic and adipose tissue glucocorticoid receptor expression with antisense oligonucleotides improves hyperglycemia and hyperlipidemia in diabetic rodents without causing systemic glucocorticoid antagonism. Diabetes 2005;54(6):1846–53.
44. Smith GD, Ben Shlomo Y, Beswick A, et al. Cortisol, testosterone, and coronary heart disease: prospective evidence from the Caerphilly study. Circulation 2005;112(3):332–40.
45. Viau V. Functional cross-talk between the hypothalamic-pituitary-gonadal and -adrenal axes. J Neuroendocrinol 2002;14(6):506–13.
46. Born J, Ditschuneit I, Schreiber M, et al. Effects of age and gender on pituitary-adrenocortical responsiveness in humans. Eur J Endocrinol 1995;132(6):705–11.
47. Rubin RT, Sekula LK, O'Toole S, et al. Pituitary-adrenal cortical responses to low-dose physostigmine and arginine vasopressin administration in normal women and men. Neuropsychopharmacology 1999;20(5):434–46.
48. Heuser IJ, Gotthardt U, Schweiger U, et al. Age-associated changes of pituitary-adrenocortical hormone regulation in humans: importance of gender. Neurobiol Aging 1994;15(2):227–31.

49. Roelfsema F, van den Berg G, Frolich M, et al. Sex-dependent alteration in cortisol response to endogenous adrenocorticotropin. J Clin Endocrinol Metab 1993;77:234–40.
50. Horrocks PM, Jones AF, Ratcliffe WA, et al. Patterns of ACTH and cortisol pulsatility over twenty-four hours in normal males and females. Clin Endocrinol (Oxf) 1990;32(1):127–34.
51. Kirschbaum C, Kudielka BM, Gaab J, et al. Impact of gender, menstrual cycle phase, and oral contraceptives on the activity of the hypothalamus-pituitary-adrenal axis. Psychosom Med 1999;61(2):154–62.
52. Heaney JL, Phillips AC, Carroll D. Ageing, physical function, and the diurnal rhythms of cortisol and dehydroepiandrosterone. Psychoneuroendocrinology 2012;37(3):341–9.
53. Van Cauter E, Plat L, Leproult R, et al. Alterations of circadian rhythmicity and sleep in aging: endocrine consequences. Horm Res 1998;49(3–4):147–52.
54. Deuschle M, Gotthardt U, Schweiger U, et al. With aging in humans the activity of the hypothalamus-pituitary-adrenal system increases and its diurnal amplitude flattens. Life Sci 1997;61(22):2239–46.
55. Mazzoccoli G, Vendemiale G, La VM, et al. Circadian variations of cortisol, melatonin and lymphocyte subpopulations in geriatric age. Int J Immunopathol Pharmacol 2010;23(1):289–96.
56. Struder HK, Hollmann W, Platen P, et al. Neuroendocrine system and mental function in sedentary and endurance-trained elderly males. Int J Sports Med 1999;20(3):159–66.
57. Pace-Schott EF, Spencer RM. Age-related changes in the cognitive function of sleep. Prog Brain Res 2011;191:75–89.
58. Espiritu JR. Aging-related sleep changes. Clin Geriatr Med 2008;24(1):1–14.
59. Vgontzas AN, Zoumakis M, Bixler EO, et al. Impaired nighttime sleep in healthy old versus young adults is associated with elevated plasma interleukin-6 and cortisol levels: physiologic and therapeutic implications. J Clin Endocrinol Metab 2003;88(5):2087–95.
60. Heaney JL, Phillips AC, Carroll D. Ageing, depression, anxiety, social support and the diurnal rhythm and awakening response of salivary cortisol. Int J Psychophysiol 2010;78(3):201–8.
61. Lai JC, Chong AM, Siu OT, et al. Humor attenuates the cortisol awakening response in healthy older men. Biol Psychol 2010;84(2):375–80.
62. Strahler J, Berndt C, Kirschbaum C, et al. Aging diurnal rhythms and chronic stress: distinct alteration of diurnal rhythmicity of salivary alpha-amylase and cortisol. Biol Psychol 2010;84(2):248–56.
63. Kumari M, Badrick E, Chandola T, et al. Measures of social position and cortisol secretion in an aging population: findings from the Whitehall II study. Psychosom Med 2010;72(1):27–34.
64. Wrosch C, Miller GE, Schulz R. Cortisol secretion and functional disabilities in old age: importance of using adaptive control strategies. Psychosom Med 2009;71(9):996–1003.
65. Ferrari E, Cravello L, Falvo F, et al. Neuroendocrine features in extreme longevity. Exp Gerontol 2008;43(2):88–94.
66. Kripke DF, Elliott JA, Youngstedt SD, et al. Circadian phase response curves to light in older and young women and men. J Circadian Rhythms 2007;5:4.
67. Lavoie HB, Marsh EE, Hall JE. Absence of apparent circadian rhythms of gonadotropins and free alpha-subunit in postmenopausal women: evidence

for distinct regulation relative to other hormonal rhythms. J Biol Rhythms 2006;21(1):58–67.
68. Copinschi G, van Reeth O, Van Cauter E. Biologic rhythms. Effect of aging on the desynchronization of endogenous rhythmicity and environmental conditions. Presse Med 1999;28(17):942–6 [in French].
69. Wolf OT, Dziobek I, McHugh P, et al. Subjective memory complaints in aging are associated with elevated cortisol levels. Neurobiol Aging 2005;26(10):1357–63.
70. Buckley TM, Schatzberg AF. Aging and the role of the HPA axis and rhythm in sleep and memory-consolidation. Am J Geriatr Psychiatry 2005;13(5):344–52.
71. Yehuda R, Golier JA, Harvey PD, et al. Relationship between cortisol and age-related memory impairments in Holocaust survivors with PTSD. Psychoneuroendocrinology 2005;30(7):678–87.
72. Ferrari E, Cravello L, Muzzoni B, et al. Age-related changes of the hypothalamic-pituitary-adrenal axis: pathophysiological correlates. Eur J Endocrinol 2001;144(4):319–29.
73. Magri F, Locatelli M, Balza G, et al. Changes in endocrine circadian rhythms as markers of physiological and pathological brain aging. Chronobiol Int 1997;14(4):385–96.
74. Ferrari E, Magri F, Locatelli M, et al. Chrono-neuroendocrine markers of the aging brain. Aging (Milano) 1996;8(5):320–7.
75. Agarwal AK, Simha V, Oral EA, et al. Phenotypic and genetic heterogeneity in congenital generalized lipodystrophy. J Clin Endocrinol Metab 2003;88(10):4840–7.
76. Burgess LH, Handa RJ. Chronic estrogen-induced alterations in adrenocorticotropin and corticosterone secretion, and glucocorticoid receptor-mediated functions in female rats. Endocrinology 1992;131(3):1261–9.
77. Viau V, Meaney MJ. Variations in the hypothalamic-pituitary-adrenal response to stress during the estrous cycle in the rat. Endocrinology 1991;129(5):2503–11.
78. Bowman RE, MacLusky NJ, Sarmiento Y, et al. Sexually dimorphic effects of prenatal stress on cognition, hormonal responses and central neurotransmitters. Endocrinology 2004;145(8):3778–87.
79. Patchev VK, Almeida OF. Gender specificity in the neural regulation of the response to stress: new leads from classical paradigms. Mol Neurobiol 1998;16(1):63–77.
80. Viau V, Soriano L, Dallman MF. Androgens alter corticotropin releasing hormone and arginine vasopressin mRNA within forebrain sites known to regulate activity in the hypothalamic-pituitary-adrenal axis. J Neuroendocrinol 2001;13(5):442–52.
81. Viau V, Meaney MJ. The inhibitory effect of testosterone on hypothalamic-pituitary-adrenal responses to stress is mediated by the medial preoptic area. J Neurosci 1996;16(5):1866–76.
82. Young EA, Altemus M, Parkison V, et al. Effects of estrogen antagonists and agonists on the ACTH response to restraint stress in female rats. Neuropsychopharmacology 2001;25(6):881–91.
83. Le Mevel JC, Abitbol S, Beraud G, et al. Temporal changes in plasma adrenocorticotropin concentration after repeated neurotropic stress in male and female rats. Endocrinology 1979;105(3):812–7.
84. Bingaman EW, Magnuson DJ, Gray TS, et al. Androgen inhibits the increases in hypothalamic corticotropin-releasing hormone (CRH) and CRH-immunoreactivity following gonadectomy. Neuroendocrinology 1994;59(3):228–34.

85. Lee HC, Chang DE, Yeom M, et al. Gene expression profiling in hypothalamus of immobilization-stressed mouse using cDNA microarray. Brain Res Mol Brain Res 2005;135(1–2):293–300.
86. Canny BJ, O'Farrell KA, Clarke IJ, et al. The influence of sex and gonadectomy on the hypothalamo-pituitary-adrenal axis of the sheep. J Endocrinol 1999; 162(2):215–25.
87. Turner AI, Canny BJ, Hobbs RJ, et al. Influence of sex and gonadal status of sheep on cortisol secretion in response to ACTH and on cortisol and LH secretion in response to stress: importance of different stressors. J Endocrinol 2002; 173(1):113–22.
88. Lado-Abeal J, Robert-McComb JJ, Qian XP, et al. Sex differences in the neuroendocrine response to short-term fasting in rhesus macaques. J Neuroendocrinol 2005;17(7):435–44.
89. Roy BN, Reid RL, van Vugt DA. The effects of estrogen and progesterone on corticotropin-releasing hormone and arginine vasopressin messenger ribonucleic acid levels in the paraventricular nucleus and supraoptic nucleus of the rhesus monkey. Endocrinology 1999;140(5):2191–8.
90. Young EA. The role of gonadal steroids in hypothalamic-pituitary-adrenal axis regulation. Crit Rev Neurobiol 1995;9(4):371–81.
91. Raven PW, Taylor NF. Sex differences in the human metabolism of cortisol. Endocr Res 1996;22(4):751–5.
92. Pomara N, Willoughby LM, Ritchie JC, et al. Sex-related elevation in cortisol during chronic treatment with alprazolam associated with enhanced cognitive performance. Psychopharmacology (Berl) 2005;2:1–6.
93. Carey MP, Deterd CH, De Koning J, et al. The influence of ovarian steroids on hypothalamic-pituitary-adrenal regulation in the female rat. J Endocrinol 1995; 144(2):311–21.
94. Wagner CK, Morrell JI. Distribution and steroid hormone regulation of aromatase mRNA expression in the forebrain of adult male and female rats: a cellular-level analysis using *in situ* hybridization. J Comp Neurol 1996; 370(1):71–84.
95. Arai Y, Gorski RA. Critical exposure time for androgenization of the developing hypothalamus in the female rat. Endocrinology 1968;82(5):1010–4.
96. Seale JV, Wood SA, Atkinson HC, et al. Organisational role for testosterone and estrogen on adult HPA axis activity in the male rat. Endocrinology 2005;146(4): 1973–82.
97. Vamvakopoulos NC, Chrousos GP. Evidence of direct estrogenic regulation of human corticotropin-releasing hormone gene expression. Potential implications for the sexual dimorphism of the stress response and immune/inflammatory reaction. J Clin Invest 1993;92:1896–902.
98. Peiffer A, Lapointe B, Barden N. Hormonal regulation of type II glucocorticoid receptor messenger ribonucleic acid in rat brain. Endocrinology 1991;129(4): 2166–74.
99. Burgess LH, Handa RJ. Estrogen-induced alterations in the regulation of mineralcorticorticoid and glucocorticoid receptor messenger RNA expression in the female rat anterior pituitary gland and brain. Mol Cell Neurosci 1993;4: 191–8.
100. Paulmyer-Lacroix O, Hery M, Pugeat M, et al. The modulatory role of estrogens on corticotropin-releasing factor gene expression in the hypothalamic paraventricular nucleus of ovariectomized rats: role of the adrenal gland. J Neuroendocrinol 1996;8(7):515–9.

101. Patchev VK, Hayashi S, Orikasa C, et al. Implications of estrogen-dependent brain organization for gender differences in hypothalamo-pituitary-adrenal regulation. FASEB J 1995;9(5):419–23.
102. Nappi RE, Rivest S. Ovulatory cycle influences the stimulatory effect of stress on the expression of corticotropin-releasing factor receptor messenger ribonucleic acid in the paraventricular nucleus of the female rat hypothalamus. Endocrinology 1995;136(9):4073–83.
103. Bohler HC Jr, Zoeller RT, King JC, et al. Corticotropin releasing hormone mRNA is elevated on the afternoon of proestrus in the parvocellular paraventricular nuclei of the female rat. Brain Res Mol Brain Res 1990;8(3):259–62.
104. Ellison ET, Burch JC. The effect of estrogenic substances upon the pituitary, adrenals and ovaries. Endocrinology 1936;20:746–52.
105. Kitay JI. Sex differences in adrenal cortical secretion in the rat. Endocrinology 1961;68:818–24.
106. Critchlow V, Liebelt RA, Bar-Sela M, et al. Sex difference in resting pituitary-adrenal function in the rat. Am J Physiol 1963;205(5):807–15.
107. Gompertz D. The effect of sex hormones on the adrenal gland of the male rat. Endocrinology 1958;17:107–13.
108. Adan RA, Burbach JP. Regulation of vasopressin and oxytocin gene expression by estrogen and thyroid hormone. Prog Brain Res 1992;92:127–36.
109. Viau V, Chu A, Soriano L, et al. Independent and overlapping effects of corticosterone and testosterone on corticotropin-releasing hormone and arginine vasopressin mRNA expression in the paraventricular nucleus of the hypothalamus and stress-induced adrenocorticotropic hormone release. J Neurosci 1999; 19(15):6684–93.
110. Lund TD, Munson DJ, Haldy ME, et al. Androgen inhibits, while oestrogen enhances, restraint-induced activation of neuropeptide neurones in the paraventricular nucleus of the hypothalamus. J Neuroendocrinol 2004;16(3):272–8.
111. Miller MA, Vician L, Clifton DK, et al. Sex differences in vasopressin neurons in the bed nucleus of the stria terminalis by in situ hybridization. Peptides 1989; 10(3):615–9.
112. DeLeon KR, Grimes JM, Melloni RH Jr. Repeated anabolic-androgenic steroid treatment during adolescence increases vasopressin V(1A) receptor binding in Syrian hamsters: correlation with offensive aggression. Horm Behav 2002; 42(2):182–91.
113. Handa RJ, Nunley KM, Lorens SA, et al. Androgen regulation of adrenocorticotropin and corticosterone secretion in the male rat following novelty and foot shock stressors. Physiol Behav 1994;55(1):117–24.
114. Miller MA, Urban JH, Dorsa DM. Steroid dependency of vasopressin neurons in the bed nucleus of the stria terminalis by in situ hybridization. Endocrinology 1989;125(5):2335–40.
115. De Vries GJ, Duetz W, Buijs RM, et al. Effects of androgens and estrogens on the vasopressin and oxytocin innervation of the adult rat brain. Brain Res 1986;399(2):296–302.
116. Moore RJ, Gazak JM, Wilson JD. Regulation of cytoplasmic dihydrotestosterone binding in dog prostate by 17 beta-estradiol. J Clin Invest 1979;63(3):351–7.
117. Rance NE, Max SR. Modulation of the cytosolic androgen receptor in striated muscle by sex steroids. Endocrinology 1984;115(3):862–6.
118. Lindheim SR, Legro RS, Bernstein L, et al. Behavioral stress responses in premenopausal and postmenopausal women and the effects of estrogen. Am J Obstet Gynecol 1992;167(6):1831–6.

119. Dayas CV, Xu Y, Buller KM, et al. Effects of chronic oestrogen replacement on stress-induced activation of hypothalamic-pituitary-adrenal axis control pathways. J Neuroendocrinol 2000;12(8):784–94.
120. Seeman MV. Psychopathology in women and men: focus on female hormones. Am J Psychiatry 1997;154(12):1641–7.
121. Jenkins R. Sex differences in depression. Br J Hosp Med 1987;38(5):485–6.
122. Seeman TE, Singer B, Wilkinson CW, et al. Gender differences in age-related changes in HPA axis reactivity. Psychoneuroendocrinology 2001;26(3):225–40.
123. Vierhapper H, Nowotny P, Waldhausl W. Sex-specific differences in cortisol production rates in humans. Metabolism 1998;47(8):974–6.
124. Vierhapper H, Nowotny P, Waldhausl W. Production rates of cortisol in men with hypogonadism. Metabolism 2004;53(9):1174–6.
125. Van Cauter E, Leproult R, Kupfer DJ. Effects of gender and age on the levels and circadian rhythmicity of plasma cortisol. J Clin Endocrinol Metab 1996; 81(7):2468–73.
126. Keenan DM, Roelfsema F, Veldhuis JD. Endogenous ACTH concentration-dependent drive of pulsatile cortisol secretion in the human. Am J Physiol Endocrinol Metab 2004;287(4):E652–61.
127. Kraan GP, Dullaart RP, Pratt JJ, et al. The daily cortisol production reinvestigated in healthy men. The serum and urinary cortisol production rates are not significantly different. J Clin Endocrinol Metab 1998;83(4):1247–52.
128. Baumann G. Estrogens and the hypothalamo-pituitary-adrenal axis in man: evidence for normal feedback regulation by corticosteroids. J Clin Endocrinol Metab 1983;57(6):1193–7.
129. Mizuno TM, Kleopoulos SP, Bergen HT, et al. Hypothalamic pro-opiomelanocortin mRNA is reduced by fasting and [corrected] in ob/ob and db/db mice, but is stimulated by leptin. Diabetes 1998;47(2):294–7.
130. Purnell JQ, Brandon DD, Isabelle LM, et al. Association of 24-hour cortisol production rates, cortisol-binding globulin, and plasma-free cortisol levels with body composition, leptin levels, and aging in adult men and women. J Clin Endocrinol Metab 2004;89(1):281–7.
131. Genazzani AR, Lemarchand-Beraud T, Aubert ML, et al. Pattern of plasma ACTH, hGH, and cortisol during menstrual cycle. J Clin Endocrinol Metab 1975;41(3):431–7.
132. Marinari KT, Leshner AI, Doyle MP. Menstrual cycle status and adrenocortical reactivity to psychological stress. Psychoneuroendocrinology 1976;1(3): 213–8.
133. Atkinson HC, Waddell BJ. The hypothalamic-pituitary-adrenal axis in rat pregnancy and lactation: circadian variation and interrelationship of plasma adrenocorticotropin and corticosterone. Endocrinology 1995;136(2):512–20.
134. Polderman KH, Gooren LJ, Van der Veen EA. Testosterone administration increases adrenal response to adrenocorticotrophin. Clin Endocrinol (Oxf) 1994;40(5):595–601.
135. Arvat E, Di Vito L, Lanfranco F, et al. Stimulatory effect of adrenocorticotropin on cortisol, aldosterone, and dehydroepiandrosterone secretion in normal humans: dose-response study. J Clin Endocrinol Metab 2000;85(9):3141–6.
136. Greenspan SL, Rowe JW, Maitland LA, et al. The pituitary-adrenal glucocorticoid response is altered by gender and disease. J Gerontol 1993;48(3):M72–7.
137. Luisi S, Tonetti A, Bernardi F, et al. Effect of acute corticotropin releasing factor on pituitary-adrenocortical responsiveness in elderly women and men. J Endocrinol Invest 1998;21(7):449–53.

138. Gallucci WT, Baum A, Laue L, et al. Sex differences in sensitivity of the hypothalamic-pituitary-adrenal axis. Health Psychol 1993;12(5):420–5.
139. Bloch M, Rubinow DR, Schmidt PJ, et al. Cortisol response to ovine corticotropin-releasing hormone in a model of pregnancy and parturition in euthymic women with and without a history of postpartum depression. J Clin Endocrinol Metab 2005;90(2):695–9.
140. Liu JH, Rasmussen DD, Rivier J, et al. Pituitary responses to synthetic corticotropin-releasing hormone: absence of modulatory effects by estrogen and progestin. Am J Obstet Gynecol 1987;157(6):1387–91.
141. Kirschbaum C, Schommer N, Federenko I, et al. Short-term estradiol treatment enhances pituitary-adrenal axis and sympathetic responses to psychosocial stress in healthy young men. J Clin Endocrinol Metab 1996;81(10):3639–43.
142. Rubinow DR, Roca CA, Schmidt PJ, et al. Testosterone suppression of CRH-stimulated cortisol in men. Neuropsychopharmacology 2005;30(10):1906–12.
143. Diamond MP, Jones T, Caprio S, et al. Gender influences counterregulatory hormone responses to hypoglycemia. Metabolism 1993;42:1568–72.
144. Rubin RT, Rhodes ME, O'Toole S, et al. Sexual diergism of hypothalamo-pituitary-adrenal cortical responses to low-dose physotigmine in elderly vs. young women and men. Neuropsychopharmacology 2002;26(5):672–81.
145. Stroud LR, Salovey P, Epel ES. Sex differences in stress responses: social rejection versus achievement stress. Biol Psychiatry 2002;52(4):318–27.
146. Earle TL, Linden W, Weinberg J. Differential effects of harassment on cardiovascular and salivary cortisol stress reactivity and recovery in women and men. J Psychosom Res 1999;46(2):125–41.
147. Deuster PA, Petrides JS, Singh A, et al. High intensity exercise promotes escape of adrenocorticotropin and cortisol from suppression by dexamethasone: sexually dimorphic responses. J Clin Endocrinol Metab 1998;83(9):3332–8.
148. Wilkinson CW, Petrie EC, Murray SR, et al. Human glucocorticoid feedback inhibition is reduced in older individuals: evening study. J Clin Endocrinol Metab 2001;86(2):545–50.
149. Boscaro M, Paoletta A, Scarpa E, et al. Age-related changes in glucocorticoid fast feedback inhibition of adrenocorticotropin in man. J Clin Endocrinol Metab 1998;83(4):1380–3.
150. Veldhuis JD, Keenan DM, Roelfsema F, et al. Aging-related adaptations in the corticotropic axis: modulation by gender. Endocrinol Metab Clin North Am 2005;34:993–1014.
151. O'Brien JT, Schweitzer I, Ames D, et al. Cortisol suppression by dexamethasone in the healthy elderly: effects of age, dexamethasone levels, and cognitive function. Biol Psychiatry 1994;36(6):389–94.
152. Oxenkrug GF, Pomara N, McIntyre IM, et al. Aging and cortisol resistance to suppression by dexamethasone: a positive correlation. Psychiatry Res 1983;10(2):125–30.
153. Ortiz-Alonso FJ, Galecki A, Herman WH, et al. Hypoglycemia counterregulation in elderly humans: relationship to glucose levels. Am J Physiol 1994;267(4 Pt 1):E497–506.
154. Pavlov EP, Harman SM, Chrousos GP, et al. Responses of plasma adrenocorticotropin, cortisol, and dehydroepiandrosterone to ovine corticotropin-releasing hormone in healthy aging men. J Clin Endocrinol Metab 1986;62(4):767–72.

155. Wilkinson CW, Peskind ER, Raskind MA. Decreased hypothalamic-pituitary-adrenal axis sensitivity to cortisol feedback inhibition in human aging. Neuroendocrinology 1997;65(1):79–90.
156. Reynolds RM, Walker BR, Syddall HE, et al. Is there a gender difference in the associations of birthweight and adult hypothalamic-pituitary-adrenal axis activity? Eur J Endocrinol 2005;152(2):249–53.
157. Won JG, Jap TS, Chang SC, et al. Evidence for a delayed, integral, and proportional phase of glucocorticoid feedback on ACTH secretion in normal human volunteers. Metabolism 1996;35:254–9.
158. Reader SC, Alaghband-Zadeh J, Daly JR, et al. Negative rate-sensitive feedback effects on adrenocorticotrophin secretion by cortisol in normal subjects. J Endocrinol 1982;92(3):443–8.
159. Mason BL, Pariante CM, Thomas SA. A revised role for P-glycoprotein in the brain distribution of dexamethasone, cortisol, and corticosterone in wild type and ABCB1A/B-deficient mice. Endocrinology 2008;149(10):5244–53.
160. Lentjes EG, Romijn F, Maassen RJ, et al. Free cortisol in serum assayed by temperature-controlled ultrafiltration before fluorescence polarization immunoassay. Clin Chem 1993;39(12):2518–21.
161. Slaunwhite WR Jr, Lockle GN, Back N, et al. Inactivity *in vivo* of transcortin-bound cortisol. Science 1962;135:1062–3.
162. Schwarz S, Pohl P. Steroid hormones and steroid hormone binding globulins in cerebrospinal fluid studied in individuals with intact and with disturbed blood-cerebrospinal fluid barrier. Neuroendocrinology 1992;55(2):174–82.
163. Viau V, Sharma S, Meaney MJ. Changes in plasma adrenocorticotropin, corticosterone, corticosteroid-binding globulin, and hippocampal glucocorticoid receptor occupancy/translocation in rat pups in response to stress. J Neuroendocrinol 1996;8(1):1–8.
164. Kawai A, Yates FE. Interference with feedback inhibition of adrenocorticotropin release by protein binding of corticosterone. Endocrinology 1966;79(6):1040–6.
165. Keenan DM, Veldhuis JD. Cortisol feedback state governs adrenocorticotropin secretory-burst shape, frequency and mass in a dual-waveform construct: time-of-day dependent regulation. Am J Physiol 2003;285(5):R950–61.
166. Veldhuis JD, Iranmanesh A, Lizarralde G, et al. Amplitude modulation of a burst-like mode of cortisol secretion subserves the circadian glucocorticoid rhythm in man. Am J Physiol 1989;257:E6–14.
167. Bright GM. Corticosteroid-binding globulin influences kinetic parameters of plasma cortisol transport and clearance. J Clin Endocrinol Metab 1995;80(3):770–5.
168. Fernandez-Real JM, Pugeat M, Grasa M, et al. Serum corticosteroid-binding globulin concentration and insulin resistance syndrome: a population study. J Clin Endocrinol Metab 2002;87(10):4686–90.
169. de Lacerda L, Kowarski A, Migeon CJ. Diurnal variation of the metabolic clearance rate of cortisol. Effect on measurement of cortisol production rate. J Clin Endocrinol Metab 1973;36(6):1043–9.
170. Besser GM, Orth DN, Nicholson WE, et al. Dissociation of the disappearance of bioactive and radioimmunoreactive ACTH from plasma in man. J Clin Endocrinol Metab 1971;32:595–603.
171. Veldhuis JD, Iranmanesh A, Naftolowitz D, et al. Corticotropin secretory dynamics in humans under low glucocorticoid feedback. J Clin Endocrinol Metab 2001;86(11):5554–63.

172. Iranmanesh A, Lizarralde G, Veldhuis JD. Coordinate activation of the corticotropic axis by insulin-induced hypoglycemia: simultaneous estimates of B-endorphin, ACTH, and cortisol secretion and disappearance in normal men. Acta Endocrinol (Copenh) 1993;128:521–8.
173. Iranmanesh A, Short D, Lizarralde G, et al. Intensive venous sampling paradigms disclose high-frequency ACTH release episodes in normal men. J Clin Endocrinol Metab 1990;71:1276–83.
174. Veldhuis JD, Iranmanesh A, Johnson ML, et al. Amplitude, but not frequency, modulation of ACTH secretory bursts gives rise to the nyctohemeral rhythm of the corticotropic axis in man. J Clin Endocrinol Metab 1990;71:452–63.
175. Keenan DM, Licinio J, Veldhuis JD. A feedback-controlled ensemble model of the stress-responsive hypothalamo-pituitary-adrenal axis. Proc Natl Acad Sci U S A 2001;98(7):4028–33.
176. Keenan DM, Alexander SL, Irvine CH, et al. Reconstruction of *in vivo* time-evolving neuroendocrine dose-response properties unveils admixed deterministic and stochastic elements. Proc Natl Acad Sci U S A 2004;101(17): 6740–5.
177. Keenan DM, Alexander S, Irvine CH, et al. Quantifying nonlinear interactions within the hypothalamo-pituitary-adrenal axis in the conscious horse. Endocrinology 2009;150:1941–51.
178. Keenan DM, Roelfsema F, Carroll BJ, et al. Sex defines the age dependence of endogenous ACTH-cortisol dose responsiveness. Am J Physiol Regul Integr Comp Physiol 2009;297(2):R515–23.
179. Veldhuis JD, Roemmich JN, Richmond EJ, et al. Somatotropic and gonadotropic axes linkages in infancy, childhood, and the puberty-adult transition. Endocr Rev 2006;27(2):101–40.
180. Milad MA, Jusko WJ. Pharmacodynamic interpretation of adrenocorticotropin stimulation tests. Ann Pharmacother 1993;27(10):1195–7.
181. Pacak K, Palkovits M. Stressor specificity of central neuroendocrine responses: implications for stress-related disorders. Endocr Rev 2001;22(4):502–48.
182. Sawchenko PE, Swanson LW. Central noradrenergic pathways for the integration of hypothalamic neuroendocrine and autonomic responses. Science 1981;214(4521):685–7.
183. Lopez JF, Akil H, Watson SJ. Neural circuits mediating stress. Biol Psychiatry 1999;46(11):1461–71.
184. Liu J, Bisschop PH, Eggels L, et al. Intrahypothalamic estradiol modulates hypothalamus-pituitary-adrenal-axis activity in female rats. Endocrinology 2012;153(7):3337–44.
185. Workel JO, Oitzl MS, Fluttert M, et al. Differential and age-dependent effects of maternal deprivation on the hypothalamic-pituitary-adrenal axis of brown Norway rats from youth to senescence. J Neuroendocrinol 2001;13(7):569–80.
186. O'Brien JT, Lloyd A, McKeith I, et al. A longitudinal study of hippocampal volume, cortisol levels, and cognition in older depressed subjects. Am J Psychiatry 2004;161(11):2081–90.
187. Berghard A, Hagglund AC, Bohm S, et al. Lhx2-dependent specification of olfactory sensory neurons is required for successful integration of olfactory, vomeronasal, and GnRH neurons. FASEB J 2012;26(8):3464–72.
188. Marin P, Darin N, Amemiya T, et al. Cortisol secretion in relation to body fat distribution in obese premenopausal women. Metabolism 1992;41(8):882–6.
189. Herbert J. Cortisol and depression: three questions for psychiatry. Psychol Med 2013;43:449–69.

190. Cocchi D. Age-related alterations in gonadotropin, adrenocorticotropin and growth hormone secretion. Aging (Milano) 1992;4(2):103–13.
191. Swaab DF, Bao AM. (Re-)activation of neurons in aging and dementia: lessons from the hypothalamus. Exp Gerontol 2011;46:178–84.
192. van Coevorden A, Mockel J, Laurent E, et al. Neuroendocrine rhythms and sleep in aging men. Am J Physiol 1991;260:E651–61.
193. Martin CG, Bruce J, Fisher PA. Racial and ethnic differences in diurnal cortisol rhythms in preadolescents: the role of parental psychosocial risk and monitoring. Horm Behav 2012;61(5):661–8.
194. Sharma M, Palacios-Bois J, Schwartz G, et al. Circadian rhythms of melatonin and cortisol in aging. Biol Psychiatry 1989;25(3):305–19.
195. Sherman B, Wysham C, Pfohl B. Age-related changes in the circadian rhythm of plasma cortisol in man. J Clin Endocrinol Metab 1985;61(3):439–43.
196. Halbreich U, Asnis GM, Zumoff B, et al. Effect of age and sex on cortisol secretion in depressives and normals. Psychiatry Res 1984;13(3):221–9.
197. Touitou Y, Sulon J, Bogdan A, et al. Adrenocortical hormones, ageing and mental condition: seasonal and circadian rhythms of plasma 18-hydroxy-11-deoxycorticosterone, total and free cortisol and urinary corticosteroids. J Endocrinol 1983; 96(1):53–64.
198. Milcu SM, Bogdan C, Nicolau GY, et al. Cortisol circadian rhythm in 70–100-year-old subjects. Endocrinologie 1978;16(1):29–39.
199. Deuschle M, Weber B, Colla M, et al. Effects of major depression, aging and gender upon calculated diurnal free plasma cortisol concentrations: a re-evaluation study. Stress 1998;2(4):281–7.
200. Bergendahl M, Iranmanesh A, Mulligan T, et al. Impact of age on cortisol secretory dynamics basally and as driven by nutrient-withdrawal stress. J Clin Endocrinol Metab 2000;85(6):2203–14.
201. Montanini V, Simoni M, Chiossi G, et al. Age-related changes in plasma dehydroepiandrosterone sulphate, cortisol, testosterone and free testosterone circadian rhythms in adult men. Horm Res 1988;29(1):1–6.
202. Zhou JN, Hofman MA, Swaab DF. VIP neurons in the human SCN in relation to sex, age, and Alzheimer's disease. Neurobiol Aging 1995;16(4):571–6.
203. Zhou JN, Swaab DF. Activation and degeneration during aging: a morphometric study of the human hypothalamus. Microsc Res Tech 1999;44(1):36–48.
204. Aiba M, Fujibayashi M. Alteration of subcapsular adrenocortical zonation in humans with aging: the progenitor zone predominates over the previously well-developed zona glomerulosa after 40 years of age. J Histochem Cytochem 2011;59(5):557–64.
205. Ferrari M, Mantero F. Male aging and hormones: the adrenal cortex. J Endocrinol Invest 2005;28(11 Suppl Proceedings):92–5.
206. Tanaka H, Akama H, Ichikawa Y, et al. Glucocorticoid receptors in normal leukocytes: effects of age, gender, season, and plasma cortisol concentrations. Clin Chem 1991;37(10 Pt 1):1715–9.
207. Morano MI, Vazquez DM, Akil H. The role of the hippocampal mineralocorticoid and glucocorticoid receptors in the hypothalamo-pituitary-adrenal axis of the aged Fisher rat. Mol Cell Neurosci 1994;5(5):400–12.
208. Hauger RL, Thrivikraman KV, Plotsky PM. Age-related alterations of hypothalamic-pituitary-adrenal axis function in male Fischer 344 rats. Endocrinology 1997;134:1528–36.
209. Meaney MJ, Aitken DH, Sharma S, et al. Basal ACTH, corticosterone and corticosterone-binding globulin levels over the diurnal cycle, and age-related

changes in hippocampal type I and type II corticosteroid receptor binding capacity in young and aged, handled and nonhandled rats. Neuroendocrinology 1992;55(2):204–13.
210. Issa AM, Rowe W, Gauthier S, et al. Hypothalamic-pituitary-adrenal activity in aged, cognitively impaired and cognitively unimpaired rats. J Neurosci 1990; 10(10):3247–54.
211. Gust DA, Wilson ME, Stocker T, et al. Activity of the hypothalamic-pituitary-adrenal axis is altered by aging and exposure to social stress in female rhesus monkeys. J Clin Endocrinol Metab 2000;85(7):2556–63.
212. Haus E, Nicolau G, Lakatua DJ, et al. Circadian rhythm parameters of endocrine functions in elderly subjects during the seventh to the ninth decade of life. Chronobiologia 1989;16(4):331–52.
213. Ferrari E, Magri F, Dori D, et al. Neuroendocrine correlates of the aging brain in humans. Neuroendocrinology 1995;61(4):464–70.
214. Blichert-Toft M, Hummer L. Serum immunoreactive corticotrophin and response to metyrapone in old age in man. Gerontology 1977;23:236–43.
215. da Silva RM, Pinto E, Goldman SM, et al. Children with Cushing's syndrome: primary pigmented nodular adrenocortical disease should always be suspected. Pituitary 2011;14(1):61–7.
216. Ambrosio MR, Campo M, Zatelli MC, et al. Unexpected activation of pituitary-adrenal axis in healthy young and elderly subjects during somatostatin infusion. Neuroendocrinology 1998;68(2):123–8.
217. Seeman TE, Singer B, Charpentier P. Gender differences in patterns of HPA axis response to challenge. Macarthur studies of successful aging. Psychoneuroendocrinology 1995;20(7):711–25.
218. Gelfin Y, Lerer B, Lesch KP, et al. Complex effects of age and gender on hypothermic, adrenocorticotrophic hormone and cortisol responses to ipsapirone challenge in normal subjects. Psychopharmacology 1995;120(3):356–64.
219. Peskind ER, Raskind MA, Wingerson D, et al. Hypothalamic-pituitary-adrenocortical axis responses to physostigmine: effects of Alzheimer's disease and gender. Biol Psychiatry 1996;40(1):61–8.
220. Lovallo WR, King AC, Farag NH, et al. Naltrexone effects on cortisol secretion in women and men in relation to a family history of alcoholism: studies from the Oklahoma Family Health Patterns Project. Psychoneuroendocrinology 2012; 37:1922–8.
221. Giordano R, Bo M, Pellegrino M, et al. Hypothalamus-pituitary-adrenal hyperactivity in human aging is partially refractory to stimulation by mineralocorticoid receptor blockade. J Clin Endocrinol Metab 2005;90(10):5656–62.
222. Heuser I, Deuschle M, Weber A, et al. The role of mineralocorticoid receptors in the circadian activity of the human hypothalamus-pituitary-adrenal system: effect of age. Neurobiol Aging 2000;21(4):585–9.
223. von Bardeleben U, Holsboer F. Effect of age on the cortisol response to human corticotropin-releasing hormone in depressed patients pretreated with dexamethasone. Biol Psychiatry 1991;29(10):1042–50.
224. Martens EA, Lemmens SG, Adam TC, et al. Sex differences in HPA axis activity in response to a meal. Physiol Behav 2012;106(2):272–7.
225. Heaney JL, Phillips AC, Carroll D. Aging, health behaviors, and the diurnal rhythm and awakening response of salivary cortisol. Exp Aging Res 2012; 38(3):295–314.
226. Olbrich D, Dittmar M. The cortisol awakening response is related with PERIOD1 clock gene expression in older women. Exp Gerontol 2012;47(7):527–33.

227. Brandtstadter J, Baltes-Gotz B, Kirschbaum C, et al. Developmental and personality correlates of adrenocortical activity as indexed by salivary cortisol: observations in the age range of 35 to 65 years. J Psychosom Res 1991; 35(2–3):173–85.
228. Evans P, Hucklebridge F, Loveday C, et al. The cortisol awakening response is related to executive function in older age. Int J Psychophysiol 2012;84(2):201–4.
229. Almela M, van der Meij L, Hidalgo V, et al. The cortisol awakening response and memory performance in older men and women. Psychoneuroendocrinology 2012;37:1929–40.
230. Nicolson N, Storms C, Ponds R, et al. Salivary cortisol levels and stress reactivity in human aging. J Gerontol A Biol Sci Med Sci 1997;52(2):M68–75.
231. Roelfsema F, Pijl H, Keenan DM, et al. Diminished adrenal sensitivity and adrenocorticotropin efficacy in obese premenopausal women. Eur J Endocrinol 2012;167:633–42.
232. Otte C, Yassouridis A, Jahn H, et al. Mineralocorticoid receptor-mediated inhibition of the hypothalamic-pituitary-adrenal axis in aged humans. J Gerontol A Biol Sci Med Sci 2003;58(10):B900–5.
233. Hatzinger M, Brand S, Herzig N, et al. In healthy young and elderly adults, hypothalamic-pituitary-adrenocortical axis reactivity (HPA AR) varies with increasing pharmacological challenge and with age, but not with gender. J Psychiatr Res 2011;45(10):1373–80.
234. Bjorntorp P. Alterations in the ageing corticotropic stress-response axis. Novartis Found Symp 2002;242:46–58.
235. Altemus M, Redwine L, Leong YM, et al. Reduced sensitivity to glucocorticoid feedback and reduced glucocorticoid receptor mRNA expression in the luteal phase of the menstrual cycle. Neuropsychopharmacology 1997;17(2):100–9.
236. Coiro V, Passeri M, Volpi R, et al. Different effects of aging on the opioid mechanisms controlling gonadotropin and cortisol secretion in man. Horm Res 1989; 32(4):119–23.
237. Berardelli R, Margarito E, Ghiggia F, et al. Neuroendocrine effects of citalopram, a selective serotonin re-uptake inhibitor, during lifespan in humans. J Endocrinol Invest 2010;33(9):657–62.
238. Komesaroff PA, Esler MD, Sudhir K. Estrogen supplementation attenuates glucocorticoid and catecholamine responses to mental stress in perimenopausal women. J Clin Endocrinol Metab 1999;84(2):606–10.
239. Lavoie JM, Dionne N, Helie R, et al. Menstrual cycle phase dissociation of blood glucose homeostasis during exercise. J Appl Physiol 1987;62(3):1084–9.
240. Roca CA, Schmidt PJ, Altemus M, et al. Differential menstrual cycle regulation of hypothalamic-pituitary-adrenal axis in women with premenstrual syndrome and controls. J Clin Endocrinol Metab 2003;88(7):3057–63.
241. Altemus M, Roca C, Galliven E, et al. Increased vasopressin and adrenocorticotropin responses to stress in the midluteal phase of the menstrual cycle. J Clin Endocrinol Metab 2001;86(6):2525–30.
242. Kripke DF, Youngstedt SD, Elliott JA, et al. Circadian phase in adults of contrasting ages. Chronobiol Int 2005;22(4):695–709.
243. Mazzoccoli G, Carughi S, Sperandeo M, et al. Alteration of circadian rhythmicity of CD3+CD4+ lymphocyte subpopulation in healthy aging. J Biol Regul Homeost Agents 2011;25(3):405–16.
244. Prinz PN, Bailey SL, Woods DL. Sleep impairments in healthy seniors: roles of stress, cortisol, and interleukin-1 beta. Chronobiol Int 2000;17(3):391–404.

Endogenous Sex Steroid Levels and Cardiovascular Disease in Relation to the Menopause

A Systematic Review

Carolyn J. Crandall, MD, MS[a,*], Elizabeth Barrett-Connor, MD[b]

KEYWORDS

• Coronary heart disease • Coronary artery disease • Endogenous estrogen
• Hormone therapy • Menopause • Estradiol • Sex hormone-binding globulin

KEY POINTS

- Favorable effects of oral estrogen therapy on increases in high-density lipoprotein and decreases in low-density lipoprotein did not translate to demonstrable decreases in coronary heart disease (CHD) events in randomized controlled trials of postmenopausal hormone therapy (HT) for women.
- Nearly all large HT trials with CHD outcomes used pharmacologic doses of oral conjugated equine estrogen.
- Endogenous estrogen levels are more relevant to the true associations between postmenopausal estrogen and CHD risk factors or clinical outcomes.

INTRODUCTION

Heart disease remains a major cause of death among women in the United States.[1] In 2008, 1 in 31 deaths in US women was attributable to breast cancer, whereas 1 in 6.6 deaths was attributable to coronary heart disease (CHD).[2] The remaining lifetime risk for CHD (acute myocardial infarction [MI], angina pectoris, and chronic ischemic heart disease) among US women at age 40 is 1 in 3.[2]

For many years, researchers and clinicians have observed gender differences in the patterns of CHD. Because the incidence of CHD in women lags behind that of men by 10 years,[2] it was hypothesized that changes in the endogenous estrogen milieu during or after the menopause transition explains most of these gender differences in CHD

[a] Department of Medicine, David Geffen School of Medicine, University of California at Los Angeles, UCLA Medicine/GIM, 911 Broxton Avenue, 1st Floor, Los Angeles, CA 90024, USA;
[b] Department of Family and Preventive Medicine, University of California, 9500 Gilman Drive, San Diego, La Jolla, CA 92093-0607, USA
* Corresponding author.
E-mail address: ccrandall@mednet.ucla.edu

Endocrinol Metab Clin N Am 42 (2013) 227–253
http://dx.doi.org/10.1016/j.ecl.2013.02.003 endo.theclinics.com
0889-8529/13/$ – see front matter

prevalence. In support of this hypothesis, the severity of coronary artery disease (CAD) in women referred to coronary angiography is correlated with measures of exposure to endogenous estrogen (time since menopause, age at menopause), independently of age.[3] Also, a cohort study reported that older age at menopause is related to reduced cardiovascular disease (CVD) mortality over 20 years of follow-up.[4] In the Multi-Ethnic Study of Atherosclerosis, early menopause (before age 46 years) was associated with shorter CHD-free survival over 4.8 years of follow-up, even after adjustment for other coronary risk factors.[5] The large Nurses' Health Study did not find this association except in women without ovaries.[6]

The menopause transition is associated with adverse changes in lipoprotein pattern; postmenopausal women have higher total cholesterol, low-density lipoprotein (LDL), and triglycerides, and lower high-density lipoproteins (HDL), than do premenopausal women.[7–9] In the Study of Women's Health Across the Nation, SWAN, a large prospective study of the menopause transition, only total cholesterol, LDL, and apolipoprotein-B showed substantial increases within the 1-year interval before and after the final menstrual period, consistent with menopause-induced changes.[10] Other CHD risk factors were consistent with a linear model, indicating chronologic aging.

Based on adverse menopause-related changes in lipoprotein profiles and gender differences in CHD incidence, one might predict that CHD risk would be decreased by menopausal hormone therapy (HT). Indeed, in the Postmenopausal Estrogen/Progestin Interventions (PEPI) Trial, conjugated equine estrogen (CEE), either alone or in combination with medroxyprogesterone acetate (MPA) or micronized progesterone) increased HDL and decreased LDL.[11] However, the favorable effects of oral estrogen therapy on increases in HDL and decreases in LDL did not translate to demonstrable decreases in CHD events in randomized controlled trials of postmenopausal women (**Table 1**). Instead, primary and secondary prevention trials of CEE 0.625 mg/d plus MPA 2.5 mg/d (CEE + MPA) versus placebo showed adverse effects on CHD events.[12,13] In the Heart and Estrogen/progestin Replacement Study (HERS), a secondary prevention trial, CEE + MPA for a mean of 4.1 years did not reduce the rate of CHD events in postmenopausal women with established CHD and there was a pattern of early increase in risk of CHD events in the CEE + MPA group compared with the group assigned to placebo, despite beneficial effects of CEE + MPA on serum lipoproteins.[12] The Women's Health Initiative (WHI), a primary prevention trial of CEE + MPA versus placebo among women aged 50 to 79 years old at baseline, was terminated early (after a mean follow-up of 5.2 years) due to a 24% increase in the risk of CHD in the CEE + MPA group compared with the placebo group (nominal 95% CI 1.00–1.54).[13] As in the HERS study, the WHI also demonstrated an early increase in the risk of CHD in the CEE + MPA group compared with the placebo group (hazard ratio [HR] at 1 year 1.81, 95% CI 1.09–3.01). Even among women who had initiated CEE + MPA within 10 years of menopause, CEE + MPA was not associated with a significantly decreased risk for CHD.[14,15]

In the WHI Estrogen-Alone Trial (comparing CEE without MPA with placebo) in women without a uterus, the risk of CHD events after a mean of 6.8 years of follow-up was similar among women assigned to CEE and women assigned to placebo.[16] In a post hoc analysis, women assigned to CEE who were aged 50 to 59 years at baseline had lower CHD risk than women assigned to placebo in this age group (HR 0.55, nominal 95% CI 0.35–0.86).[16] A subset of participants of that trial were assessed by cardiac CT.[17] Among participants 50 to 59 years old at enrollment, very few had a clinically significant coronary artery calcified plaque burden in the coronary arteries after trial completion; the difference was slightly but significantly lower among these younger women who were assigned to estrogen than in those assigned to placebo.[17]

Table 1
Major clinical trials testing the effects of estrogen (with or without progestogen) on CHD risk

Trial	Number of Participants	Intervention	Duration of Intervention	Main Intention-to-Treat Result	Reference
Heart and Estrogen/progestin Replacement Study (HERS)	2763 postmenopausal women with CAD, aged <80 y	Daily CEE 0.625 mg + MPA 2.5 mg vs placebo	Mean 4.1 y	No significant difference in 1° outcome (nonfatal MI or CHD death)	12
Women's Health Initiative (WHI) Estrogen Plus Progestin Trial	16,608 postmenopausal women aged 50–70 y	Daily CEE 0.625 mg + MPA 2.5 mg vs placebo	Mean 5.2 y	HT increased risk of 1° outcome (nonfatal MI or CHD death), HR 1.24 (1.00–1.54)	13
Women's Health Initiative (WHI) Estrogen-Alone Trial	10,739 postmenopausal women aged 50–70 y with prior hysterectomy	Daily CEE 0.625 mg/d vs placebo	Mean 6.8 y	No significant difference in 1° outcome (nonfatal MI or CHD death)	16
Danish Osteoporosis Prevention Study[a]	1006 health perimenopausal or postmenopausal women aged 45–58 y	Triphasic E_2 + norethisterone acetate (or E_2 alone for women with hysterectomy) vs no treatment	Mean 10.1 y	HT associated with decreased risk of 1° outcome (death, admission to hospital for heart failure, or MI) HR was 0.48 (0.26–0.87)	18
Kronos Early Estrogen Prevention study (KEEPS)[b]	727 women aged 42–58 y, within 3 y of final menstrual period	Cyclical micronized progesterone with one of the following: CEE 0.45 mg/d, transdermal 0.05 mg/d, or placebo	4 y	No significant difference among groups in risk of MI, but number of events in all 3 groups was very small	19

[a] This trial did not include a placebo group.
[b] Results of this study are not yet published.

The possibility that younger early postmenopausal women may derive benefit from HT is also suggested by a recent Danish report[18]: 1006 participants, who were, on average, 50 years-old at baseline, were randomly assigned to receive HT (a triphasic regimen of estradiol [E_2] plus norethisterone acetate, or E_2 2 mg/d if they had undergone previous hysterectomy) or no treatment. The primary endpoint was a combined outcome of all-cause mortality, heart failure, or MI. After 10 years of follow-up, participants who were assigned to HT and were aged less than 50 years at baseline had a 65% lower risk of the primary endpoint (HR 0.35, 95% CI 0.13–0.89), whereas women aged 50 years or more at baseline who were assigned to HT did not have a significant reduction in the primary outcome.[18] Unfortunately, there was no placebo and the trial was not blinded.

Recently, initial results of the Kronos Early Estrogen Prevention Study (KEEPS), a 4-year clinical trial of estrogen (either daily CEE 0.45 mg/d or E_2 patch 50 μg/d, combined with micronized progesterone 300 mg/d for 12 days monthly) or placebo reported no difference in rates of MI or subclinical disease (coronary artery calcium or carotid artery intima-media thickness) among the three treatment groups.[19,20] Participants were healthy women aged 42 to 58 years within 3 years of their last menstrual period.[19,20] Because no older women were included in this study, this study does not provide information about HT in younger versus older women.

These pharmacologic intervention trials, almost entirely without CVD benefit despite favorable changes in lipoproteins, may reflect the large estrogen (pharmacologic) doses, the oral route of administration (with first pass liver effects explaining the lipoprotein changes), or the diversity of postmenopausal women, although nearly all trials were conducted in women of European ancestry. Despite effects of HT on serum inflammatory marker, homocysteine, and lipoprotein (a) levels, evidence is lacking to show that changes in these marker levels alter CVD risk.[21,22] It is not clear that effects vary according to whether estrogen is given with progestogen or according to age. Some experts believe that HT may have beneficial effects on CVD risk if it is initiated in early menopause, but not if it is initiated in late menopause, the "timing hypothesis."[16,23] Of note, interaction testing among prespecified subgroup analyses in the WHI Estrogen Plus Progestin trial and the Estrogen-Alone trial found no significant differences in effects of HT on CVD risk according to age or years since menopause.[24] Observed differences in CVD risk among women taking estrogen alone (given to women who have undergone hysterectomy) and women taking estrogen plus progestogen (given to women who have not undergone hysterectomy) may reflect the underlying differences in CVD risk related to undergoing hysterectomy and/or oophorectomy.

Therefore, this article focuses on physiologic endogenous estrogen levels with a systematic review of literature related to endogenous sex steroid levels and CAD among postmenopausal women with natural or surgical menopause.

METHODS

In October 2012, the authors performed a systematic PubMed review using the following keywords (limiting to female humans and English language): serum estradiol AND cardiovascular disease AND menopause (218 references), endogenous estrogen AND cardiovascular disease (310 references), and androgen AND cardiovascular disease (309 references). We retained for inclusion in this article the publications that assessed endogenous serum levels of estrogens, androgens, and/or sex hormone binding-globulins (SHBGs) in relation to CAD (n = 20 articles, **Table 2**) or traditional clinical CAD risk factors among postmenopausal women not taking exogenous HT (n = 18 articles, **Table 3**). Four publications met criteria for inclusion in both **Tables 2** and **3**.[25–28]

RESULTS

The study design, numbers of participants, and findings of the studies are presented in **Table 2** (CHD outcome) and **Table 3** (CHD risk factors). Wherever possible, 95% CIs are displayed; *P* values are substituted if corresponding 95% CIs were not described in an article.

Associations Between Serum Sex Steroid and SHBG Levels and CVD Among Postmenopausal Women

Study outcomes

Study outcomes varied considerably according to how CAD was assessed and the study design (see **Table 2**). Of the 20 studies, 14 were cross-sectional[25,28–40] and 6 were longitudinal.[26,27,41–44] Information presented in publications was sometimes inadequate for us to determine how CAD was reported or verified (eg, self-report, medical record review).

Of the 20 articles, 3 articles used CAD assessed by coronary angiography as their key outcomes,[29,30,38] 4 articles reported joint outcomes of angioplasty, nonfatal and fatal MI, and coronary artery bypass grafting,[31,34,36,43] 4 articles reported coronary artery calcium assessed by CT,[32,33,35,41] 2 articles used self-reported CVD as outcomes without giving further detail,[25,39] 2 articles reported joint outcomes of coronary revascularization, MI, stroke death, or coronary death,[28,37] 1 article reported MI as an outcome without further details of MI ascertainment,[40] 2 articles reported ischemic heart disease death based on death certificates as an outcome,[26,27] 1 article reported medical record-based MI as an outcome,[42] and 1 article reported primary care physician-assessed CAD as the outcome without providing further criteria for diagnosis.[44]

Associations of circulating estrogens with CAD

In cross-sectional studies outcomes and potential predictors varied across the studies and circulating estrogen levels were not consistently associated with CAD (see **Table 2**). Cross-sectional studies reported no association between estrone (E_1) level and angiographic CAD,[30] positive associations of bioavailable E_2 (bioE_2) level with medical record-confirmed CHD events that disappeared after adjustment for other CAD risk factors,[31] inverse associations between E_2 level and coronary calcium score,[32] lack of association between E_2 level and coronary calcium plaques after adjustment for other risk factors,[33,35] no association of free estrogen index (FEI) with medical record-confirmed CVD,[28,37] no association of free E_2 with angiographic CAD,[38] and inverse association between high serum E_2 levels ($\geq$55 pmol/L) and self-reported CVD.[39] A study with unclear methods for ascertainment of MI reported no association between E_2 level and MI.[40]

In the only longitudinal study that confirmed CAD by angiography, death certificate, and/or medical records, bioE_2, E_2, and/or E_1 levels were not associated with ischemic heart disease death.[26]

Associations of circulating androgens with CAD

In cross-sectional studies outcomes and predictors varied across the studies and circulating androgen levels were not consistently associated with CAD (see **Table 2**). The following associations were suggested regarding testosterone (T) and CAD: positive associations of total T and/or free T and/or free androgen index (FAI)

Table 2
Characteristics of studies examining associations of serum sex steroid and SHBG levels with CVD in postmenopausal women

Cross-Sectional Analyses			
Reference	**Study Population**	**CAD Assessment**	**Results**
Braunstein et al,[29] 2008	Women's Ischemia Syndrome Evaluation Study (WISE) study 284 postmenopausal women with chest pain or suspected MI, not taking HT	CAD by coronary angiography	Significant association of total T (OR 1.03, 95% CI 1.00–1.04) and free T (OR 1.12, 95% CI 1.01–1.23) with presence of CAD after adjustment for free E_2 level, but no mention of analysis of E_2 level itself with CAD
Cauley et al,[30] 1994	87 postmenopausal women aged 50–81 y admitted for diagnostic cardiac catheterization, not taking HT (62 cases with $\geq$1 coronary artery $\geq$50% occluded, 25 controls)	Cardiac catheterization (diagnostic)	No significant difference in estrone concentrations between case and control groups in unadjusted and adjusted models
Chen et al,[31] 2011	Nested case-control study 99 postmenopausal healthy women who later had CHD event and 198 controls without CHD, not taking HT	CHD events (percutaneous transluminal coronary angioplasty, nonfatal MI, fatal MI, coronary artery bypass grafting)	Association of top tertile of bioE_2 level with increased CHD event risk (OR 2.10, 95% CI 1.13–3.90), and association of top tertile of SHBG level with decreased CHD event risk (OR 0.50, 95% CI 0.28–0.92) Associations disappeared after adjustment for BMI, cholesterol, HTN
Jeon et al,[32] 2010	436 postmenopausal women not using HT	Coronary artery calcium by CT	Women with higher serum E_2 ($\geq$20 pg/mL) had lower chance of having high coronary artery calcium score ($\geq$100) (crude OR 0.28, 95% CI 0.08–0.95), even after adjusting for age, years since menopause, cholesterol, BMI, blood pressure, HTN, DM, and glucose (adjusted OR 0.25, 95% CI 0.07–0.86)

Khatibi et al,[25] 2007	6440 women aged 50–59 y the Women's Health in the Lund Area Study, half of whom were using HT	Self-reported CVD (details not given)	Among women not using HT, median values of androstenedione, T index, T, and SHBG were similar among cases (prevalent CVD) and controls
Munir et al,[33] 2012	126 asymptomatic perimenopausal women (mean age 50 y), assessment of the Transition of Hormonal Evaluation with Noninvasive Imaging of Atherosclerosis, a substudy of the Prospective Army Coronary Calcium project, HT use not described	Calcified and noncalcified coronary artery plaques by contrast-enhanced multidetector CT angiography	Increased free T levels were significantly associated with increased number of calcified (correlation 0.21) and noncalcified (0.24) coronary artery plaque SHBG level was inversely correlated with total number of coronary artery plaques (−0.14) (associations were not independent of cardiovascular risk factors) E_2 levels were unrelated to plaque presence and extent
Naessen et al,[34] 2010	72 women 70 y old in the Vasculature in Uppsala Seniors, not taking HT	CHD (MI, angina pectoris, coronary bypass, or balloon angioplasty)	Odds of CVD were associated with levels of pregnenolone (OR 0.31, 95% CI 0.11–0.90), 17-hydroxypregnenolone (0.18, 95% CI 0.06–0.61), DHEA (OR 0.33, 95% CI 0.15–0.71), but was not associated with E_2/T or E_2/E1 ratios All associations lost statistical significance after adjustment for statin use, smoking, and BMI

(*continued on next page*)

Table 2
(*continued*)

Reference	Study Population	CAD Assessment	Results
	Cross-Sectional Analyses		
Ouyong et al,[35] 2009	1947 postmenopausal women in the Multiethnic Study of Atherosclerosis, not taking HT	Coronary calcium by CT	Serum E_2, T, bioT, and SHBG levels were not associated with coronary calcium, after adjustment for age, race/ethnicity, and BMI Among women with measurable coronary calcium, higher SHBG and lower bioT were associated with greater coronary calcium score, but E_2 levels were not associated with coronary calcium score β-coefficient for ln bioT −1.82 (95% CI −0.35 to −0.02); β-coefficient for ln SHBG level 0.30 (95% CI 0.02–0.57) After additional simultaneous adjustment for levels of all sex steroids, a 2.72-fold (1 log-unit) greater SHBG was associated with a 1.30-fold geometric mean coronary calcium score
Page-Wilson et al,[28] 2009	200 nondiabetic postmenopausal women ≥45 y old not using HT in the Women's Health Study of female health professionals, (98 with incident CVD over 2.9 y follow-up, remainder matched controls without CVD)	Composite endpoint of CVD (1st occurrence of nonfatal MI, coronary revascularization, nonfatal stroke, coronary disease, or stroke death) confirmed by medical records	Higher FAI among CVD cases (geometric mean 0.01 nmol/L) than among controls (geometric mean 0.02 nmol/L) No difference in mean FEI between case and control groups
Patel et al,[36] 2009	344 women aged 65–98 y in the Cardiovascular Health Study (included HT users but adjusted statistical models for HT use)	CHD defined as angina, MI, coronary angioplasty, or coronary artery bypass graft surgery based on medical record review	After adjustment, women with T levels in the top quartile had a 3-fold greater odds of CHD than those in the second quartile (OR 2.95, 95% CI 1.2–7.3), but free T was not significantly associated with CHD risk

Phillips et al,[38] 1997	60 postmenopausal undergoing coronary angiography	CAD by coronary angiography, expressed as % maximal luminal diameter	In models containing free T, E_2, age, BMI, systolic blood pressure, total cholesterol, smoking, and insulin, free T level, but not E_2 level, was significantly associated with extent of CAD (β-coefficient 0.38, *P*<.008) The association was almost identical after additional adjustment for SHBG and DHEA-S levels (β-coefficient 0.41, *P* = .03) SHBG and DHEA-S levels were not significantly associated with extent of CAD in fully adjusted models (containing all sex steroid levels together)
Rexrode et al,[37] 2003	200 postmenopausal women ≥45 y old not using HT in the Women's Health Study of female health professionals, (nested case-control study of 98 women with incident CVD over 2.9 y follow-up, remainder matched controls without CVD)	Composite end point of CVD, (1st occurrence of nonfatal MI, coronary revascularization, nonfatal stroke, coronary disease, or stroke death) confirmed by medical records	Among HT nonusers, E_2 and FEI were not associated with CVD risk but the lowest quartile of SHBG was associated with odds of CVD (OR 2.25, 95% CI 1.03–4.91), and the odds of CVD increased with increasing quartiles of FAI (p_{trend} 0.03) (associations were only statistically significant before adjustment for BMI, HTN, DM, and elevated cholesterol)
Shakir et al,[39] 2007	104 postmenopausal women with CVD (MI or stroke) and 208 controls, stratified by HT use	Self-reported CVD	In postmenopausal women who were not taking HT, E_2 levels ≥55 pmol/L were less frequent among cases than among controls (*P* = .04, exact frequencies not presented) Median T, E_2, androstenedione, and SHBG levels were not different in cases than controls

(*continued on next page*)

Table 2
(*continued*)

Cross-Sectional Analyses			
Reference	**Study Population**	**CAD Assessment**	**Results**
Skalba et al,[40] 2003	35 postmenopausal women (18 women with CVD, 17 women without CVD) aged 65–75 y not using HT	Myocardial infarction or coronary insufficiency in the past 5 y, details not further described	No difference in total T, free T, androstenedione, DHEA, DHEA-S, SHBG, or E_2 levels between the groups with CVD and without CVD

Longitudinal Studies			
Reference	**Study Population**	**Cardiovascular Disease Assessed**	**Results**
Barrett-Connor et al,[26] 1995	Rancho Bernardo study, 651 Caucasian postmenopausal women not using HT, 19-y follow-up	Ischemic heart disease death confirmed by death certificates	Age-adjusted bioT, bioE_2, estrone, E_2, and T levels did not predict age-adjusted ischemic heart disease death
Calderon-Margalit et al,[41] 2010	1629 women aged 18–30 at baseline in the Coronary Artery Risk Development in Young Adults (CARDIA) study, population-based cohort study, 20-y follow-up, statistical models adjusted for oral contraceptive use	Coronary artery calcified plaques by chest CT assessed at year 20	SHBG level (mean of years 2, 10, and 16) was inversely associated with the presence of coronary artery calcium (SHBG > median vs ≤ median adjusted OR 0.59, 95% CI 0.40–0.87) No association of total or free T with coronary artery calcified plaques E_2 levels not examined
Goodman-Gruen et al,[27] 1996	624 women followed for 19 y for incident ischemic heart disease death, not using HT	Ischemic heart disease death by death certificate	SHBG levels were not significantly associated with ischemic heart disease mortality either before or after adjustment for covariates
Lapidus et al,[42] 1986	253 postmenopausal women who were 54 or 60 y old at baseline, not taking HT, 12-y follow-up	Nonfatal or fatal MI, angina, or stroke confirmed by medical record review	Plot of the 12-y incidence of MI vs SHBG concentration was U-shaped Statistical analysis of the U-shaped association was not performed due to small number of participants

Laughlin et al,[43] 2010	Rancho Bernardo study, prospective population-based study, 639 white postmenopausal women 50–91 y old not using HT, median follow-up 12.3 y	Incident CHD (nonfatal MI, fatal MI, coronary revascularization)	Women in lowest quintile of T had 1.62-fold increased risk of incident CHD (95% CI 1.10–2.39), after adjustment for lifestyle, adiposity, E2, and CHD risk factors There was a U-shaped curve for association of bioT with CHD after adjustment for lifestyle, adiposity, E_2, and CHD risk factors Compared with the other quintiles, women with highest bioT quintiles had 1.79-fold higher CHD risk (95% CI 1.03–3.16) Women with lowest bioT quintiles had 1.96-fold higher CHD risk (95% CI 1.13–3.41) Associations between E_2 level and CHD events were not described
Sievers et al,[44] 2010	Prospective cohort study with 4.5-y follow-up of 2914 female patients between 18 and 75 y from representative sample of Germany primary care practices, 1394 of the 2914 women were postmenopausal analyses among women not taking HT were performed	CAD as ascertained by patient's primary care physician	Patients with total T in the lowest quintile had higher risk of cardiovascular events during follow-up compared with the higher quintiles (quintiles 2–5 vs quintile 1 crude HR 0.54, 95% CI 0.38–0.77; adjusted HR 0.68, 95% CI 0.48–0.97) E2 levels were not examined

Abbreviations: bioE_2, bioavailable E_2; bioT, bioavailable testosterone; DHEA, dehydroepiandrosterone; DHEA-S, DHEA sulfate; FAI, free androgen index; FEI, free estrogen index; OR, odds ratio; P_{trend}, P values for test of trend; T, testosterone.

Table 3
Characteristics of studies examining associations of serum sex steroid and sex hormone-binding globulin levels with cardiovascular risk factors in postmenopausal women

Reference	Study Population	Cardiac Risk Factors Examined	Results
Cross-Sectional Studies			
Barrett-Connor et al,[26] 1995	Rancho Bernardo study, 651 white postmenopausal women not using HT, 19-y follow-up	SBP, DBP, fasting glucose, BMI, smoking	After adjustment for age, and BMI, mean levels of the hormones (androstenedione, T, E_1, E_2, bioE, and bioT) did not vary significantly by category of risk factors (SBP, DBP, cholesterol, fasting glucose, BMI, history of smoking)
Goodman-Gruen et al,[45] 2000	Rancho Bernardo study, 633 white postmenopausal women ≥55 y old not using HT	IGT, type 2 DM, fasting glucose, BMI, physical activity, smoking	After adjustment for age and BMI, women with IGT had significantly higher bioT (0.18 nmol/L vs 0.15 nmol/L), total E_2 (23.3 pol/L vs 20.6 pmol/L) and bioE_2 (11.4 pmol/L vs 10.3 pmol/L) levels than women with normal glucose tolerance After adjustment for age and BMI, women with type 2 DM had significantly higher bioT (0.18 nmol/L vs 0.15 nmol/L), total E2 (25.4 pmol/L vs 20.6 pmol/L) and bioE_2 (15.0 pmol/L vs 10.3 pmol/L) levels than women with normal glucose tolerance After adjustment for age, median values of total E_2 were higher above vs below median BMI (27.6 vs 21.2 pmol/L), higher above vs below median waist-to-hip ratio (24.2 vs 22.5 pmol/L), and higher with physical activity less than 3 times weekly (22.6 vs 21.4 pmol/L) After adjustment for age, median values of bioE_2 were higher above vs below median BMI (16.3 vs 11.1 pmol/L), higher above vs below median waist-to-hip ratio (13.6 vs 12.1 pmol/L), and higher with physical activity less than 3 times weekly (14.6 vs 11.9 pmol/L) Median values of total T and bioT did not differ according to categories of waist-to-hip ratio, smoking, or physical activity Median bioT level was higher above vs below the median BMI (0.19 vs 0.16 nmol/L) Median values of total T did not differ according to BMI above vs below median

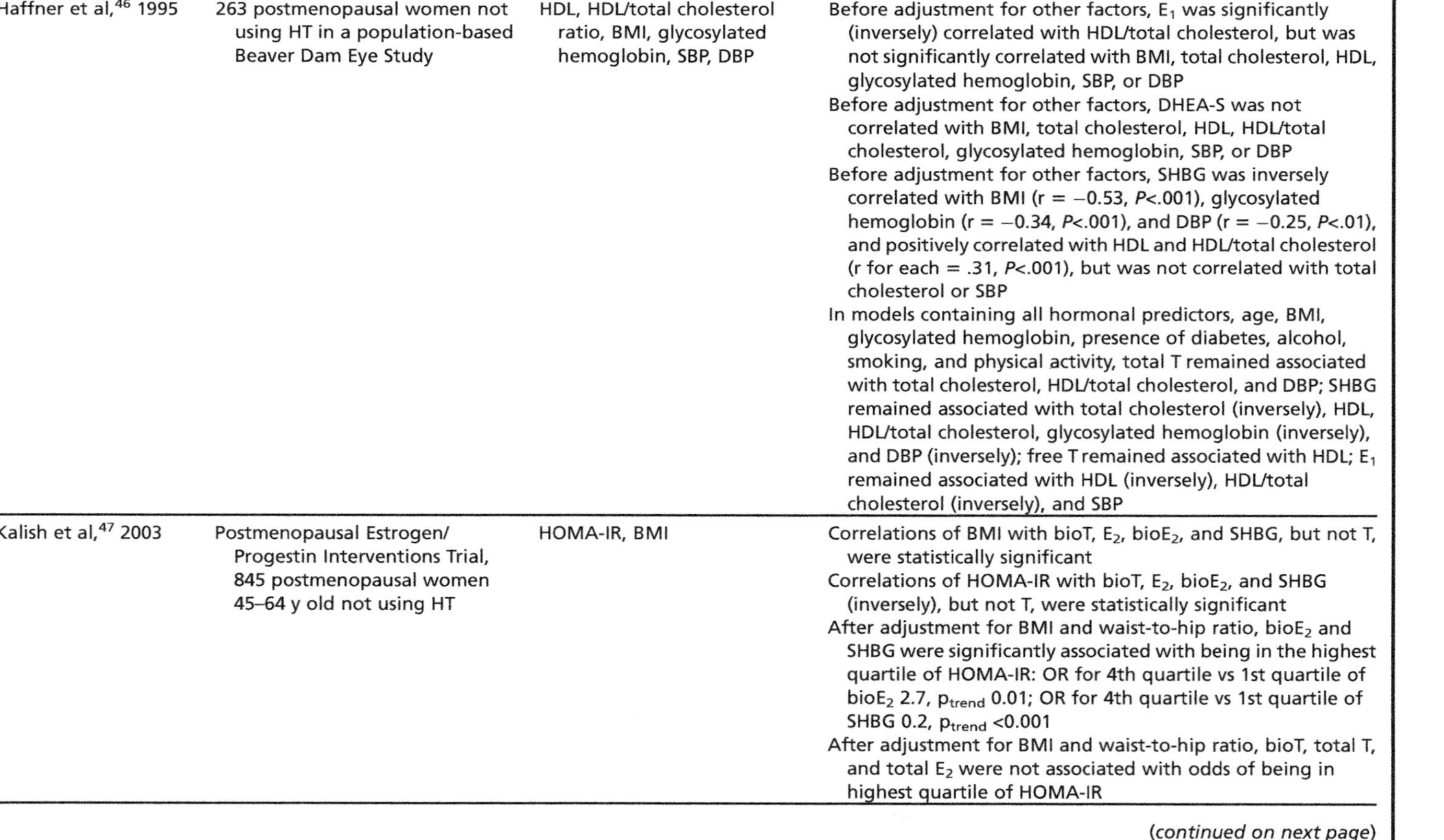

Haffner et al,[46] 1995	263 postmenopausal women not using HT in a population-based Beaver Dam Eye Study	HDL, HDL/total cholesterol ratio, BMI, glycosylated hemoglobin, SBP, DBP	Before adjustment for other factors, E_1 was significantly (inversely) correlated with HDL/total cholesterol, but was not significantly correlated with BMI, total cholesterol, HDL, glycosylated hemoglobin, SBP, or DBP Before adjustment for other factors, DHEA-S was not correlated with BMI, total cholesterol, HDL, HDL/total cholesterol, glycosylated hemoglobin, SBP, or DBP Before adjustment for other factors, SHBG was inversely correlated with BMI ($r = -0.53$, $P<.001$), glycosylated hemoglobin ($r = -0.34$, $P<.001$), and DBP ($r = -0.25$, $P<.01$), and positively correlated with HDL and HDL/total cholesterol (r for each = .31, $P<.001$), but was not correlated with total cholesterol or SBP In models containing all hormonal predictors, age, BMI, glycosylated hemoglobin, presence of diabetes, alcohol, smoking, and physical activity, total T remained associated with total cholesterol, HDL/total cholesterol, and DBP; SHBG remained associated with total cholesterol (inversely), HDL, HDL/total cholesterol, glycosylated hemoglobin (inversely), and DBP (inversely); free T remained associated with HDL; E_1 remained associated with HDL (inversely), HDL/total cholesterol (inversely), and SBP
Kalish et al,[47] 2003	Postmenopausal Estrogen/Progestin Interventions Trial, 845 postmenopausal women 45–64 y old not using HT	HOMA-IR, BMI	Correlations of BMI with bioT, E_2, bioE_2, and SHBG, but not T, were statistically significant Correlations of HOMA-IR with bioT, E_2, bioE_2, and SHBG (inversely), but not T, were statistically significant After adjustment for BMI and waist-to-hip ratio, bioE_2 and SHBG were significantly associated with being in the highest quartile of HOMA-IR: OR for 4th quartile vs 1st quartile of bioE_2 2.7, p_{trend} 0.01; OR for 4th quartile vs 1st quartile of SHBG 0.2, p_{trend} <0.001 After adjustment for BMI and waist-to-hip ratio, bioT, total T, and total E_2 were not associated with odds of being in highest quartile of HOMA-IR

(*continued on next page*)

Table 3
(continued)

Cross-Sectional Studies			
Reference	**Study Population**	**Cardiac Risk Factors Examined**	**Results**
Khatibi et al,[25] 2007	6440 women aged 50–59 y the Women's Health in the Lund Area Study, half of whom were using HT	Total cholesterol, TG, LDL, HDL	Among HT nonusers, after adjustment for age, smoking, and BMI, T was significantly associated with total cholesterol (β-coefficient 0.029, $P<.05$), TG (β-coefficient −0.152, $P<.001$), LDL (β-coefficient 0.031, $P<.05$), and HDL (β-coefficient 0.41, $P<.001$) After adjustment for age, smoking, and BMI, SHBG was significantly associated with HDL (β-coefficient, $P<.01$), but was not associated with total cholesterol, TG, or LDL After adjustment for age, smoking, and BMI, E_2 was significantly associated with total cholesterol (β-coefficient −0.001, $P<.001$) and LDL (β-coefficient −0.001, $P<.001$), but was not significantly associated with TG or HDL Androstenedione was not significantly associated with cholesterol, TG, LDL, or HDL
Lambrinoudaki et al,[48] 2006	598 postmenopausal women not taking HT	HOMA-IR, HDL, LDL, TG	Mean levels of TG were significantly higher in women with highest quartile of T and FAI, and significantly lower in women with highest quartile of SHBG, compared with lower quartiles, but did not differ by quartile of E_2, androstenedione, DHEA-S, or FEI Mean TC levels were higher in women with T or FAI values in the highest quartile compared with other quartiles, but did not differ by quartile of E_2, androstenedione, DHEA-S, SHBG, or FEI Mean LDL was higher in higher quartiles of E_2, T and FAI compared with lower quartiles, but did not differ by quartile of androstenedione, DHEA-S, SHBG, or FEI Mean HDL was higher in higher quartiles of SHBG and in lower quartiles of E_2, T, FEI, and FAI compared with lower quartiles, but did not differ by quartile of androstenedione or DHEA-S

			Mean HOMA-IR was higher in lower quartiles of SHBG and in higher quartiles of E_2, T, FEI, and FAI compared with lower quartiles, but did not differ by quartile of androstenedione or DHEA-S After adjustment for age, BMI, smoking, alcohol, and physical activity, only certain associations persisted: FAI and T with total cholesterol; T, SHBG (inversely), and FAI with TG; T, androstenedione, and FAI with LDL; E_2 (inversely), T (inversely), SHBG, FAI (inversely), and FEI (inversely) with HDL; T, SHBG (inversely), FAI, and FEI with HOMA-IR
Masi et al,[49] 2009	52 women postmenopausal women aged 55–69 y in Illinois, not using HT	SBP	Out of 14 estrogen metabolites measured by mass spectrometry, after adjustment for age, BMI, race or ethnicity, and vasoactive medications, 2 of them were independently (inversely) associated with SBP: ln 16α-hydroxyestrone (β-coefficient −5.3, $P<.05$) and ln 16-ketoestradiol (β-coefficient −4.7, $P<.05$ No significant association between serum E_2 and SBP
Mesch et al,[50] 2008	124 women, of whom 31 were postmenopausal, none using HT	HOMA, TG, HDL, LDL, waist circumference	SHBG was inversely correlated with waist circumference (r = −0.34, P = .006), HOMA-IR (r = −0.41, P = .0002), LDL (r = −0.28, P = .02), TG (r = −0.40, P = .0005), and positively correlated with HDL (r = 0.36, P = .003) FAI was correlated with waist circumference (r = 0.40, P = .001), HOMA-IR (r = 0.33, P = .003), and TG (r = 0.31, P = .01) and inversely correlated with HDL (r = −0.25, P = .04), but not significantly associated with LDL After adjustment for waist circumference, inverse correlation persisted between SHBG and HOMA-IR, but correlations between SHBG and lipoproteins, and correlations of FAI with HOMA-IR, TG and HDL were lost

(*continued on next page*)

Table 3
(continued)

Cross-Sectional Studies			
Reference	**Study Population**	**Cardiac Risk Factors Examined**	**Results**
Mudali et al,[51] 2005	172 postmenopausal women without carotid atherosclerosis, not taking HT	Total cholesterol, TG, HDL, LDL	After adjustment for age, race, smoking, alcohol intake, physical activity, SBP, fasting glucose, and presence of diabetes, SHBG was positively associated with HDL level (β-coefficient 3.11 per SD in SHBG, $P = .004$) and inversely associated with total cholesterol (β-coefficient −9.28 per SD in SHBG, $P = .007$), TG (β-coefficient −20.5 per SD in SHBG, $P<.0001$), and LDL level (β-coefficient −7.87 per SD in SHBG, $P = .01$) No significant associations of E1, total T, or FAI with total cholesterol, TG, HDL, or LDL after adjustment
Phillips et al,[52] 1997	24 hypertensive and 19 healthy postmenopausal women not taking HT	Systolic blood pressure	Mean values of free T were higher in the hypertensive than control group (1.23 vs 0.83 pg/mL, $P = .01$), but mean levels of T, E_2, androstenedione, SHBG and DHEA-S were not statistically different between hypertensive and control groups
Shelley et al,[53] 1998	363 Australian nondiabetic women 45–56 y old not taking HT	HDL, LDL, TG, DBP	HDL was higher with increasing quartiles of E_2 (p_{trend} 0.03), and lower with increasing quartiles of FAI (p_{trend} 0.0007) LDL was higher with increasing quartile of FAI (p_{trend} 0.002) was not significantly related to quartile of E_2 TG levels were lower with increasing quartile of E_2 (p_{trend} 0.02) and higher with increasing quartiles of FAI (p_{trend} 0.0003) After adjustment for age, BMI, smoking, alcohol intake, and physical activity, the only association that remained was a positive association between log FAI and LDL (β-coefficient 1.74, standard error 0.49) Neither FAI nor E_2 level was significantly associated with DBP

Tufano et al,[54] 2004	24 normal-weight premenopausal women, 24 normal-weight postmenopausal women, 24 obese premenopausal women, 20 obese postmenopausal women, all free of HTN and DM	Waist-to-hip ratio, BMI, cholesterol, HDL, LDL, TG, HOMA, SBP, DBP	Significant inverse correlations of waist-to-hip ratio with T (r = −0.40, *P*<.01) and SHBG (r = −0.33, *P*<.03), but no correlation with FAI Significant inverse correlation of TG with SHBG (r = −0.31, *P*<.01) and positive correlation of TG with FAI (r = 0.47 (*P*<.003), but no correlation with T Significant inverse correlation of HOMA with SHBG (r = −0.38, *P*<.01) and positive correlation of HOMA with FAI (r = 0.77, *P*<.0001), but no correlation with T level No significant correlations of T, FAI, or SHBG with the following: BMI, cholesterol, HDL, LDL, SBP, or DBP

Longitudinal Studies

Reference	Study Population	Cardiac Risk Factors Examined	Results
Ding et al,[56] 2007	Postmenopausal women health professionals in the Women's Health Study, mean age 60 y, not taking HT, free of baseline CVD and DM, average follow-up 10 y	Incident DM confirmed by medical records	E_2, free E_2, free T, T, and DHEA-S were each strongly, positively associated with risk of type 2 DM, even after adjustment for BMI, smoking, alcohol use, exercise, blood pressure, past HT use, remainder of hormonal predictors, and other covariates RR for developing type 2 DM in the highest vs lowest quintiles were: E_2 RR 12.6 (95% CI 2.83–56.3); free E_2 RR 13.1 (95% CI 4.18–40.8), T RR 4.15 (95% CI 1.21–14.2), free T RR 14.8 (95% CI 4.44–49.2) DHEA-S was not significantly associated with risk of incident type 2 DM when adjusted for age and race

(*continued on next page*)

Table 3
(continued)

Reference	Study Population	Cardiac Risk Factors Examined	Results
Longitudinal Studies			
Goodman-Gruen et al,[27] 1996	624 women aged 50–82 in the Rancho Bernardo Study, not using HT, 19-y follow-up	Fasting glucose, HFL, BMI, SBP, DBP, cholesterol, TG	After adjustment for age, SHBG level inversely associated with BMI (r = −0.16, *P*<.005) After adjustment for age and BMI, SHBG correlated negatively with fasting glucose (r = −.08, *P*<.05) Inverse correlation between SHBG and TG (r = −0.09, *P*<.05) and positive correlation between SHBG and HDL (r = 0.18, *P*<.005) after adjustment for age, but not after additional adjustment for BMI No significant correlations between SHBG and SBP, DBP, TG, or cholesterol levels after adjustment for age or for both age and BMI E_2 not examined
Janssen et al,[57] 2008	949 participants in the Study of Women's Health Across the Nation who had never taken HT, 9-y follow-up	Metabolic syndrome by National Cholesterol Education Program Adult Treatment Panel III criteria	After adjustment for age, ethnicity, BMI, smoking, and other covariates, change in bioT level was positively associated (OR 1.10, 95% CI 1.01–1.20), and change in SHBG was inversely associated (OR 0.87, 95% CI 0.81–0.93), with odds of developing metabolic syndrome Change in E_2 level or T level were not significantly associated with odds of developing metabolic syndrome Change in E_2 level was positively associated with change in HDL, and inversely associated with change in SBP, but was not associated with change in TG or glucose level Change in bioT level was positively associated with change in waist circumference and change in fasting glucose level, but inversely associated with change in HDL

			Change in SHBG level was positively associated with change in HDL level and inversely associated with change in fasting glucose level In fully adjusted models: significant associations of change in bioT (β-coefficient 0.14, $P \leq .01$) and change in SHBG (β-coefficient −0.21, $P \leq .001$) with change in waist circumference; significant associations of change in bioT (β-coefficient −0.48, $P \leq .01$) and change in SHBG (β-coefficient 0.81, $P \leq .001$) with change in HDL; significant association of change in T with change in TG (β-coefficient 1.92, $P \leq .05$); significant associations of change in E_2 (β-coefficient −0.41, $P \leq .01$) with change in SBP In fully adjusted models: no associations of change in E_2 or T and change in waist circumference or change in HDL; no associations of change in SHBG or change in bioT with change in TG or change in SBP; no association of change in E_2 and change in TG; no association of change in T and change in SBP
Kalyani et al,[58] 2009	1612 postmenopausal participants aged 45–84 y of the Multi-Ethnic Study of Atherosclerosis (MESA), free of DM at baseline, median follow-up 4.7 y	Incident type 2 MD based on fasting glucose and/or treatment of DM	After adjustment for age, race/ethnicity, BMI, HOMA-IR, LDL, HDL, TG, SBP, smoking, physical activity, and other factors, there was a significantly greater risk of developing incident DM across higher quartiles of E_2 (HR 1.92 for quartile 4 vs quartile 1, $p_{trend} = 0.01$), and lower quartiles of SHBG (HR 0.52 for quartile 4 vs quartile 1, p_{trend} 0.02) Association between quartile of bioT and risk of incident diabetes (HR 2.45 for quartile 4 vs quartile 1, 95% CI 1.48–4.03) was no longer significant after adjustment No significant associations between DHEA and risk of developing diabetes before or after adjustment

(*continued on next page*)

Table 3
(continued)

Longitudinal Studies			
Reference	**Study Population**	**Cardiac Risk Factors Examined**	**Results**
Oh et al,[55] 2002	Rancho Bernardo study, 233 women 55–89 y old not using HT, 8-y follow-up	Fasting and after challenge glucose and insulin, incident DM	After adjustment for age, T was correlated with HDL (r = 0.20, $P<.01$) but not with BMI, waist-to-hip ratio, SBP, DBP, or HOMA-IR; bioT was correlated with BMI (r = 0.13, $P<.05$) and DBP (r = 0.16, $P<.05$) but not with waist-to-hip ratio, SBP, HDL, or HOMA-IR; E_2 was correlated with BMI (r = 0.13, $P<.05$) but not with waist-to-hip ratio, SBP, DBP, HDL, or HOMA-IR; and bioE_2 was correlated with BMI (r = 0.21, $P\leq.01$), waist-to-hip ratio (r = 0.20, $P<.01$) and TG (r = 0.22, $P<.01$), but not with SBP, DBP, or TG
Page-Wilson et al,[28] 2009	200 nondiabetic postmenopausal women ≥45 y old not using HT in the Women's Health Study of female health professionals, (98 with incident CVD over 2.9 y follow-up, remainder matched controls without CVD)	Hemoglobin A1c	After adjustment for development of CVD and age, ln FAI (β-coefficient 0.02, $P = .0004$), ln FEI (β-coefficient 0.01, $P = .0004$), and ln SHBG (β-coefficient −0.04, $P = .0003$) were significantly associated with ln hemoglobin A1c, but E_2 and T were not significantly correlated with hemoglobin A1c After further adjustment for BMI, associations between FEI and hemoglobin A1c did not persist

Abbreviations: bioE_2, bioavailable E_2; bioT, bioavailable testosterone; BMI, body mass index; DBP, diastolic blood pressure; DHEA-S, DHEA-sulfate; DM, diabetes mellitus; FAI, free androgen index; FEI, free estrogen index; HOMA-IR, homeostatic model assessing insulin resistance; HTN, hypertension; IGT, impaired glucose tolerance; ln, natural log; OR, odds ratio; r, correlation; SBP, systolic blood pressure; SHBG, sex hormone-binding globulin; T, testosterone; TG, triglycerides.

with medical record-confirmed CAD[28,29,36] and radiographically-assessed CAD,[33] no association between T and self-reported CVD,[25,39] inverse associations between bioavailable T (bioT) and radiographically-assessed CAD,[35] inverse associations between free T and angiographically-confirmed CAD.[38] A study that lacked detail regarding how MI was ascertained reported no association between T or free T level and MI.[40] Regarding androgens other than T, cross-sectional studies found no associations between androstenedione and self-reported CVD,[25,39] dehydroepiandrosterone (DHEA) level and medical record-confirmed CHD,[34] or DHEA-sulfate (DHEA-S) level and angiographic CAD.[38] A study reported no association between androstenedione, DHEA, or DHEA-S level and MI, but did not provide detail regarding how MI was ascertained.[40]

In longitudinal studies that confirmed CAD by medical records and/or death certificates, bioT levels did not predict ischemic heart disease death[26] and free T levels were not associated with radiographic coronary artery plaques,[41] but there was a U-shaped curve for the association between bioT and CHD, with the risk of CHD being higher in both the lowest and the highest quintiles of bioT, and lower in the middle quintiles.[43] This U-shaped curve may partially explain the variability in associations between circulating androgen levels and CAD in the cross-sectional studies.

Associations of SHBG level with CAD

In cross-sectional studies outcomes and potential predictors varied across the studies and SHBG levels were not consistently associated with CAD (see **Table 2**). Cross-sectional studies reported inverse association of SHBG with medical record-confirmed CHD events,[31] no association of SHBG level with self-reported CVD,[25] inverse associations between SHBG level and number of radiographic coronary artery plaques,[33] positive associations between SHBG level and coronary artery calcium score,[35] no association between SHBG level and angiographic CAD,[38] no association between SHBG level and self-reported CVD,[39] and inverse associations of SHBG level with medical record-confirmed CVD events that disappeared after adjustment for other cardiac risk factors.[37] A study with unclear methods for ascertainment of MI reported no association between SHBG level and MI.[40]

In longitudinal studies that confirmed CAD by medical records and/or death certificates, one longitudinal study described a U-shaped association between SHBG level and 12-year incidence of MI ascertained from medical records, although the number of study participants was small.[42] In another study, SHBG level was not associated with ischemic heart disease death assessed on death certificates.[27]

Associations of progesterone-related metabolites with CAD

A cross-sectional study found serum pregnenolone level and 17-hydroxypregnenolone level to be associated with significantly lower odds of medical record-confirmed CVD (see **Table 2**).[34]

Association Between Serum Sex Steroid and SHBG Levels and CVD Risk Factors Among Postmenopausal Women

Summary of cardiac risk factors

Specific cardiovascular risk factors examined varied considerably across studies, spanning glucose tolerance testing, a clinical diagnosis of diabetes mellitus (DM), fasting glucose level, body mass index, physical activity, smoking, HDL, total cholesterol, LDL cholesterol, triglycerides, glycosylated hemoglobin, systolic blood pressure, diastolic blood pressure, waist circumference, waist-to-hip ratio, and homeostasis model assessing insulin resistance (HOMA-IR) (see **Table 3**). Of the 18 studies, 12 were cross-sectional[25,26,45–54] and 6 were longitudinal.[27,28,55–58]

Associations of circulating estrogens with CAD risk factors

Because the cardiac risk factors examined varied widely across cross-sectional studies, and associations were not consistent across studies, we summarize here the results from longitudinal studies and focus on DM-related associations (see **Table 3**). With regard to studies of DM and insulin resistance, longitudinal studies reported positive associations of circulating E_2 and free E_2 levels with incident DM,[56,58] and no association between E_2 and HOMA-IR.[55] Some associations between FEI and hemoglobin A1c disappeared after adjustment for other risk factors.[28]

Associations of circulating androgens with CAD

Longitudinal studies of DM and insulin resistance reported positive associations of free T and total T with incident DM,[56] association of bioT level with increased odds of developing metabolic syndrome,[57] no correlation of T with HOMA-IR,[55] and positive association between FAI and hemoglobin A1c level (see **Table 3**).[28] However, one longitudinal study reported that associations between bioT level and incident DM disappeared after adjustment for other risk factors.[58]

Associations of SHBG level with CAD

Longitudinal studies of DM and insulin resistance showed inverse correlations of SHBG level with fasting glucose level,[27] a protective association of increases in SHBG level with decreased odds of developing metabolic syndrome,[57] an inverse association of SHBG level with incident diabetes risk,[58] or an inverse association between SHBG level and hemoglobin A1c level (see **Table 3**).[28]

DISCUSSION

In this review, six longitudinal studies reported circulating sex steroid and SHBG levels in relation to incident CAD in postmenopausal women. In these longitudinal studies, circulating estrogen levels were usually not associated with ischemic heart disease death. In one longitudinal study each, associations of bioT with CHD and associations of SHBG level with incidence of MI were U-shaped. The six longitudinal studies did not consistently find associations between estrogen levels and incident DM or insulin resistance, but circulating androgen levels (free T, bioT) were associated with incident DM and metabolic syndrome. In four out of four longitudinal studies, SHBG level was inversely related to both the incidence of metabolic syndrome and the incidence of DM. Many longitudinal studies reported that associations of circulating sex steroid levels and CAD or CAD risk factors disappeared after adjustment for other CAD risk factors, highlighting the difficulty of generalizing results across studies, and raising questions about mechanisms for associations and possible over-adjustment.

We encountered challenges in interpretation of results because of substantial heterogeneity across studies regarding how CAD outcomes were ascertained or defined and tremendous diversity regarding which sex steroid levels were measured (eg, free, total, bioavailable). Moreover, many older studies used assays that did not have adequate sensitivity to detect the very low E_2 levels characteristic of postmenopausal women, obscuring the ability to detect associations between very low E_2 levels and subsequent development of CAD. Finally, serum sex steroid levels do not capture the entire hormonal milieu at the tissue level. Many, if not most, publications did not address the influence of body fat or fat distribution on hormone levels and CVD risk.

Despite these caveats, there is adequate reason to seek evidence for associations of circulating estrogen levels and CAD. Estrogen receptors (ERs) exist in the vascular endothelium, vascular smooth muscle, and adventitial cells of humans.[59] This localization of ERs may explain why brachial artery flow-mediated dilation (assessed by ultrasound) is inversely associated with years since menopause.[60] Moreover, in postmenopausal women, brachial artery flow-mediated dilation was positively associated with serum E_2 level.[61]

Estrogen has both genomic and nongenomic effects on endothelial and vascular smooth muscle cells.[62] Estrogen stimulates gene transcription and estrogen-regulated genes themselves encode transcription factors.[59] Adding yet another layer of complexity to the study of endogenous estrogen's link with CAD, the vascular endothelium contains polymorphisms in the genes encoding ERs and truncated forms of ERα and ERβ.[59] These polymorphisms may influence the development of CHD by influencing ER binding. Also, polymorphisms in ER may also influence development of CHD by influencing E_2 levels themselves. For example, in the Framingham Heart Study, postmenopausal carriers of the ESR2 (CA)n long allele (vs short/long or short/short allele), and the rs1256031C allele (vs T/T), had moderately higher E_2 levels.[63] Finally, ERα polymorphisms have been linked with lipoprotein metabolism in postmenopausal women.[64] ERβ expression is increased in women with CAD.[59]

Beyond the genes themselves, modification of genes, such as occurs with gene methylation, should be considered as potential factors influencing the effects of endogenous estrogen on the heart such that the same genetic code can result in different phenotypic effects depending on the degree of gene methylation. In human right atrium, there is an age-related increase in ERα gene methylation, and human internal mammary arteries contain significant levels of ERα gene methylation.[65] Moreover, ERα gene methylation is increased in coronary atherosclerotic plaques compared with normal proximal aortic tissue.[65]

In the future, even if ovarian senescence-associated hormonal changes are confirmed to be associated with CAD in cohort studies of postmenopausal women, there may be other components explaining the gender differences in CAD patterns. Theoretically, gender differences in heart disease mortality rates with age could be due to adverse influences of menopause, or to protective effects of the premenopausal circulating hormonal milieu. To explore this question, a recent study analyzed ischemic heart disease mortality in England, Wales, and the United States among three birth cohorts: 1916 to 1925, 1926 to 1935, and 1936 to 1945.[66] The study compared associations between mortality rates and age modeled under two alternative assumptions: a linear relationship, or a proportional (logarithmically-associated) relationship. The proportional age-related changes in ischemic heart disease mortality fit the longitudinal mortality data better than absolute age-related changes in mortality did, suggesting that acceleration in heart disease mortality among men ceased at around age 45, whereas the CHD association in women did not change at the age of menopause—although the expected postmenopausal decrease in breast cancer risk after age 50 was readily apparent. These observations suggest that the reason postmenopausal women have CVD risks more like those of older men is not explained by female estrogen deficiency but by the decreasing risk in surviving old men.[66] This paper also shows similar decreases in CVD mortality in both sexes during the past three decades despite the ongoing obesity epidemic, which could be due to behavior change and medication use. This will certainly make it more difficult to understand hormones and women's health in the future, and suggests the potential added value of previous cohort studies when data were collected before widespread medical or lifestyle interventions.

SUMMARY

In conclusion, the associations of circulating androgens and SHBG with CHD, incident DM, and metabolic syndrome in longitudinal studies of postmenopausal women are of great interest and are clearly worthy of future study. Unfortunately, limited information exists regarding the biologic mechanisms underlying these associations. The few longitudinal studies did not support the existence of notable associations between circulating estrogen levels and CAD incidence in postmenopausal women.

REFERENCES

1. Kochanek K, Xu J, Murphy S, et al. Deaths: final data for 2009. Hyattsville (MD): National Center for Health Statistics; 2012.
2. Roger VL, Go AS, Lloyd-Jones DM, et al. Heart disease and stroke statistics—2012 update: a report from the American Heart Association. Circulation 2012; 125(1):e2–220.
3. Saltiki K, Doukas C, Kanakakis J, et al. Severity of cardiovascular disease in women: relation with exposure to endogenous estrogen. Maturitas 2006;55(1): 51–7.
4. de Kleijn MJ, van der Schouw YT, Verbeek AL, et al. Endogenous estrogen exposure and cardiovascular mortality risk in postmenopausal women. Am J Epidemiol 2002;155(4):339–45.
5. Wellons M, Ouyang P, Schreiner PJ, et al. Early menopause predicts future coronary heart disease and stroke: the Multi-Ethnic Study of Atherosclerosis. Menopause 2012;19(10):1081–7.
6. Hu FB, Grodstein F, Hennekens CH, et al. Age at natural menopause and risk of cardiovascular disease. Arch Intern Med 1999;159(10):1061–6.
7. Tremollieres FA, Pouilles JM, Cauneille C, et al. Coronary heart disease risk factors and menopause: a study in 1684 French women. Atherosclerosis 1999; 142(2):415–23.
8. de Aloysio D, Gambacciani M, Meschia M, et al. The effect of menopause on blood lipid and lipoprotein levels. The Icarus Study Group. Atherosclerosis 1999;147(1):147–53.
9. Sultan N, Nawaz M, Sultan A, et al. Effect of menopause on serum HDL-cholesterol level. J Ayub Med Coll Abbottabad 2003;15(3):24–6.
10. Matthews KA, Crawford SL, Chae CU, et al. Are changes in cardiovascular disease risk factors in midlife women due to chronological aging or to the menopausal transition? J Am Coll Cardiol 2009;54(25):2366–73.
11. Effects of estrogen or estrogen/progestin regimens on heart disease risk factors in postmenopausal women. The Postmenopausal Estrogen/Progestin Interventions (PEPI) Trial. The Writing Group for the PEPI Trial. JAMA 1995;273(3): 199–208.
12. Hulley S, Grady D, Bush T, et al. Randomized trial of estrogen plus progestin for secondary prevention of coronary heart disease in postmenopausal women. Heart and Estrogen/progestin Replacement Study (HERS) Research Group. JAMA 1998;280(7):605–13.
13. Manson JE, Hsia J, Johnson KC, et al. Estrogen plus progestin and the risk of coronary heart disease. N Engl J Med 2003;349(6):523–34.
14. Toh S, Hernandez-Diaz S, Logan R, et al. Coronary heart disease in postmenopausal recipients of estrogen plus progestin therapy: does the increased risk ever disappear? A randomized trial. Ann Intern Med 2010;152(4):211–7.
15. Rossouw JE, Prentice RL, Manson JE, et al. Postmenopausal hormone therapy and risk of cardiovascular disease by age and years since menopause. JAMA 2007;297(13):1465–77.

16. Hsia J, Langer RD, Manson JE, et al. Conjugated equine estrogens and coronary heart disease: the Women's Health Initiative. Arch Intern Med 2006;166(3):357–65.
17. Manson JE, Allison MA, Rossouw JE, et al. Estrogen therapy and coronary-artery calcification. N Engl J Med 2007;356(25):2591–602.
18. Schierbeck LL, Rejnmark L, Tofteng CL, et al. Effect of hormone replacement therapy on cardiovascular events in recently postmenopausal women: randomised trial. BMJ 2012;345:e6409.
19. Kronos Longevity Research Institute. Hormone therapy has many favorable effects in newly menopausal women: initial findings of the Kronos Early Estrogen Prevention study (KEEPS). 2012. Available at: http://www.keepstudy.org/news/pr_100312_a.pdf. Accessed November 8, 2012.
20. Harman SM, Brinton EA, Cedars M, et al. KEEPS: the Kronos Early Estrogen Prevention Study. Climacteric 2005;8(1):3–12.
21. Farish E, Rolton HA, Barnes JF, et al. Lipoprotein(a) and postmenopausal oestrogen. Acta Endocrinol (Copenh) 1993;129(3):225–8.
22. Davison S, Davis SR. New markers for cardiovascular disease risk in women: impact of endogenous estrogen status and exogenous postmenopausal hormone therapy. J Clin Endocrinol Metab 2003;88(6):2470–8.
23. Manson JE, Bassuk SS. Invited commentary: hormone therapy and risk of coronary heart disease why renew the focus on the early years of menopause? Am J Epidemiol 2007;166(5):511–7.
24. Barrett-Connor E. Hormones and heart disease in women: the timing hypothesis. Am J Epidemiol 2007;166(5):506–10.
25. Khatibi A, Agardh CD, Shakir YA, et al. Could androgens protect middle-aged women from cardiovascular events? A population-based study of Swedish women: the Women's Health in the Lund Area (WHILA) Study. Climacteric 2007;10(5):386–92.
26. Barrett-Connor E, Goodman-Gruen D. Prospective study of endogenous sex hormones and fatal cardiovascular disease in postmenopausal women. BMJ 1995;311(7014):1193–6.
27. Goodman-Gruen D, Barrett-Connor E. A prospective study of sex hormone-binding globulin and fatal cardiovascular disease in Rancho Bernardo men and women. J Clin Endocrinol Metab 1996;81(8):2999–3003.
28. Page-Wilson G, Goulart AC, Rexrode KM. Interrelation between sex hormones and plasma sex hormone-binding globulin and hemoglobin A1c in healthy postmenopausal women. Metab Syndr Relat Disord 2009;7(3):249–54.
29. Braunstein GD, Johnson BD, Stanczyk FZ, et al. Relations between endogenous androgens and estrogens in postmenopausal women with suspected ischemic heart disease. J Clin Endocrinol Metab 2008;93(11):4268–75.
30. Cauley JA, Gutai JP, Glynn NW, et al. Serum estrone concentrations and coronary artery disease in postmenopausal women. Arterioscler Thromb 1994;14(1):14–8.
31. Chen Y, Zeleniuch-Jacquotte A, Arslan AA, et al. Endogenous hormones and coronary heart disease in postmenopausal women. Atherosclerosis 2011;216(2):414–9.
32. Jeon GH, Kim SH, Yun SC, et al. Association between serum estradiol level and coronary artery calcification in postmenopausal women. Menopause 2010;17(5):902–7.
33. Munir JA, Wu H, Bauer K, et al. The perimenopausal atherosclerosis transition: relationships between calcified and noncalcified coronary, aortic, and carotid atherosclerosis and risk factors and hormone levels. Menopause 2012;19(1):10–5.

34. Naessen T, Sjogren U, Bergquist J, et al. Endogenous steroids measured by high-specificity liquid chromatography-tandem mass spectrometry and prevalent cardiovascular disease in 70-year-old men and women. J Clin Endocrinol Metab 2010;95(4):1889–97.
35. Ouyang P, Vaidya D, Dobs A, et al. Sex hormone levels and subclinical atherosclerosis in postmenopausal women: the Multi-Ethnic Study of Atherosclerosis. Atherosclerosis 2009;204(1):255–61.
36. Patel SM, Ratcliffe SJ, Reilly MP, et al. Higher serum testosterone concentration in older women is associated with insulin resistance, metabolic syndrome, and cardiovascular disease. J Clin Endocrinol Metab 2009;94(12):4776–84.
37. Rexrode KM, Manson JE, Lee IM, et al. Sex hormone levels and risk of cardiovascular events in postmenopausal women. Circulation 2003;108(14):1688–93.
38. Phillips GB, Pinkernell BH, Jing TY. Relationship between serum sex hormones and coronary artery disease in postmenopausal women. Arterioscler Thromb Vasc Biol 1997;17(4):695–701.
39. Shakir YA, Samsioe G, Khatibi EA, et al. Health hazards in middle-aged women with cardiovascular disease: a case-control study of Swedish women. The women's health in the Lund area (WHILA) study. J Womens Health (Larchmt) 2007;16(3):406–14.
40. Skalba P, Wojtowicz M, Sikora J. Androgen and SHBG serum concentrations in late post-menopause women. Med Sci Monit 2003;9(3):CR152–6.
41. Calderon-Margalit R, Schwartz SM, Wellons MF, et al. Prospective association of serum androgens and sex hormone-binding globulin with subclinical cardiovascular disease in young adult women: the "Coronary Artery Risk Development in Young Adults" women's study. J Clin Endocrinol Metab 2010;95(9):4424–31.
42. Lapidus L, Lindstedt G, Lundberg PA, et al. Concentrations of sex-hormone binding globulin and corticosteroid binding globulin in serum in relation to cardiovascular risk factors and to 12-year incidence of cardiovascular disease and overall mortality in postmenopausal women. Clin Chem 1986;32(1 Pt 1):146–52.
43. Laughlin GA, Goodell V, Barrett-Connor E. Extremes of endogenous testosterone are associated with increased risk of incident coronary events in older women. J Clin Endocrinol Metab 2010;95(2):740–7.
44. Sievers C, Klotsche J, Pieper L, et al. Low testosterone levels predict all-cause mortality and cardiovascular events in women: a prospective cohort study in German primary care patients. Eur J Endocrinol 2010;163(4):699–708.
45. Goodman-Gruen D, Barrett-Connor E. Sex differences in the association of endogenous sex hormone levels and glucose tolerance status in older men and women. Diabetes Care 2000;23(7):912–8.
46. Haffner SM, Newcomb PA, Marcus PM, et al. Relation of sex hormones and dehydroepiandrosterone sulfate (DHEA-SO4) to cardiovascular risk factors in postmenopausal women. Am J Epidemiol 1995;142(9):925–34.
47. Kalish GM, Barrett-Connor E, Laughlin GA, et al. Association of endogenous sex hormones and insulin resistance among postmenopausal women: results from the Postmenopausal Estrogen/Progestin Intervention Trial. J Clin Endocrinol Metab 2003;88(4):1646–52.
48. Lambrinoudaki I, Christodoulakos G, Rizos D, et al. Endogenous sex hormones and risk factors for atherosclerosis in healthy Greek postmenopausal women. Eur J Endocrinol 2006;154(6):907–16.
49. Masi CM, Hawkley LC, Xu X, et al. Serum estrogen metabolites and systolic blood pressure among middle-aged and older women and men. Am J Hypertens 2009;22(11):1148–53.

50. Mesch VR, Siseles NO, Maidana PN, et al. Androgens in relationship to cardiovascular risk factors in the menopausal transition. Climacteric 2008;11(6):509–17.
51. Mudali S, Dobs AS, Ding J, et al. Endogenous postmenopausal hormones and serum lipids: the atherosclerosis risk in communities study. J Clin Endocrinol Metab 2005;90(2):1202–9.
52. Phillips GB, Jing TY, Laragh JH. Serum sex hormone levels in postmenopausal women with hypertension. J Hum Hypertens 1997;11(8):523–6.
53. Shelley JM, Green A, Smith AM, et al. Relationship of endogenous sex hormones to lipids and blood pressure in mid-aged women. Ann Epidemiol 1998;8(1): 39–45.
54. Tufano A, Marzo P, Enrini R, et al. Anthropometric, hormonal and biochemical differences in lean and obese women before and after menopause. J Endocrinol Invest 2004;27(7):648–53.
55. Oh JY, Barrett-Connor E, Wedick NM, et al. Endogenous sex hormones and the development of type 2 diabetes in older men and women: the Rancho Bernardo study. Diabetes Care 2002;25(1):55–60.
56. Ding EL, Song Y, Manson JE, et al. Plasma sex steroid hormones and risk of developing type 2 diabetes in women: a prospective study. Diabetologia 2007; 50(10):2076–84.
57. Janssen I, Powell LH, Crawford S, et al. Menopause and the metabolic syndrome: the Study of Women's Health Across the Nation. Arch Intern Med 2008;168(14): 1568–75.
58. Kalyani RR, Franco M, Dobs AS, et al. The association of endogenous sex hormones, adiposity, and insulin resistance with incident diabetes in postmenopausal women. J Clin Endocrinol Metab 2009;94(11):4127–35.
59. Vitale C, Fini M, Speziale G, et al. Gender differences in the cardiovascular effects of sex hormones. Fundam Clin Pharmacol 2010;24(6):675–85.
60. Vitale C, Mercuro G, Cerquetani E, et al. Time since menopause influences the acute and chronic effect of estrogens on endothelial function. Arterioscler Thromb Vasc Biol 2008;28(2):348–52.
61. Li XP, Zhou Y, Zhao SP, et al. Effect of endogenous estrogen on endothelial function in women with coronary heart disease and its mechanism. Clin Chim Acta 2004;339(1–2):183–8.
62. Qiao X, McConnell KR, Khalil RA. Sex steroids and vascular responses in hypertension and aging. Gend Med 2008;5(Suppl A):S46–64.
63. Peter I, Kelley-Hedgepeth A, Fox CS, et al. Variation in estrogen-related genes associated with cardiovascular phenotypes and circulating estradiol, testosterone, and dehydroepiandrosterone sulfate levels. J Clin Endocrinol Metab 2008;93(7):2779–85.
64. Demissie S, Cupples LA, Shearman AM, et al. Estrogen receptor-alpha variants are associated with lipoprotein size distribution and particle levels in women: the Framingham Heart Study. Atherosclerosis 2006;185(1):210–8.
65. Post WS, Goldschmidt-Clermont PJ, Wilhide CC, et al. Methylation of the estrogen receptor gene is associated with aging and atherosclerosis in the cardiovascular system. Cardiovasc Res 1999;43(4):985–91.
66. Vaidya D, Becker DM, Bittner V, et al. Ageing, menopause, and ischaemic heart disease mortality in England, Wales, and the United States: modelling study of national mortality data. BMJ 2011;343:d5170.

Reproductive Aging in Men

Shehzad Basaria, MD

KEYWORDS

- Late-onset hypogonadism • Androgen deficiency • Andropause • Frailty
- Sexual dysfunction

KEY POINTS

- In aging men, associations between serum testosterone levels and health-related outcomes are weak and confounded by the colinearity of age-related comorbidities and low testosterone levels.
- Obesity, illness, and medications also significantly contribute to low testosterone levels.
- Weight reduction, treatment of comorbidities, and discontinuation of offending medications may prevent or attenuate age-related declines in gonadal hormones.

INTRODUCTION

For centuries, the importance of the testes for the maintenance of male phenotype, psychosexual behavior, and physical power has been recognized. Indeed, testicular extracts have been used for the treatment of impotence[1] and, even during the early part of the last century, castration was used as a punishment for sexual offenders. Brown-Sequard, considered by many the Father of Andrology, was so convinced that the age-associated decline in sexual function and frailty was a result of decreased production of "a chemical" from the testes, that in 1885, he self-injected aqueous extracts of guinea pig and dog testes and reported an improvement in his virility and well-being at the Societé de Biologie de Paris meeting in 1889.[2] Although the improvements that Brown-Sequard experienced were due to the "placebo effect," his work ultimately led to the isolation of testosterone, the major testicular androgen, by Butennandt and colleagues[3] almost a century later.

Unlike female menopause, which is accompanied by an abrupt and permanent cessation of ovarian function (both folliculogenesis and estradiol production), male aging does not result in either *cessation* of testosterone production nor infertility. Although the circulating serum testosterone concentration does decline with aging, in most men this decrease is small, resulting in levels that are generally within the normal range. However, testosterone deficiency does occur in some aging men,

Section of Men's Health, Aging and Metabolism, Brigham and Women's Hospital, Harvard Medical School, 221 Longwood Avenue, 5th Floor, Boston, MA 02115, USA
E-mail address: sbasaria@partners.org

Endocrinol Metab Clin N Am 42 (2013) 255–270
http://dx.doi.org/10.1016/j.ecl.2013.02.012 **endo.theclinics.com**

resulting in symptoms that are reminiscent of "organic hypogonadism," such as caused by testicular or hypothalamic-pituitary disease. Age-related hypogonadism has been referred to as andropause, viropause, partial androgen deficiency of the aging male, and late-onset hypogonadism (LOH), with LOH considered to be the most suitable term for this condition. Although symptoms such as sexual dysfunction, muscle weakness, loss of bone mass, fatigue, cognitive decline, and mood changes are seen in organic hypogonadism, they also occur as part-and-parcel of aging. The similarities between organic hypogonadism and LOH have resulted in a growing interest in testosterone replacement therapy in aging men. This interest is mainly driven by the following 2 factors: (1) lack of understanding among clinicians to differentiate LOH from organic hypogonadism (that may occur at any age), and (2) the robust marketing campaign of testosterone products by the industry toward physicians and the general public. This campaign has been effective because the marketing volume of testosterone preparations has increased more than 15-fold over the past 2 decades.[4]

The uncertainty surrounding LOH has triggered numerous recommendations for its diagnosis and treatment by various organizations.[5,6] To some extent, these recommendations are based on insufficient scientific evidence because large, adequately powered randomized controlled trials of testosterone replacement are lacking. A large randomized controlled efficacy trial, The T-Trial, is underway and should provide valuable data on the efficacy (and risks) of testosterone replacement in LOH.

This review summarizes the current concepts of the prevalence, pathophysiology, and diagnostic criteria of LOH and evaluates possible associations of LOH with various organ systems.

ANDROGEN PHYSIOLOGY IN MEN

Testosterone is the predominant and biologically most important circulating androgen in men and is secreted almost exclusively by the testes. The other androgens include dihydrotestosterone, androstenedione, dehydroepiandrosterone (DHEA), and dehydroepiandrosterone sulfate (DHEAS). Most dihydrotestosterone (80%) is derived from 5-α reduction of testosterone in peripheral tissues (by the enzyme 5-α reductase), whereas the remaining 20% is secreted directly from the testes.[7] Approximately 85% of serum androstenedione levels are contributed equally by the testes and the adrenal glands, whereas the remainder originates from peripheral conversion of testosterone (via 17β-hydroxysteroid dehydrogenase) and DHEA (via 3β-hydroxysteroid dehydrogenase).[8] Both DHEA and DHEAS are produced almost exclusively from the adrenal glands.

Testosterone is largely bound to plasma proteins with approximately 40% loosely bound to albumin and 58% tightly bound to the sex hormone binding globulin (SHBG),[9] which leaves only 1% to 2% of testosterone unbound, the moiety considered to be "biologically active." The free testosterone diffuses passively through lipophilic cell membranes into the target cell, where it binds to the androgen receptor and is carried to the nucleus, where it binds to androgen response elements in the DNA to initiate transcription.[10] Due to loose binding, the albumin-bound testosterone dissociates during tissue transit, whereas SHBG-bound testosterone does not.[11] Therefore, the combination of free and albumin-bound testosterone (non-SHBG-bound testosterone) is referred to as the "bioavailable testosterone." Dihydrotestosterone also exerts its effects via binding to the androgen receptor, whereas androstenedione, DHEA, and DHEAS do not bind substantially to the androgen receptor as they exert their effects via conversion to testosterone.

TESTOSTERONE LEVELS IN AGING MEN

In healthy adult men, rate of testosterone production ranges between 3 and 10 mg/d, which approximately translates into serum levels of 300 to 1000 ng/dL.[12] Testosterone is secreted in a circadian fashion with the highest levels occurring in the morning and nadir levels seen in the evening.[13] It has been known for more than half a century that testosterone levels decline with age, when reduced testosterone concentrations were found in the spermatic veins of elderly men (compared with young men).[14] Since then, both cross-sectional and longitudinal studies have confirmed an age-related decline in serum testosterone levels.[15–17] Although total testosterone levels are lower in older men, there is no clear age-based inflection point at which there is an abrupt cessation of testosterone production. Longitudinal studies have confirmed that testosterone levels peak in the second and the third decade of life and then decline gradually throughout life (at a rate of 1%–1.5% per year) (**Fig. 1**).[18] This age-related decline in serum testosterone is due to a decreased rate of production,[19] which is significant considering that the rate of metabolic clearance of testosterone also decreases with aging.[20] At the same time as testosterone levels are declining, there is an age-associated increase in serum SHBG levels (1.0% per year), resulting in an even steeper decline in free and bioavailable fractions (2%–3% per year).[16,17] Indeed, studies show that at age 75 years, mean total serum testosterone level is about two-thirds of the level at age 25, whereas mean serum FT level is only about

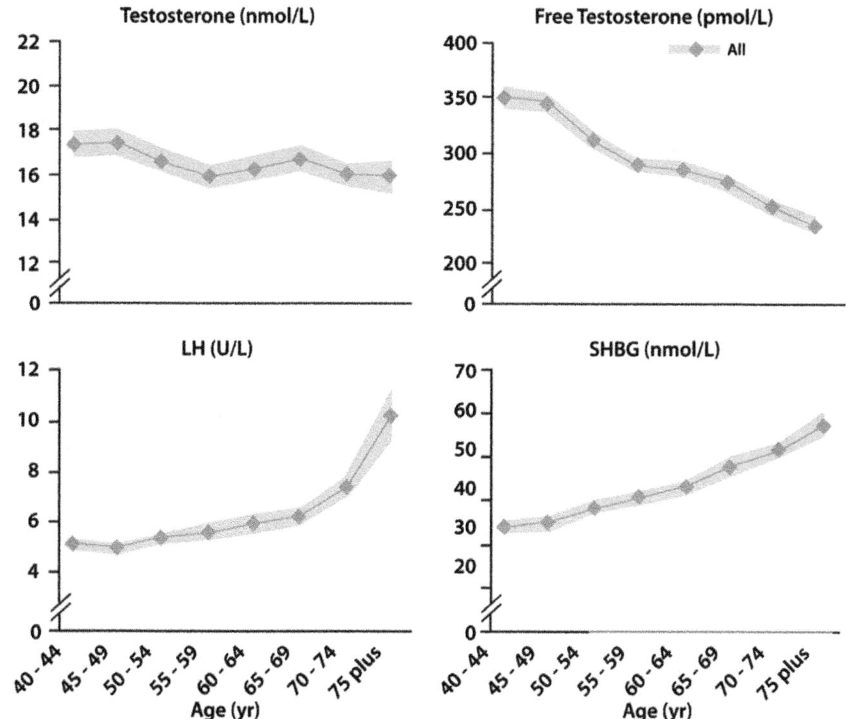

Fig. 1. Influence of aging on the changes in total testosterone, free testosterone, LH, and SHBG levels. (*Data from* Wu FC, Tajar A, Pye SR, et al. Hypothalamic-pituitary-testicular axis disruptions in older men are differentially linked to age and modifiable risk factors: the European Male Aging Study. J Clin Endocrinol Metab 2008;93:2737–45.)

one-half of that in young men. In the Baltimore Longitudinal Study of Aging (BLSA),[15] 19%, 28%, and 49% of men greater than 60, 70, and 80 years of age, respectively, had total testosterone levels below the young reference range (325 ng/dL), whereas 34%, 68%, and 91% had subnormal free testosterone index (T/SHBG) (**Fig. 2**).

The trajectory of age-related decline of testosterone is affected by adiposity, comorbid conditions, medications, and some genetic factors.[21,22] The European Male Aging Study (EMAS) is the first population study that has proposed a "syndromic" definition of LOH whereby a constellation of symptoms are associated with androgen deficiency.[23] In EMAS, symptoms of poor morning erections, low sexual desire, and erectile dysfunction were associated with total testosterone levels less than 317 ng/dL.

Contrary to the decline in sex hormones, a man remains fertile throughout his entire postpubertal life. However, the testicular volume of an older man is lower compared with a young man, reflecting some degree of tubular atrophy.[24] Similarly, there is some decline in the volume of seminal fluid and sperm motility.[25]

PREVALENCE OF ANDROGEN DEFICIENCY

Estimates of the prevalence of low testosterone concentrations vary among epidemiologic studies. These variations are due to differences in the study population, numeric thresholds for defining low testosterone levels, ethnic composition of the population, and the assays used to measure testosterone levels. In the BLSA,[15] 30% of men over the age of 60 years age and 50% over the age of 70 years age had total testosterone concentrations less than the lower limit of the normal range for healthy young men (<325 ng/dL). In the Massachusetts Male Aging Study,[16] 4% of community-dwelling men, 40 to 70 years of age, had a serum total testosterone concentration less than 150 ng/dL in association with an elevated luteinizing hormone (LH) concentration. As androgen deficiency is a syndrome (not simply a low numerical value) characterized by a cluster of signs and symptoms,[5] the presence of low testosterone levels by itself is not diagnostic of androgen deficiency. In the EMAS, although 23.5% of community-dwelling men 40 to 70 years of age had low testosterone levels, only 2.1% had

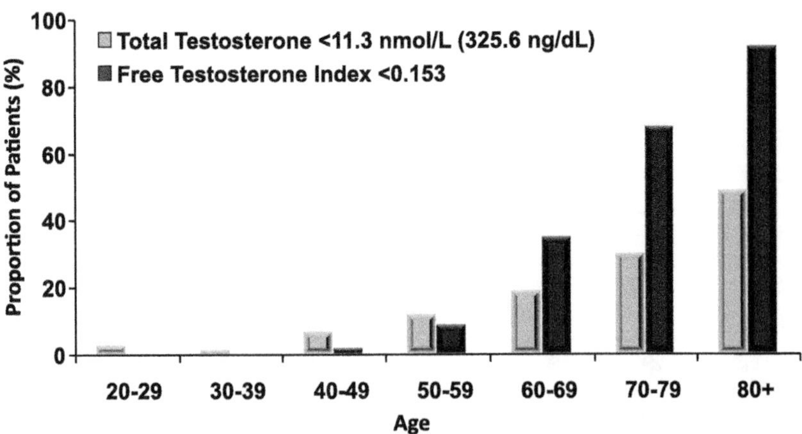

Fig. 2. Prevalence of age-related hypogonadism based on total testosterone and free testosterone index. (*Data from* Harman SM, Metter EJ, Tobin JD, et al. Longitudinal effects of aging on serum total and free testosterone levels in healthy men. Baltimore Longitudinal Study of Aging. J Clin Endocrinol Metab 2001;86:724–31.)

symptomatic androgen deficiency,[23] showing that the prevalence of symptomatic androgen deficiency is substantially lower than numerically low testosterone levels.[26]

In addition to the effect of biologic age, the prevalence of androgen deficiency is also influenced by the degree of adiposity and comorbidities (diabetes, cardiac failure, renal disease, chronic obstructive lung disease).[27,28] Similarly, use of medications, such as glucocorticoids and opioids, that suppress testosterone levels also contribute to this decrease in testosterone levels. Among all of these factors, obesity has the most potent effect on androgen levels.[18] The data from EMAS show that irrespective of age, an obese man (body mass index [BMI] >30 kg/m^2) has a 30% lower serum testosterone level than a man with a normal BMI (BMI <25 kg/m^2) (**Fig. 3**). Less than 1.0% of men with normal weight have LOH compared with 1.6% of overweight men and 5.2% of obese men. Indeed, data from the Massachusetts Male Aging Study show that the trajectory of age-related decline in serum testosterone is much steeper if a person becomes obese during the course of the follow-up (**Fig. 4**).[21] Although the exact mechanism remains unclear, negative feedback to the hypothalamic-pituitary unit by hyperestrogenemia has been posited because compensatory increases in gonadotropins are not seen in these men.[18]

The EMAS also showed that the prevalence of LOH is increased with poor general health and is 10-fold higher in men with at least 2 comorbid conditions compared with men with none.[18] These findings are supported by data from The Healthy Man Study, whereby men aged 40 years and older who described themselves to be in very good or excellent health did not display an age-related decline in testosterone levels.[29] Interestingly, some studies have shown a secular population-level decline in serum testosterone levels across all age groups.[30,31]

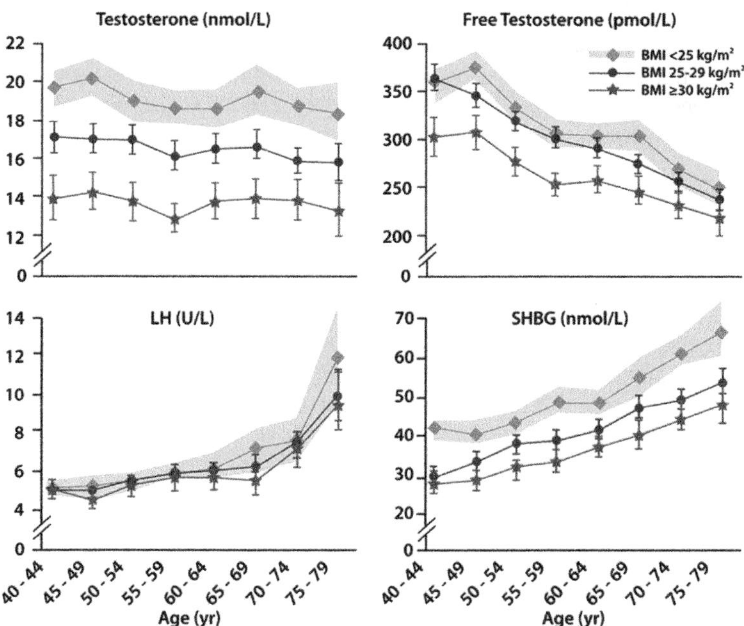

Fig. 3. Influence of body mass index on age-related decline in gonadal hormones. (*Data from* Wu FC, Tajar A, Pye SR, et al. Hypothalamic-pituitary-testicular axis disruptions in older men are differentially linked to age and modifiable risk factors: the European Male Aging Study. J Clin Endocrinol Metab 2008;93:2737–45.)

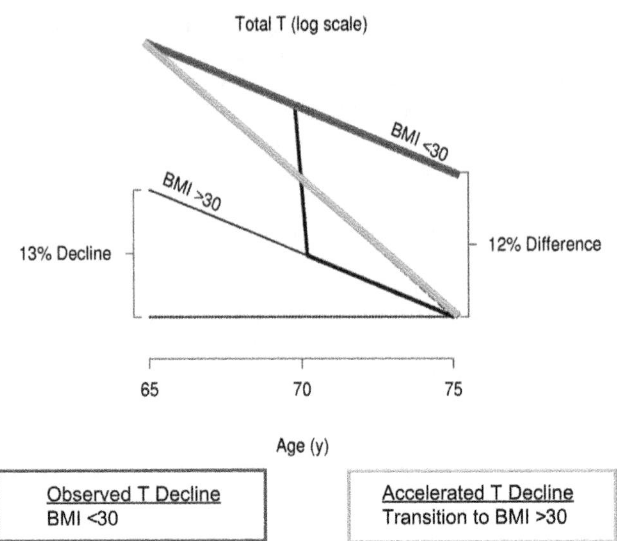

Fig. 4. Effect of obesity on the trajectory of age-related decrease in total testosterone. (*Data from* Travison TG, Araujo AB, Kupelian V, et al. The relative contributions of aging, health, and lifestyle factors to serum testosterone decline in men. J Clin Endocrinol Metab 2007;92:549–55.)

PATHOPHYSIOLOGIC BASIS OF AGE-RELATED DECLINE IN TESTOSTERONE LEVELS

Studies show that the age-related decline in serum testosterone levels occurs as a result of changes at the level of both the testes and the hypothalamic-pituitary unit, as there is diminished testicular secretory capacity and alterations in the pulsatility of the GnRH neurons (pulse-generator).[32]

Testicular Changes

Aging is associated with attrition in the testicular Leydig cells (**Fig. 5**).[33,34] This decrease in Leydig cell number is reflected in the observation that older men display a diminished secretory capacity compared with young men when their testes are stimulated with human chorionic gonadotropin or via pulsatile GnRH.[35–37] In addition to attrition of the Leydig cells, there is also atrophy, to some extent, of the seminiferous tubules as the average testicular volume of older men in their eighth decade of life is approximately 30% compared with their younger counterparts.[24] Aging is associated with stable serum inhibin-B levels and elevated FSH levels, suggesting compensated Sertoli cell function under maximum stimulation by FSH.[38]

Neuroendocrine Changes

The loss of negative feedback that occurs as a result of decreased testosterone production due to Leydig cell failure results in a modest increase in mean serum LH levels with age. However, this increase is not a universal phenomenon because many older men do not have elevated LH levels even though their testosterone levels are low,[39,40] highlighting the inability of the hypothalamic-pituitary unit to maintain a robust LH drive to stimulate the testes. Stimulation with synthetic GnRH has revealed a normal or even a slightly increased LH response in older men compared

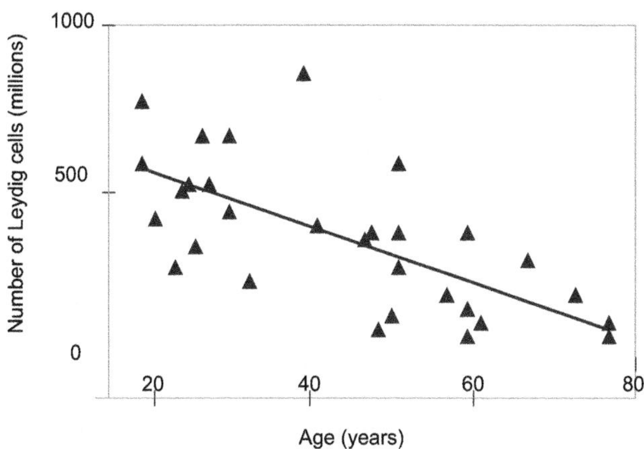

Fig. 5. Age-related attrition of human Leydig cells. (*Data from* Neaves WB, Johnson L, Porter JC, et al. Leydig cell numbers, daily sperm production, and serum gonadotropin levels in aging men. J Clin Endocrinol Metab 1984;59:756–63.)

with their younger counterparts, suggesting that the secretory capacity of the pituitary gonadotropes is preserved.[41,42] This preservation of the pituitary gonadotropes suggests that the inadequate increase in serum LH levels in response to hypoandrogenemia is a result of hypothalamic dysfunction as the pulsatile secretion of GnRH governs the release of LH. This is somewhat supported by studies showing that LH secretory pattern in the elderly displays low pulse amplitude and increased pulse frequency (**Fig. 6**).[43] It has been posited that these secretory dynamics are a consequence of a reduced number of functional GnRH neurons secreting a weaker bolus of GnRH into the hypothalamic portal system. Indeed, animal studies have shown that the GnRH content and the number of neurons expressing prepro-GnRH mRNA are lower in older compared with younger rats.[44] Some studies have suggested that elderly men have an increased responsiveness to negative feedback from androgens.[45,46]

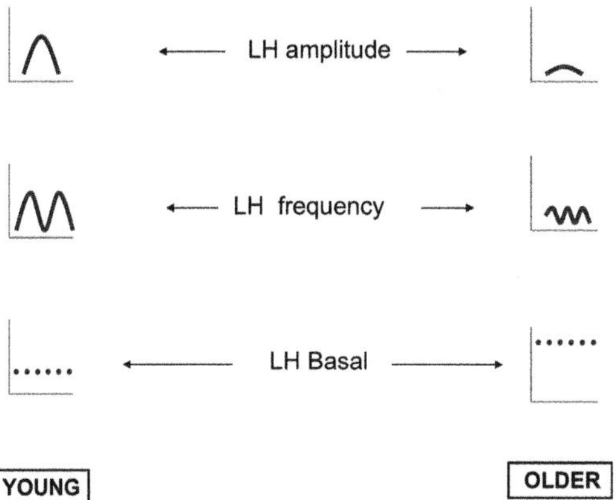

Fig. 6. Characteristics of LH secretion in older men compared with their younger counterparts reveals decreased pulse amplitude, increased pulse frequency, and elevated basal LH levels.

DIAGNOSIS OF LATE-ONSET HYPOGONADISM

Unlike men with organic hypogonadism in whom serum testosterone levels are profoundly and permanently suppressed, testosterone levels in LOH are only marginally low and often fluctuate toward the lower limit of the normal range. The diagnosis of LOH is further complicated by the fact that older men with symptoms indicative of LOH often have normal testosterone levels, whereas some men with low serum testosterone concentrations do not manifest hypogonadal symptoms, making it difficult to attribute their symptoms to testosterone deficiency. This difference poses a challenge to identify men whose symptoms are in fact caused by androgen deficiency, who are a minority compared with either men with isolated symptoms or asymptomatic men with low testosterone.

Previous epidemiologic studies have generally defined LOH only based on low serum testosterone levels, some using less reliable assays. The EMAS used objective criteria for the diagnosis of LOH by identifying symptoms that display a statistically significant inverse correlation with serum testosterone levels and attempted to determine the inflection point of testosterone below which the frequency of these presumed hypogonadal symptoms increase significantly.[23] In this multicenter study, more than 3000 men (age 40–79 years) were administered questionnaires and asked about 32 symptoms suggested by previous studies to be related to androgen deficiency. Importantly, serum testosterone was measured using gas chromatography tandem mass spectrometry, and free testosterone level was calculated. Detailed analysis revealed significant syndromic association only between serum testosterone levels and 3 sexual symptoms (decreased sexual thoughts, weak morning erections, and erectile dysfunction). The remaining 29 symptoms, including symptoms commonly attributed to androgen deficiency, such as difficulty in climbing stairs or performing daily domestic tasks and impaired concentrating ability, were not correlated with testosterone levels. The authors suggested that the diagnosis of LOH can be made in a man with these sexual symptoms and serum total testosterone level less than 230 ng/dL or serum total testosterone level of 230 to 317 ng/dL and free testosterone level less than 63 pg/mL. Using these criteria, LOH diagnosis was diagnosed in only 2.1% of the EMAS participants, suggesting that the prevalence of LOH is much less common than previous estimates of 6% to 12%.[26,47]

CLINICAL EVALUATION OF A PATIENT WITH LOH

Before diagnosing a patient with LOH, it is important to ensure that all the organic (pathologic) causes of androgen deficiency have been excluded because older men may also encounter testicular injury, pituitary lesions, and infiltrative diseases. Diagnosis of LOH should be avoided during an acute illness and one must exclude systemic illness, and use of opioid analgesics, glucocorticoids, and spironolactone. The signs and symptoms of LOH, such as decreased vitality, depressed mood, impaired memory, and diminished exercise tolerance, are nonspecific because these symptoms are also common in normal aging. Testosterone is secreted in a circadian fashion with peaks in the morning; however, this rhythmicity is lost in older men (**Fig. 7**).[13] However, recent data suggest that this circadian rhythm is maintained in healthy, fit older men.[48] Therefore, testosterone levels should be measured in the morning using a reliable assay. The best screening test for the diagnosis of hypogonadism is serum total testosterone.[5] Low levels should be confirmed by repeat measurement because testosterone levels are inherently variable and repeat levels may end up being normal.[49] In many commercial laboratories, the lower range of testosterone is 280 to 300 ng/dL. Because the threshold testosterone level below

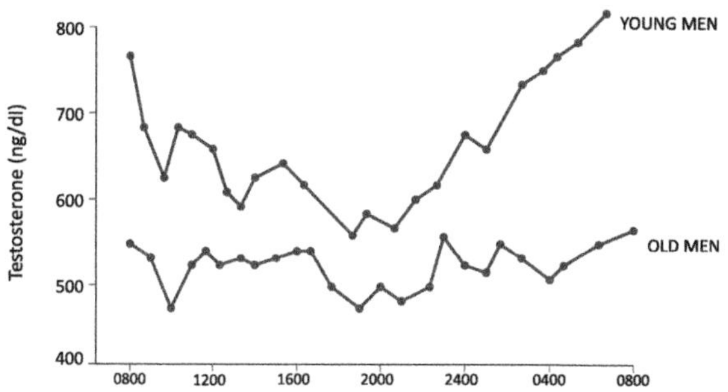

Fig. 7. Diurnal rhythm of testosterone secretion in young and old men. (*Data from* Bremner WJ, Vitiello MV, Prinz PN. Loss of circadian rhythmicity in blood testosterone levels with aging in normal men. J Clin Endocrinol Metab 1983;56:1278–81.)

which hypogonadal symptoms occur remains unclear, the thresholds suggested by EMAS and some other studies may provide some guidance to the clinician.[23,50,51] If SHBG abnormalities are suspected in a patient, free or bioavailable testosterone should be measured by equilibrium dialysis or ammonium-sulfate precipitation, respectively.[52] As these methods are cumbersome and not widely available in commercial laboratories, free and bioavailable testosterone concentrations can be calculated from the law of mass action equations that use total testosterone, SHBG, and albumin concentrations.[53,54] Tracer analogue displacement assays are inaccurate and should not be used to make the diagnosis of LOH.[55]

Once the diagnosis of LOH is ascertained, gonadotropins should be measured. Data from EMAS suggest that only a minority of men will present with elevated gonadotropins (usually very old men); therefore, most of the men will have either low or inappropriately normal gonadotropins. These patients should undergo measurements of serum prolactin, iron studies, and, if indicated, other pituitary hormones. Hyperprolactinemia, symptoms of mass effect (headaches, peripheral vision disturbances), and panhypopituitarism should be evaluated with sellar imaging. Men with morbid obesity (BMI >40 kg/m^2), in addition to having low total testosterone (due to low SHBG levels), may also have low free testosterone and gonadotropins[56,57] presumably secondary to hyperestrogenemia. Most of these men have a normal sellar magnetic resonance image. Therefore, hypopituitarism, hyperprolactinemia, and features of mass effect are the main indications for sellar imaging.

POPULATION SCREENING AND CASE DETECTION

Population-level screening for LOH is not recommended because its cost-effectiveness and impact on public health remain unclear. Many screening questionnaires have been developed, such as the Androgen Deficiency in Aging Male,[58] Massachusetts Male Aging Study Scale,[59] Aging Males Symptom Scale,[60] and New England Research Institutes Hypogonadism Screener,[61] although their performance characteristics have not been rigorously established.

ASSOCIATION BETWEEN LOW TESTOSTERONE AND HEALTH OUTCOMES

Sexual Function

Circulating testosterone levels have been associated with several health outcomes in middle-aged and older men. In the Massachusetts Male Aging Study, decreased libido was associated with low testosterone levels; however, no association was found with erectile dysfunction.[62] In the EMAS, men with low testosterone levels were more likely to report decreased morning erections, erectile dysfunction, and decreased frequency of sexual thoughts.[23] Unlike older men, the prevalence of low testosterone levels is not significantly different in middle-aged men with erectile dysfunction and those without erectile dysfunction.[63]

Body Composition and Physical Function

Low testosterone levels have been associated with decreased self-reported (subjective) as well as performance-based (objective) measures of physical function, such as gait speed.[64] Population studies have shown that men with low free testosterone levels, compared with those with normal free testosterone levels, are more likely to suffer from incident mobility limitation, frailty, and falls.[65,66] Low testosterone levels have also been associated with decreased appendicular skeletal muscle mass and decreased muscle strength.[67]

Cognition

Studies have shown weak associations of verbal memory, visuospatial memory, and executive function with testosterone levels.[68–70] Low total and bioavailable testosterone levels have also been associated with increased risk of mild cognitive impairment and Alzheimer disease.[71,72] The association of testosterone levels and depression has been inconsistent.[73,74] Testosterone levels are lower in older men with dysthymic disorder than in those without any depressive symptoms.[75]

Skeletal Health

Testosterone levels have been associated with bone mineral density, bone geometry, and bone quality.[76–78] In the Osteoporotic Fractures in Men Study, the odds of osteoporosis in men with a total testosterone less than 200 ng/dL were approximately 4-fold higher than in men with a normal testosterone level.[79,80] Similarly, free testosterone levels were an independent predictor of prevalent osteoporotic fractures.[79] Interestingly, bioavailable testosterone and estradiol levels are more strongly associated with these outcomes than total testosterone.[81]

Cardiometabolic Outcomes

In many studies, serum total testosterone levels have been associated with the risk of prevalent diabetes mellitus and metabolic syndrome.[82,83] Interestingly, the association of total testosterone with diabetes is attenuated after adjusting for SHBG concentrations.[84] In one longitudinal analysis, SHBG was significantly associated with diabetes risk, but neither total nor free testosterone levels were associated.[84] As SHBG concentrations are influenced by obesity, insulin resistance, and inflammation, it is conceivable that SHBG is a marker of metabolic health. The role of SHBG as a marker or a contributor to metabolic risk needs to be clarified.

Numerous cross-sectional studies have found no difference in serum testosterone levels between men who had coronary artery disease and those who did not, whereas other studies have reported lower testosterone levels in men with coronary artery disease compared with men without coronary artery disease.[85–87] Some epidemiologic studies have reported higher all-cause mortality and cardiovascular mortality in men with low testosterone levels.[88,89] In the Rancho Bernardo Study, men in the lowest quartile of testosterone levels (<241 ng/dL) were 40% more likely to die over the next 20 years than those in the higher quartiles, even after adjusting for various confounders.[89]

SUMMARY

The global annual prescription sales of testosterone are skyrocketing. Clinicians continue to be confronted, with growing pressure from patients and the industry alike, to prescribe testosterone therapy in older men for nonspecific symptoms that may not be a direct consequence of LOH. Associations between serum testosterone levels and health-related outcomes are weak and confounded by the colinearity of age-related comorbidities and low testosterone levels. Furthermore, just as causality cannot be inferred from cross-sectional studies, reverse causality also cannot be excluded. Recent data show that the prevalence of LOH in middle-aged and older men is approximately 2%. Furthermore, multiple end-organ dysfunction in LOH is only encountered in a minority of patients, particularly those with total testosterone less than 230 ng/dL.[90] Obesity, other comorbidities, and medications also significantly contribute to low testosterone levels. Hence, it remains unclear whether LOH is a cause or a consequence (biomarker of health) of age-related comorbidities. Therefore, practicing clinicians must exercise caution and only initiate testosterone replacement in older men with unequivocal hypogonadism based on symptoms and multiple testosterone levels that are measured using a reliable assay. Based on the recent data that men who are in excellent health do not experience age-related decrease in sex hormones[29] and that treatment of obesity results in restoration of serum testosterone levels,[91] weight reduction, treatment of comorbidities, and discontinuation of offending medications may prevent or attenuate age-related declines in gonadal hormones.

REFERENCES

1. Basaria S, Wahlstrom JT, Dobs AS. Anabolic-androgenic steroid therapy in the treatment of chronic diseases. J Clin Endocrinol Metab 2001;86:5108–17.
2. Brown-Sequard CE. Note on the effects produced on man by subcutaneous injections of a liquid obtained from the testicles of animals. Lancet 1889;2:105–7.
3. Freeman ER, Bloom DA, McGuire EJ. A brief history of testosterone. J Urol 2001; 165:371–3.
4. Handelsman DJ. Trends and regional differences in testosterone prescribing in Australia, 1991-2001. Med J Aust 2004;181:419–22.
5. Bhasin S, Cunningham GR, Hayes FJ, et al. Testosterone therapy in adult men with androgen deficiency syndromes: an endocrine society clinical practice guideline. J Clin Endocrinol Metab 2010;95:2536–59.
6. Wang C, Nieschlag E, Swerdloff R, et al. Investigation, treatment and monitoring of late-onset hypogonadism in males: ISA, ISSAM, EAU, EAA and ASA recommendations. Eur J Endocrinol 2008;159:507–14.
7. Hammond GL, Ruokonen A, Kontturi M, et al. Simultaneous radioimmunoassay of 7 steroids in human spermatic and peripheral venous-blood. J Clin Endocrinol Metab 1977;45:16–24.
8. Horton R, Tait J. The in vivo conversion of dehydroisoandrosterone to plasma androstenedione and testosterone. J Clin Endocrinol Metab 1967;27:79.
9. Dunn JF, Nisula BC, Rodbard D. Transport of steroid-hormones-binding of 21 endogenous steroids to both testosterone binding globulin and corticosteroid-binding globulin in human plasma. J Clin Endocrinol Metab 1981;53:58–68.
10. Chan L, O'Malley BW. Mechanism of action of the sex steroid hormones. N Engl J Med 1976;294:1322–8.
11. Pardridge WM. Serum bioavailability of sex steroid hormones. Clin Endocrinol Metab 1986;15:259–78.

12. Vermeulen A. Androgen replacement therapy in the aging male. A critical evaluation. J Clin Endocrinol Metab 2001;86:2380–90.
13. Bremner WJ, Vitiello MV, Prinz PN. Loss of circadian rhythmicity in blood testosterone levels with aging in normal men. J Clin Endocrinol Metab 1983;56:1278–81.
14. Hollander N, Hollander VP. The microdetermination of testosterone in human spermatic vein blood. J Clin Endocrinol Metab 1958;19:966–70.
15. Harman SM, Metter EJ, Tobin JD, et al. Longitudinal effects of aging on serum total and free testosterone levels in healthy men. Baltimore Longitudinal Study of Aging. J Clin Endocrinol Metab 2001;86:724–31.
16. Feldman HA, Longcope C, Derby CA, et al. Age trends in the level of serum testosterone and other hormones in middle-aged men: longitudinal results from the Massachusetts male aging study. J Clin Endocrinol Metab 2002;87:589–98.
17. Ferrini RL, Barrett-Connor E. Sex hormones and age: a cross-sectional study of testosterone and estradiol and their bioavailable fractions in community-dwelling men. Am J Epidemiol 1998;147:750–4.
18. Wu FC, Tajar A, Pye SR, et al. Hypothalamic-pituitary-testicular axis disruptions in older men are differentially linked to age and modifiable risk factors: the European Male Aging Study. J Clin Endocrinol Metab 2008;93:2737–45.
19. Giusti G, Gonnelli P, Borrelli D, et al. Age-related secretion of androstenedione, testosterone and dihydrotestosterone by human testis. Exp Gerontol 1975;10: 241–5.
20. Vermeulen A, Verdonck L, Rubens R. Testosterone secretion and metabolism in male senescence. J Clin Endocrinol Metab 1972;34:730–5.
21. Travison TG, Araujo AB, Kupelian V, et al. The relative contributions of aging, health, and lifestyle factors to serum testosterone decline in men. J Clin Endocrinol Metab 2007;92:549–55.
22. Tajar A, Forti G, O'Neill TW, et al. Characteristics of secondary, primary, and compensated hypogonadism in aging men: evidence from the European Male Ageing Study. J Clin Endocrinol Metab 2010;95:1810–8.
23. Wu FC, Tajar A, Beynon JM, et al. Identification of late-onset hypogonadism in middle-aged and elderly men. N Engl J Med 2010;363:123–35.
24. Mahmoud AM, Goemaere S, El-Garem Y, et al. Testicular volume in relation to hormonal indices of gonadal function in community-dwelling elderly men. J Clin Endocrinol Metab 2003;88:179–84.
25. Kidd SA, Eskenazi B, Wyrobek AJ. Effects of male age on semen quality and fertility: a review of the literature. Fertil Steril 2001;75:237–48.
26. Araujo AB, Esche GR, Kupelian V, et al. Prevalence of symptomatic androgen deficiency in men. J Clin Endocrinol Metab 2007;92:4241–7.
27. Handelsman DJ, Dong Q. Hypothalamo-pituitary gonadal axis in chronic renal failure. Endocrinol Metab Clin North Am 1993;22:145–61.
28. Jankowska EA, Biel B, Majda J, et al. Anabolic deficiency in men with chronic heart failure: prevalence and detrimental impact on survival. Circulation 2006; 114:1829–37.
29. Sartorius G, Spasevska S, Idan A, et al. Serum testosterone, dihydrotestosterone and estradiol concentrations in older men self-reporting very good health: the healthy man study. Clin Endocrinol (Oxf) 2012;77:755–63.
30. Travison TG, Araujo AB, O'Donnell AB, et al. A population-level decline in serum testosterone levels in American men. J Clin Endocrinol Metab 2007;92:196–202.
31. Andersson AM, Jensen TK, Juul A, et al. Secular decline in male testosterone and sex hormone binding globulin serum levels in Danish population surveys. J Clin Endocrinol Metab 2007;92:4696–705.

32. Vermeulen A. Androgens in the aging male. J Clin Endocrinol Metab 1991;73:221–4.
33. Neaves WB, Johnson L, Porter JC, et al. Leydig cell numbers, daily sperm production, and serum gonadotropin levels in aging men. J Clin Endocrinol Metab 1984;59:756–63.
34. Neaves WB, Johnson L, Petty CS. Age-related change in numbers of other interstitial cells in testes of adult men. Evidence bearing on the fate of Leydig cells lost with increasing age. Biol Reprod 1985;33:259–69.
35. Rubens R, Dhont M, Vermeule A. Further studies on Leydig cell function in old-age. J Clin Endocrinol Metab 1974;39:40–5.
36. Longcope C. Effect of human chorionic gonadotropin on plasma steroid levels in young and old men. Steroids 1973;21:583–90.
37. Nankin HR, Lin T, Murono EP, et al. The aging Leydig cell. Gonadotropin stimulation in men. J Androl 1981;2:181–9.
38. Mahmoud AM, Goemaere S, De Bacquer D, et al. Serum inhibin B levels in community-dwelling elderly men. Clin Endocrinol (Oxf) 2000;53:141–7.
39. Urban RJ, Veldhuis JD, Blizzard RM, et al. Attenuated release of biologically active luteinizing hormone in healthy aging men. J Clin Invest 1988;81:1020–9.
40. Pincus SM, Veldhuis JD, Mulligan T, et al. Effects of age on the irregularity of LH and FSH serum concentrations in women and men. Am J Physiol 1997;273:E989–95.
41. Mulligan T, Iranmanesh A, Kerzner R, et al. Two-week pulsatile gonadotropin releasing hormone infusion unmasks dual (hypothalamic and Leydig cell) defects in the healthy aging male gonadotropic axis. Eur J Endocrinol 1999;141:257–66.
42. Kaufman JM, Giri M, Deslypere JM, et al. Influence of age on the responsiveness of the gonadotrophs to luteinizing-hormone-releasing hormone in males. J Clin Endocrinol Metab 1991;72:1255–60.
43. Veldhuis JD, Urban RJ, Lizarralde G, et al. Attenuation of luteinizing hormone secretory burst amplitude as a proximate basis for the hypoandrogenism of healthy aging in men. J Clin Endocrinol Metab 1992;75:707–13.
44. Bonavera JJ, Swerdloff RS, Sinha Hakim AP, et al. Aging results in attenuated gonadotropin releasing hormone-luteinizing hormone axis responsiveness to glutamate receptor agonist N-methyl-D-aspartate. J Neuroendocrinol 1998;10:93–9.
45. Winters SJ, Sherins RJ, Troen P. The gonadotropin-suppressive activity of androgen is increased in elderly men. Metabolism 1984;33:1052–9.
46. Winters SJ, Atkinson L. Serum LH concentrations in hypogonadal men during transdermal testosterone replacement through scrotal skin: further evidence that ageing enhances testosterone negative feedback. Clin Endocrinol (Oxf) 1997;47:317–22.
47. Araujo AB, O'Donnell AB, Brambilla DJ, et al. Prevalence and incidence of androgen deficiency in middle-aged and older men: estimates from the Massachusetts Male Aging Study. J Clin Endocrinol Metab 2004;89:5920–6.
48. Diver MJ, Imtiaz KE, Ahmad AM, et al. Diurnal rhythms of serum total, free and bioavailable testosterone and of SHBG in middle-aged men compared with those in young men. Clin Endocrinol (Oxf) 2003;58:710–7.
49. Brambilla DJ, Matsumoto AM, Araujo AB, et al. The effect of diurnal variation on clinical measurement of serum testosterone and other sex hormone levels in men. J Clin Endocrinol Metab 2009;94:907–13.
50. Zitzmann M, Faber S, Nieschlag E. Association of specific symptoms and metabolic risks with serum testosterone in older men. J Clin Endocrinol Metab 2006;91:4335–43.

51. Kelleher S, Conway AJ, Handelsman DJ. Blood testosterone threshold for androgen deficiency symptoms. J Clin Endocrinol Metab 2004;89:3813–7.
52. Manni A, Pardridge WM, Cefalu W, et al. Bioavailability of albumin-bound testosterone. J Clin Endocrinol Metab 1985;61:705–71.
53. Vermeulen A, Verdonck L, Kaufman JM. A critical evaluation of simple methods for the estimation of free testosterone in serum. J Clin Endocrinol Metab 1999; 84:3666–72.
54. Mazer NA. A novel spreadsheet method for calculating the free serum concentrations of testosterone, dihydrotestosterone, estradiol, estrone and cortisol: with illustrative examples from male and female populations. Steroids 2009;74:512–9.
55. Winters SJ, Kelley DE, Goodpaster B. The analog free testosterone assay: are the results in men clinically useful? Clin Chem 1998;44:2178–82.
56. Vermeulen A, Kaufman JM, Giagulli VA. Influence of some biological indexes on sex hormone-binding globulin and androgen levels in aging or obese males. J Clin Endocrinol Metab 1996;81:1821–6.
57. Glass AR, Swerdloff RS, Bray GA, et al. Low serum testosterone and sex-hormone-binding-globulin in massively obese men. J Clin Endocrinol Metab 1977;45:1211–9.
58. Morley JE, Charlton E, Patrick P, et al. Validation of a screening questionnaire for androgen deficiency in aging males. Metabolism 2000;49:1239–42.
59. Smith KW, Feldman HA, McKinlay JB. Construction and field validation of a self-administered screener for testosterone deficiency (hypogonadism) in ageing men. Clin Endocrinol (Oxf) 2000;53:703–11.
60. Moore C, Huebler D, Zimmermann T, et al. The Aging Males' Symptoms scale (AMS) as outcome measure for treatment of androgen deficiency. Eur Urol 2004;46:80–7.
61. Rosen RC, Araujo AB, Connor MK, et al. The NERI Hypogonadism Screener: psychometric validation in male patients and controls. Clin Endocrinol (Oxf) 2011;74:248–56.
62. Travison TG, Morley JE, Araujo AB, et al. The relationship between libido and testosterone levels in aging men. J Clin Endocrinol Metab 2006;91:2509–13.
63. Korenman SG, Morley JE, Mooradian AD, et al. Secondary hypogonadism in older men: its relation to impotence. J Clin Endocrinol Metab 1990;71:963–9.
64. Orwoll E, Lambert LC, Marshall LM, et al. Endogenous testosterone levels, physical performance, and fall risk in older men. Arch Intern Med 2006;166:2124–31.
65. Cawthon PM, Ensrud KE, Laughlin GA, et al. Sex hormones and frailty in older men: the osteoporotic fractures in men (MrOS) study. J Clin Endocrinol Metab 2009;94:3806–15.
66. Krasnoff JB, Basaria S, Pencina MJ, et al. Free testosterone levels are associated with mobility limitation and physical performance in community-dwelling men: the Framingham Offspring Study. J Clin Endocrinol Metab 2010;95:2790–9.
67. Roy TA, Blackman MR, Harman SM, et al. Interrelationships of serum testosterone and free testosterone index with FFM and strength in aging men. Am J Physiol Endocrinol Metab 2002;283:E284–94.
68. Hier DB, Crowley WF Jr. Spatial ability in androgen-deficient men. N Engl J Med 1982;306:1202–5.
69. Janowsky JS, Oviatt SK, Orwoll ES. Testosterone influences spatial cognition in older men. Behav Neurosci 1994;108:325–32.
70. Alexander GM, Swerdloff RS, Wang C, et al. Androgen-behavior correlations in hypogonadal men and eugonadal men. II. Cognitive abilities. Horm Behav 1998;33:85–94.

71. Moffat SD, Zonderman AB, Metter EJ, et al. Longitudinal assessment of serum free testosterone concentration predicts memory performance and cognitive status in elderly men. J Clin Endocrinol Metab 2002;87:5001–7.
72. Moffat SD, Resnick SM. Long-term measures of free testosterone predict regional cerebral blood flow patterns in elderly men. Neurobiol Aging 2007; 28:914–20.
73. Barrett-Conner E, Von Muhlen DG, Kritz-Silverstein D. Bioavailable testosterone and depressed mood in older men: the Rancho Bernardo study. J Clin Endocrinol Metab 1999;84:573–7.
74. Seidman SN, Araujo AB, Roose SP, et al. Testosterone level, androgen receptor polymorphism, and depressive symptoms in middle-aged men. Biol Psychiatry 2001;50:371–6.
75. Seidman SN, Araujo AB, Roose SP, et al. Low testosterone levels in elderly men with dysthymic disorder. Am J Psychiatry 2002;159:456–9.
76. Greendale GA, Edelstein S, Barrett-Connor E. Endogenous sex steroids and bone mineral density in older women and men: the Rancho Bernardo Study. J Bone Miner Res 1997;12:1833–43.
77. Khosla S, Melton LJ 3rd, Robb RA, et al. Relationship of volumetric BMD and structural parameters at different skeletal sites to sex steroid levels in men. J Bone Miner Res 2005;20:730–40.
78. Benito M, Vasilic B, Wehrli FW, et al. Effect of testosterone replacement on trabecular architecture in hypogonadal men. J Bone Miner Res 2005;20:1785–91.
79. Mellstrom D, Johnell O, Ljunggren O, et al. Free testosterone is an independent predictor of BMD and prevalent fractures in elderly men: MrOS Sweden. J Bone Miner Res 2006;21:529–35.
80. Fink HA, Ewing SK, Ensrud KE, et al. Association of testosterone and estradiol deficiency with osteoporosis and rapid bone loss in older men. J Clin Endocrinol Metab 2006;91:3908–15.
81. Khosla S, Melton LJ III, Atkinson EJ, et al. Relationship of serum sex steroid levels and bone turnover markers with bone mineral density in men and women: a key role for bioavailable estrogen. J Clin Endocrinol Metab 1998;83:2266–74.
82. Ding EL, Song Y, Malik VS, et al. Sex differences of endogenous sex hormones and risk of type 2 diabetes: a systematic review and meta-analysis. JAMA 2006;295:1288–99.
83. Brand JS, van der Tweel I, Grobbee DE, et al. Testosterone, sex hormone-binding globulin and the metabolic syndrome: a systematic review and meta-analysis of observational studies. Int J Epidemiol 2011;40:189–207.
84. Lakshman KM, Bhasin S, Araujo AB. Sex hormone-binding globulin as an independent predictor of incident type 2 diabetes mellitus in men. J Gerontol A Biol Sci Med Sci 2010;65:503–9.
85. Wu FC, von Eckardstein A. Androgens and coronary artery disease. Endocr Rev 2003;24:183–217.
86. Barrett-Connor E, Khaw KT. Endogenous sex hormones and cardiovascular disease in men. A prospective population-based study. Circulation 1988;78: 539–45.
87. Shores MM, Matsumoto AM, Sloan KL, et al. Low serum testosterone and mortality in male veterans. Arch Intern Med 2006;166:1660–5.
88. Araujo AB, Kupelian V, Page ST, et al. Sex steroids and all-cause and cause-specific mortality in men. Arch Intern Med 2007;167:1252–60.
89. Laughlin GA, Barrett-Connor E, Bergstrom J. Low serum testosterone and mortality in older men. J Clin Endocrinol Metab 2008;93:68–75.

90. Tajar A, Huhtaniemi IT, O'Neill TW, et al. Characteristics of androgen deficiency in late-onset hypogonadism: results from the European Male Aging Study (EMAS). J Clin Endocrinol Metab 2012;97:1508–16.
91. Hammoud A, Gibson M, Hunt SC, et al. Effect of Roux-en-Y gastric bypass surgery on the sex steroids and quality of life in obese men. J Clin Endocrinol Metab 2009;94:1329–32.

Testosterone Administration in Older Men

Alvin M. Matsumoto, MD[a,b,*]

KEYWORDS

• Hypogonadism • Aging • Diagnosis • Testosterone • Treatment

KEY POINTS

- In older men, consider the potential contribution of comorbidities and medications on clinical manifestations and their impact on the diagnosis and management of male hypogonadism.
- The goals of testosterone treatment in older hypogonadal men should be patient-centered and include potential improvements in quality of life and functional status.
- The choice testosterone formulations in older men is based both on pharmacologic considerations and patient preferences.
- In older hypogonadal men, appropriate monitoring of efficacy and safety should be performed during testosterone administration.

INTRODUCTION

The only indication for testosterone (T) administration in older men is replacement therapy for male hypogonadism, which is defined as a syndrome consisting of symptoms and signs of androgen deficiency in the presence of consistently low serum T levels.[1] Male hypogonadism is common, occurring in 2% to 6% of community-dwelling middle-aged to older men and its prevalence and incidence increases with age.[2–4] Compared with young hypogonadal men, the diagnosis and optimal management of male hypogonadism in older men presents greater challenges.

Clinical manifestations of androgen deficiency in older adults are nonspecific, and serum T levels decline progressively with increasing age, such that an increasing proportion of men have T levels in the hypogonadal range with age.[5,6] Both symptoms and signs of androgen deficiency and low T levels may be caused or modified by comorbid illnesses that occur commonly as men age and by medications that are taken more frequently by older men.[7,8] As result, there is an increasing likelihood of

[a] Geriatric Research, Education and Clinical Center and Clinical Research Unit, VA Puget Sound Health Care System, 1660 South Columbian Way (S-182-GRECC), Seattle, WA 98108, USA; [b] Division of Gerontology and Geriatric Medicine, Department of Medicine, University of Washington School of Medicine, 1959 NE Pacific Street, Seattle, WA 98195, USA

* VA Puget Sound Health Care System, 1660 South Columbian Way (S-182-GRECC), Seattle, WA 98108.

E-mail address: alvin.matsumoto@va.gov

Endocrinol Metab Clin N Am 42 (2013) 271–286
http://dx.doi.org/10.1016/j.ecl.2013.02.011 **endo.theclinics.com**
0889-8529/13/$ – see front matter Published by Elsevier Inc.

overdiagnosis of male hypogonadism and subsequent inappropriate use of T administration and inadequate response to treatment in older men.

Therefore, it is important to use a systematic, holistic clinical approach to the diagnosis and management of older men with clinical findings and low serum T levels that could be caused by androgen deficiency. In older men, the approach should include the following elements:

- Considering the potential contribution of comorbidities and medications on clinical manifestations and their impact on the diagnosis and management of male hypogonadism
- Setting patient-specific or patient-centered goals of treatment, including improvements in quality of life and functional status
- Choosing T formulations based both on pharmacologic considerations and patient preferences
- Using appropriate monitoring for efficacy and adverse effects during T therapy

Before initiating T treatment, endocrinologists should consider the following questions in older men with hypogonadism:

- Has the diagnosis of hypogonadism been established and, if so, what is the cause of hypogonadism?
- Should older men with hypogonadism be treated with T replacement therapy?
- What T formulation should be used for treatment in older men?
- What monitoring is appropriate in older men treated with T?

DIAGNOSIS

The Endocrine Society clinical practice guidelines recommend that the diagnosis of male hypogonadism be made only in men with symptoms and signs of androgen deficiency and consistently low serum T levels (on at least 2 occasions).[1] For endocrinologists in a referral practice, it is not uncommon for older patients to be referred with a "presumptive diagnosis" of hypogonadism based on a single low total T level without complete consideration of the clinical manifestations of androgen deficiency and without an evaluation to determine the cause of hypogonadism. Therefore, it is important for an endocrine specialist to ask first whether a diagnosis of hypogonadism has been established and to investigate its cause.

Clinical Diagnosis

The clinical manifestations of hypogonadism may be classified into 3 domains: sexual, behavioral, and physical (**Box 1**). In the European Male Ageing Study, although sexual symptoms were nonspecific (ie, they occurred in men with normal T levels as well as those with low T levels), decreased frequency of sexual thoughts (low libido) and morning erections, and erectile dysfunction (ED) were found to cluster most strongly with low T levels.[4] These findings suggested that compared with behavioral and physical manifestations, sexual symptoms were more prominently associated with hypogonadism in older men.

The clinical diagnosis of male hypogonadism in adults is challenging because the symptoms and signs of androgen deficiency (including sexual symptoms) are nonspecific and, in older men, age-associated comorbid illness and/or medications may produce some of the same symptoms as androgen deficiency. For example, depression may cause diminished libido and sexual activity, ED, diminished energy and vitality, depressed mood, irritability, difficulty concentrating, and sleep disturbance. Heart disease, type 2 diabetes mellitus, and use of antihypertensive or cardiovascular

Box 1
Clinical manifestations of androgen deficiency

Sexual

- Diminished libido and sexual activity
- Reduced morning erections
- ED
- Infertility, small testes

Behavioral

- Diminished energy and vitality
- Depressed mood, irritability
- Difficulty concentrating
- Increased sleep, hot flashes, and sweats

Physical

- Gynecomastia
- Reduced male hair
- Decreased muscle bulk, strength, and activity
- Low bone mineral density [BMD], osteoporosis

medications that are common in older men may cause diminished libido and sexual activity, ED, diminished energy and vitality, and depression.

The clinical manifestations of androgen deficiency in older men also may be less prominent than in young hypogonadal men. Young men with classical severe hypogonadism (eg, due to idiopathic hypogonadotropic hypogonadism) demonstrate most if not all of the symptoms and signs of androgen deficiency. In older men with hypogonadism, the manifestations may be less prominent, in large part because androgen deficiency may be less severe. Older men who undergo androgen deprivation therapy to induce medical castration (eg, with gonadotropin-releasing hormone agonist treatment) for prostate cancer, however, develop classical symptoms and signs similar to those demonstrated by young men with severe hypogonadism. Finally, it is important to appreciate that prior T treatment may attenuate some manifestations of androgen deficiency (eg, male body hair) for some time after cessation of therapy and that often prominent manifestations of comorbid illness may mask or take clinical precedence over those of androgen deficiency.

Biochemical Diagnosis

If a patient's clinical presentation suggests androgen deficiency, male hypogonadism is confirmed if serum T levels are consistently low. Biochemical confirmation of male hypogonadism is often difficult, however, because (1) T measurements in various immunoassays are highly variable and may be inaccurate; (2) circulating T levels exhibit circadian and day-to-day biologic variability; (3) clinical conditions that alter sex hormone–binding globulin (SHBG) and, therefore, total T levels occur commonly, particularly in older men; and (4) T levels may be suppressed transiently with illness, nutritional deficiency, and certain medications.[1]

Because endocrinologists rely on hormone measurements to confirm diagnoses, it is essential that they use the most accurate, precise, and reliable assays available to make clinical decisions. Practitioners should be aware that various T immunoassays differ considerably in absolute levels measured and in accuracy. The extreme variability in T assays was highlighted in a recent comparison of T measurements made on the same external quality control sample in different immunoassays that reported T levels that ranged from 160 ng/dL to 508 ng/dL (ie, from the hypogonadal to eugonadal range).[9] Therefore, T assay variability may affect an endocrinologist's ability to confidently confirm the biochemical diagnosis of hypogonadism.

In addition to assay variability, serum T levels also exhibit a circadian variability with highest values in the morning.[10,11] Circadian variability of T levels is blunted in older men. In one study, however, more than half of men over 65 years who had low T levels in the afternoon were found to have repeatedly normal T levels in the morning,[12] supporting guideline recommendations to measure serum T levels in the morning. There is also considerable day-to-day biologic variability in T levels,[13] and a single low T level may be normal on repeat testing in up to 30% to 35% of men.[14] Therefore, it is important that T levels be measured on at least 2 occasions and be consistently low to confirm the diagnosis of hypogonadism prior to considering T treatment.

Compared with younger individuals, older men are more likely to have clinical conditions or take medications that decrease or increase SHBG concentrations (**Box 2**) and, therefore, decrease or increase total T levels, respectively, without altering free T levels.[1] With regard to the diagnosis of hypogonadism, conditions that lower SHBG and total T levels without affecting free T levels, such as obesity, are particularly noteworthy. In men with a high prevalence of obesity and comorbidity, more than 60% of men who had low total T levels were reported to have normal free T levels.[15] Total T levels less than 350 ng/dL were not sufficiently sensitive to exclude hypogonadism and, except when levels were less than 150 ng/dL, total T had low specificity for the biochemical diagnosis of hypogonadism (defined as low calculated free T <34 pg/mL). Therefore, if conditions that alter SHBG levels are present or suspected or if total T levels are close to the lower limit of the normal reference range, it is recommended that accurate measurements of free T (eg, calculated free T or free T by equilibrium dialysis) be used to confirm the diagnosis of hypogonadism.[1]

Finally, T levels may be suppressed transiently during and sometime after an acute illness and/or nutritional deficiency or while taking certain medications (eg, opioids or glucocorticoids).[1] Therefore, before T treatment is considered, it is important to

Box 2
Causes of alterations in sex hormone–binding globulin

Causes of decreased SHBG

- Moderate obesity, type 2 diabetes mellitus
- Glucocorticoids, progestins, and androgens
- Nephrotic syndrome
- Hypothyroidism
- Acromegaly

Causes of increased SHBG

- Aging
- Anticonvulsants and estrogens
- Liver disease (hepatitis and cirrhosis)
- Hyperthyroidism
- HIV disease

confirm that low T levels were not measured during these situations and, if they were, o repeat a biochemical evaluation after complete recovery from illness and nutritional deficiency and discontinuation of offending medications.

Etiology

When serum T levels are repeated to confirm that they are low, they are usually measured in conjunction with serum gonadotropin, luteinizing hormone and follicle-stimulating hormone, measurements to ascertain whether is hypogonadism is (1) primary hypogonadism due to a disorder of the testes (characterized by low T with elevated gonadotropin levels), (2) secondary hypogonadism due to a disorder of the pituitary and/or hypothalamus (characterized by low T with low or inappropriately normal gonadotropin levels), or (3) combined primary and secondary hypogonadism characterized by low T with mid-normal to slightly high gonadotropin levels).[1] Subsequently, it is important to pursue the cause of hypogonadism because, with treatment or discontinuation of a medication, some functional causes of hypogonadism may be reversible and not necessarily require T treatment.

From the standpoint of management, it is useful to classify the cause of hypogonadism as having organic or functional origins (**Box 3**). Organic causes of hypogonadism are due to congenital, developmental, destructive, or pathologic conditions of the hypothalamic-pituitary-testicular axis that are not reversible. Most causes of primary and some causes of secondary hypogonadism are organic. Functional causes of hypogonadism are due to nondestructive suppression of the hypothalamic-pituitary-testicular axis by conditions that are potentially reversible, if they can be treated or offending medications can be discontinued and, therefore, may not require T treatment. Many causes of secondary and combined primary and secondary hypogonadism are functional.

TREATMENT

Considerations Before Staring T Treatment

Once clinical hypogonadism is diagnosed in older men, several issues need to be considered before T treatment is started:

- The severity of clinical and biochemical androgen deficiency
- The contribution of comorbidities and medications to clinical manifestations
- Treatment of potentially reversible functional causes of hypogonadism
- Potential clinical benefits and risks of T treatment
- Patient-centered goals of T treatment
- Contraindications and precautions to T treatment

Severity of androgen deficiency

The severity of clinical and biochemical hypogonadism affects the decision to start T replacement therapy. Older men with reduced libido, spontaneous erections and energy, ED, and loss of male body hair associated with very low serum total T levels and free T levels and very high gonadotropin levels (primary hypogonadism) are more likely to treated with T than men with isolated ED or poor energy, low end of normal to slightly low total T levels and free T levels, and normal gonadotropin levels.

Contribution of comorbidities and medications

In older men, treatment of comorbidities (eg, depression) or discontinuation of medications (eg, antihypertensive medications that might cause fatigue, low libido, and ED)

Box 3
Organic and functional causes of hypogonadism

Organic causes

- Primary
  - Klinefelter syndrome
  - Cryptorchidism, myotonic dystrophy, and anorchia
  - Chemotherapy, irradiation, and orchidectomy
  - Orchitis
- Secondary
  - Pituitary tumor
  - Hypopituitarism (tumor, infiltrative, destructive, and surgical)
  - Hemochromatosis
  - Idiopathic hypogonadotropic hypogonadism and Kallmann syndrome

Functional causes

- Secondary
  - Hyperprolactinemia
  - Opioids, central nervous system–active medications
  - Nutritional deficiency and excessive exercise
  - Morbid obesity and sleep apnea
  - Anabolic steroids, progestins and and estrogens
- Combined primary and secondary
  - Chronic systemic illness
  - Organ failure (renal, liver, heart, and lung)
  - Aging
  - Alcohol abuse
  - Glucocorticoids

that might contribute to clinical manifestations should be considered before starting T treatment.

Treatment of functional causes of hypogonadism

Treatment of potentially reversibly functional causes of hypogonadism that might improve or resolve clinical and biochemical androgen deficiency should also be considered before initiating T treatment (eg, discontinuing medications that cause hyperprolactinemia or dopamine agonist treatment of hyperprolactinemia; discontinuing opioids, glucocorticoids, central nervous system–active medications, or progestins; correction of nutritional deficiency; weight reduction program or surgery for morbid obesity; continuous positive airway pressure [CPAP] or bilevel positive airway pressure [BPAP] therapy for obstructive sleep apnea [OSA]; or withdrawal from alcohol dependence). Although these functional causes of hypogonadism are potentially reversible with treatment, in many instances, the etiologic condition cannot be treated or managed in a reasonable time frame (eg, chronic opioid or glucocorticoid treatment of certain comorbid conditions), so that T treatment of these functional causes of hypogonadism should be considered.

Potential benefits and risks of T treatment

As with any therapeutic modality, practitioners should consider the potential benefits and risks of T treatment (**Box 4**),[1] the patient-specific goals of T therapy, and presence of contraindications or precautions to T treatment (**Table 1**)[1] prior to initiating T therapy. Unfortunately, long-term controlled trials of the effects of T treatment in older men on clinically meaningful outcomes, such as fractures, frailty, dementia, diabetes mellitus, cardiovascular events, prostate cancer, and mortality, are not available to guide clinical practice.

Based on current evidence, the potential benefits of T treatment include improvements in sexual function and activity, energy and vitality, and mood (see **Box 4**).[1,16] Therefore, T treatment has the potential to significantly improve symptoms of androgen deficiency and consequently the quality of life in older hypogonadal men. Although a reduction in the risk of fractures has not been investigated and improvement in physical function has not been demonstrated consistently in previous studies, increase in BMD and muscle strength with T treatment[1] has the potential to contribute to fracture reduction by conventional osteoporosis therapies and improve functional status in older men with hypogonadism. The most common short-term risk of T treatment is erythrocytosis or increase in hematocrit[17]; other risks are uncommon (see **Box 4**). As a consequence of increased monitoring for prostate cancer (eg, DRE and PSA levels) during T therapy, there is an increased likelihood of detecting an abnormality during monitoring that may result in a prostate biopsy that may be associated with physical discomfort or psychological distress; thus, this is a potential risk of T treatment.[17]

Patient-centered treatment goals

T treatment should be considered in older men if the potential benefits outweigh the risks of T therapy. Consistent with patient-centered care, it is critical to discuss patient-specific goals of therapy with each patient before initiating T treatment in older men with hypogonadism. A patient's treatment goals may differ from those of a practitioner. Identification of patient-specific goals and expectations is particularly important for older men with borderline hypogonadism (ie, men with limited clinical manifestations of androgen deficiency [eg, isolated ED] and low total T levels but

Box 4
Benefits and risks of testosterone treatment

Benefits

- Increased sexual function and activity
- Improved energy and vitality
- Improved mood
- Increased BMD
- Increased muscle strength

Risks

- Erythrocytosis
- Formulation-related adverse effect
- Increased prostate biopsy (related to monitoring)
- Gynecomastia (uncommon)
- Increased OSA (rare)

Table 1
Contraindications to testosterone treatment

Contraindications	Concern
• Active or metastatic prostate cancer	• Stimulation of cancer growth
• Estrogen receptor–positive breast cancer	• Stimulation of cancer growth
Precautions	**Concern**
• Unevaluated prostate nodule/induration or high prostate-specific antigen (PSA)[a]	• Increased prostate cancer risk
• High hematocrit or poorly controlled hypoxic condition[b]	• Increased risk of erythrocytosis; cardiovascular risk[e]
• Severe, untreated OSA	• Increased OSA; cardiovascular risk[e]
• Severe lower urinary tract symptoms (LUTS)[c]	• Increased risk of urinary retention
• Severe or poorly controlled CHF or edematous condition[d]	• Worsening of CHF or edema from fluid retention

[a] PSA >4 ng/mL or >3 ng/mL in men at higher risk for prostate cancer (eg, African American, family history of prostate cancer, or abnormal digital rectal examination [DRE]).
[b] Hematocrit >50% (dependent on regional normal male range); poorly controlled hypoxic conditions, such as severe chronic obstructive pulmonary disease, restrictive lung disease, or OSA.
[c] International Prostate Symptom Score (IPSS) >19.
[d] Edematous conditions, such as congestive heart failure (CHF), hepatic cirrhosis, and nephrotic syndrome.
[e] Increased erythrocytosis and worsening OSA may increase the risk of cardiovascular adverse events.

low-normal to slightly low free T levels). Often there are other causes for a patient's symptoms and alternative treatments to T therapy (eg, phosphodiesterase type 5 inhibitors for ED) in these borderline cases, and it is reasonable to not treat these men with T. If T treatment is considered, however, a suggested approach is to identify specific treatment goals with a patient, discuss alternative treatment options, lower a patient's expectation of improvement in symptoms in response to T treatment, treat with T replacement for a limited prescribed period of time (eg, 6 months), and discontinue T treatment if there is no clinical response.

Contraindications and precautions to T treatment

Metastatic prostate cancer is initially an androgen-dependent malignancy that regresses with androgen deprivation and may be stimulated by increased T levels, such as occurs initially during luteinizing hormone-releasing hormone agonist therapy without androgen receptor blockade or with T treatment.[18–20] Short-term controlled studies of T treatment have not demonstrated an increased incidence of prostate cancer in T treated older men.[17] However, sufficiently powered, long-term controlled studies, however, have not been conducted to assess the effect of T treatment on the risk of prostate cancer. Therefore, the risk of prostate cancer, most importantly, of high-grade prostate cancer, during T treatment is at present not known.

A recent 6-month randomized, placebo-controlled trial of T treatment in older men with impaired mobility and low T levels who also had a high baseline prevalence of cardiovascular disease was stopped because of an increased number of cardiovascular events in T-treated men,[21] particularly in men who achieved high serum T levels.[22] In a similar, 6-month, randomized, placebo-controlled trial of T treatment in frail and near-frail older men[23] and a recent meta-analysis of T treatment trials,[17] no increase in cardiovascular events was reported with T treatment. As with prostate cancer, however, sufficiently powered, long-term controlled trials of T treatment have not been conducted to assess the risk of T on cardiovascular events.

The prevalence and incidence of both prostate cancer and cardiovascular disease increase with aging and, as discussed previously, there is uncertainty regarding the effects of T treatment on the natural history of these common, age-associated conditions. Thus, there remain concerns that T treatment in older men may increase the risk of prostate cancer and cardiovascular events. Given this concern and lack of long-term clinical outcome studies of T treatment in older men, it is important to discuss the potential short-term benefits and risks of T therapy and the uncertainty regarding long-term benefits and risks (ie, informed consent, whether formal or informal) when considering T treatment in older men.

Because T may stimulate the growth of androgen-dependent malignancy, T treatment is contraindicated in men with active or metastatic prostate cancer (see **Table 1**).[1] Administered T is aromatized endogenously to estradiol and both T and estradiol levels increase during T treatment. Therefore, T treatment is also contraindicated in men who have breast cancer, particularly if it is estrogen receptor positive.

According to The Endocrine Society clinical practice guidelines,[1] men who are found to have a prostate nodule or induration on DRE or who have a consistently high PSA level (>4 ng/mL or >3 ng/mL in men at higher risk for prostate cancer) should undergo a urologic evaluation before starting T treatment (see **Table 1**). It is important to repeat serum PSA measurements if they are found high on initial testing because values may normalize spontaneously. The concern in older hypogonadal men is that institution of T treatment may stimulate growth of undiagnosed prostate cancer, although there is no evidence for this.

Although uncommon, T treatment may worsen OSA.[24–26] Hypoxemia associated with OSA may cause erythrocytosis and cardiovascular morbidity, such as hypertension, edema, and arrhythmias. Therefore, men with untreated, severe OSA should be treated (eg, with CPAP or BPAP) or surgery before starting T therapy. In men with benign prostatic hyperplasia (BPH) who are bothered by persistently severe LUTS, treatment with pharmacologic agents (eg, α-adrenergic receptor antagonist or 5α-reductase inhibitor therapy) or surgery should be considered before starting T therapy.[1] T treatment may increase fluid retention, and it should be used with caution in men with severe, uncontrolled edematous conditions, such as CHF, hepatic cirrhosis, or nephrotic syndrome.[1]

T Formulations

If, after a discussion of benefits and risks of T, both patient and physician decide to start T therapy and there are no contraindications to T, a decision regarding which T formulation to use needs to be made. Several T formulations are available for T replacement therapy (**Table 2**).[1] Intramuscular or transdermal T formulations, however, are used most often for T replacement therapy for hypogonadal men. The choice of a specific T formulation to use is based both on pharmacologic considerations and patient preferences (eg, related to convenience and cost) in older men with hypogonadism.

Because of uncertainties regarding the long-term risks of T therapy in hypogonadal men, The Endocrine Society clinical practice guidelines recommend a therapeutic goal in the lower part of the normal range for young men (400–500 ng/dL).[1] In older men, the clearance of T is reduced so that the dosage of T required to achieve normal T levels may be less in older than in young hypogonadal men.[27] Compared with transdermal T, the usual therapeutic dosages of intramuscular T enanthate or cypionate (200 mg every 2 weeks or 100 mg every week) result in higher average T levels and more frequent erythrocytosis.[28] Therefore, it is advisable to initially use a lower dosage (eg, 150 mg every 2 weeks or 75 mg every week) of intramuscular T or to use

Table 2
Testosterone formulations

Formulation	Advantages	Disadvantages
IM T enanathate or cypionate 150–200 mg IM every 2 wk or 75–100 mg IM every week T undecanoate[d] 1000 mg every 10–14 weeks	• Long-standing use • Effective • Reliable • Inexpensive (self-injection) • Some flexibility in dose • Less fluctuation in T levels • Convenient	• IM injections every 1–2 wk (inconvenience and discomfort) • Occasional symptomatic fluctuations in T levels • Higher T levels and more erythroctyosis vs transdermal T • Large volume (4 mL) injection • Not self-injectable • Not removable
Transdermal T gel (1%) 50[a]–100 mg Daily to shoulders, upper arms T gel (1.62%) 40.5[b]–81 mg Daily to shoulders, upper arms T gel (2%) 40[c]–70 mg Daily to thighs T solution 60[e]–120 mg to Underarms T patch (adhesive) 4[f]–6 mg (1–2 Patches) nightly	• Effective • Relatively steady T levels (T gels and solution) • Circadian T variation (T patch) • Ease and convenience (no injections) • Less erythroctyosis vs IM injections	• Daily application • More variable T absorption and lower T levels vs IM T • Dose titration, 2 patches often needed • Skin irritation/rash (T patch > gel or solution), skin dryness or stickiness; odor; poor adhesion of T patch with excessive hair or sweating • Contact transfer of T (gels and solutions) • Expensive
Transbuccal T tablet 30 mg bid placed between cheek and gums	• Relatively steady T levels	• Twice-daily application • Only single dosage • Gum irritation, poorly tolerated initially • Expensive
Implanted pellet T pellet 2–6 75-mg Pellets implanted subcutaneously every 3–6 mo	• Relatively steady T levels over 3–6 mo	• Surgical implantation • Large number of pellets • Extrusion, bleeding, and infection (uncommon) • Not removable, if adverse effect of T • Infrequent use
Oral[d] T undecanoate 40–80 mg 2 or 3 Times daily with meals	• Ease (oral)	• 2 to 3 Times daily with meals • Variable T absorption, lower T levels, and variable clinical response vs other T formulations • High dihydrotestosterone levels (unclear clinical consequence)

[a] May be adjusted down to 25 mg daily.
[b] May be adjusted down to 20.25 mg daily.
[c] May be adjusted down to 20 mg daily.
[d] Not available in United States.
[e] May be adjusted down to 30 mg.
[f] May be adjusted down to 2 mg patch.

a transdermal T formulation initially in older men. Occasionally, when using transdermal T formulations, it may be difficult achieve adequate T levels and there may be greater variability in T levels so that monitoring of T levels during therapy is critical during transdermal T therapy. Intramuscular T formulations more reliably achieve adequate T levels but cause fluctuating T levels (levels above normal shortly after an injection, which fall to the lower end of the normal range or to low levels before the next injection) that may be associated with noticeable fluctuations in symptoms (eg, libido or energy).[1] In contrast, transdermal T results in more stable T levels than intramuscular T formulations. Because subcutaneous T pellets release T over several months and are not removable, they are less desirable for the treatment of older men who might develop prostate cancer while on therapy. Outside the United States, a longer-acting intramuscular formulation, testosterone undecanoate, is available; it is given at a dosage of 1000 mg every 10–14 weeks. This formulation produces less fluctuations in T levels and symptoms, but it requires a 4 mL intramuscular injection that can't be self-administered and is not removable. Oral androgen formulations (eg, methyltestosterone) available in the United States should not be used for T replacement therapy because they are not effective and have the potential for liver toxicity. Oral T undecanoate, which is available countries outside the United States, produces highly variable T levels and clinical responses.

In addition to these pharmacologic considerations, the choice of a specific T formulation may be influenced by patient preferences.[1] Intramuscular T injections may be uncomfortable, need to be given every 1 to 2 weeks, and may be inconvenient for older men who are not able to self-inject or do not have a spouse or housemate to administer injections. Therefore, they may be less desirable than transdermal T formulations. Alternatively, some transdermal T formulations may cause skin rash, irritation, dryness, or stickiness or have a disagreeable odor, and T patches may adhere poorly in men with excessive hair or sweating. T gels and solutions have a potential risk of transferring T to a child or female partner with prolonged skin contact. Therefore, these formulations require thorough hand washing after application and covering of the application site with clothing; also, residual T at the application site may be washed off several hours after application. Finally, transdermal T formulations are more expensive than intramuscular T injections.

The need for a minor surgical procedure for subcutaneous implantation of T pellets, twice-daily application of buccal T tablets and possible gum irritation, and 2 or 3 times daily administration of T undecanoate with a meals (for adequate T absorption) make these formulations less desirable for older men with hypogonadism.

Monitoring

Efficacy

Because the evidence base for the efficacy of T treatment is based on short-term studies, the prevalence of prostate cancer and cardiovascular disease increases with aging, and the effect of T therapy on the natural history of these conditions is uncertain, it is important to monitor the efficacy and safety of T treatment shortly after starting T therapy (ie, within the first 6 months, in addition to subsequent regular monitoring during T treatment) (**Table 3**).[1]

The efficacy of T treatment is monitored by self-reported improvement of symptoms and measurement of serum T levels, initially at 3 to 6 months after starting T and subsequently on an approximately yearly basis, relative to baseline assessments. It is expected that some sexual and behavioral symptoms of androgen deficiency, such as reduced libido and energy, will improve by 3 months and be maintained by 6 months of T therapy. Physical manifestations of androgen deficiency (such as loss

Table 3
Monitoring during testosterone treatment

Efficacy Monitoring	Frequency	Management
• Clinical improvement and maintenance of improvement ○ Self-reported symptoms and physical examination	• Baseline, 3–6 mo, then yearly	• If no clinical improvement or worsening of symptoms by 6 mo or physical manifestations by 1 y ○ Assess proper administration of and compliance with T treatment ○ Assess contribution of comorbidities and medications ○ Check T level at nadir after IM T or any time after other T formulations, and if levels low, increase T dosage ○ In the absence of these explanations, consider stopping T treatment
• Serum T level ○ IM T at midinterval or nadir if worsening symptoms ○ T gel/solution—anytime ○ T patch—3–12 h after applied	• Baseline, 3–6 mo, then yearly depending on clinical change • Transdermal T—after 1 wk	• Adjust T dosage to achieve mid-normal to low-normal T level
• BMD ○ Dual-energy x-ray absorptiometry	• Baseline, then 1–2 y depending on other risks factors for bone loss and fracture	• If osteoporosis is present at baseline, calcium, vitamin D and conventional osteoporosis treatment (eg, bisphosphonates)
Safety Monitoring	**Frequency**	**Management**
• Hematocrit	• Baseline, 3–6 mo, then yearly	• If hematocrit >54%, stop T ○ Check T level at nadir after IM T or any time after other T formulations and, if levels high, decrease T dosage ○ Evaluate for hypoxic conditions, such as OSA and treat appropriately, and consider restarting T treatment at a reduced dosage
• LUTS, PSA, and DRE ○ LUTS by IPSS	• Baseline, 3–6 mo, then as per standard of care	• If IPPSS >19, PSA increase >1.4 in any 12-mo period, or abnormal DRE (new nodule or induration), consider appropriate treatment (eg, α-blocker for LUTS) and/or urologic consultation
• Gynecomastia ○ Self-reported breast pain, tenderness, or enlargement and physical examination	• Baseline, 3–6 mo, then yearly	• If new or worsening symptomatic gynecomastia, consider reducing T dosage
• Induction or worsening of OSA ○ Daytime somnolence, witnessed apnea, snoring	• Baseline, 3–6 mo, then yearly	• If new or worsening symptomatic OSA, consider sleep study and institution of CPAP or BPAP therapy or adjustment of CPAP or BPAP, respectively
• Formulation-related adverse reaction	• Baseline, 3–6 mo, then yearly	• If adverse effect, consider switching T formulation

of body hair, muscle bulk and strength, and BMD) should improve by 6 months and continue to improve over the next year or 2.

If no clinical improvement or worsening of symptoms occurs, proper use and compliance with T treatment should be reviewed, worsening of comorbid illness or change in medications that might contribute to worsening of symptoms assessed, and serum T levels measured to determine whether adequate T levels (in midrange to lower end of the normal range) are achieved with the initial dosage regimen of T.

Men on intramuscular T injections should be asked whether there is a noticeable worsening of symptoms (eg, decreased libido, energy, or vitality) just before their next injection. If this is the case, serum T measurement should be performed at the time when T levels are at their nadir, and if T levels are below the normal range, shortening the interval between T injections should be considered (eg, from every 2 weeks to every 10 days). Because absorption of T is variable and unpredictable, measurement of T levels is essential in men using transdermal T formulations. After at least 1 of week of treatment, T levels can be measured anytime after application of T gel or solution and 3 to 12 hours after application of a T patch.[1]

If symptoms of androgen deficiency improve initially but improvement is not sustained or if there is no clinical improvement by 6 months of therapy in the presence of mid-normal T levels and in the absence of problems with T administration, compliance, or change in comorbidities or medications, discontinuation of T treatment should be considered. Because physical manifestations may take longer to improve than sexual or behavioral symptoms of androgen deficiency, the assessment of clinical improvement and decision to continue with T therapy should be made at or after 1 year. Because fracture reduction has not been demonstrated with T treatment, hypogonadal older men with osteoporosis should receive calcium, vitamin D, and, if appropriate, conventional osteoporosis treatment (eg, bisphosphonates).[29] T treatment does improve BMD, however, which probably contributes to fracture reduction. Therefore, in older hypogonadal men with osteoporosis, it is reasonable to monitor BMD by dual-energy x-ray absorptiometry scan at baseline and after 1 to 2 years of T therapy.[1]

Safety

The stimulatory effect of T on hematocrit and, therefore, the risk of significant erythrocytosis on T treatment is greater in older compared with younger men.[30] Older men with hypogonadism should have hematocrit monitored initially at 3 to 6 months and then yearly during T therapy.[1] If significant erythrocytosis (eg, hematocrit >54%) occurs, T treatment should be discontinued, T levels should be measured, and an evaluation should be performed for conditions that may cause hypoxia (eg, OSA or chronic lung disease) and, therefore, induce erythrocytosis. If T levels are found to be high or if a hypoxic condition is identified and treated appropriately, it is possible to consider restarting T treatment at a lower dosage.

Prostate gland growth and development and early advanced prostate cancer are androgen dependent. The incidence of both BPH and prostate cancer increases with age as does the incidence of male hypogonadism that may in some cases require T treatment. The effect of T administration on the natural history of BPH and prostate cancer, however, is not known. In the absence of this knowledge and because of concerns related to the potential risk of T therapy in these common age-associated conditions, The Endocrine Society clinical practice guidelines recommend monitoring for LUTS and prostate cancer.[1] These guidelines recommend that older men should have LUTS assessed by self-report or, preferably, a standardized questionnaire, such as the IPSS; PSA level; and DRE at baseline and 3 to 6 months after starting T and then according to the standard of care in the practitioner's community or as recommended by existing guidelines that the practitioner uses. If older men on T therapy develop severe LUTS (IPSS score >19), a PSA level greater than 1.4 ng/mL in any 12-month period, or an abnormal DRE (new nodule or induration), appropriate treatment (eg, α-adrenergic receptor antagonists for LUTS) and/or a urologic consultation should be considered. These recommendations for PSA monitoring are controversial, however, particularly given recent findings that PSA screening results in overdiagnosis of prostate cancer and does not prevent mortality.[31,32] Because there is uncertainty related to the effect of T treatment on the natural history and prognosis of prostate cancer, however, monitoring to detect an initial change in PSA from baseline within 3 to 6 months after initiation of T treatment is not equivalent to PSA screening in the general population and is a reasonable and conservative approach for older men on T treatment.

At baseline and at each follow-up visit, monitoring for gynecomastia, OSA, and formulation-specific adverse reaction should performed. New or worsening gynecomastia (breast pain, tenderness, and/or enlargement) is uncommon but, if it occurs, a reduction in T dosage should be considered. Induction or worsening of OSA is also uncommon and usually associated with higher-dosage T treatment.[24] Older men on T treatment should be asked about new or worsening daytime somnolence (as a result of disrupted sleep associated with frequent episodes of oxygen desaturation due to apnea), witnessed apnea episodes, and excessive, loud snoring. If new, these symptoms should prompt a formal sleep study, and if OSA is documented, institution of CPAP or BPAP therapy should be considered. If a formulation-specific adverse reaction occurs, switching to another T formulation should be considered.

REFERENCES

1. Bhasin S, Cunningham GR, Hayes FJ, et al. Testosterone therapy in men with androgen deficiency syndromes: an Endocrine Society clinical practice guideline. J Clin Endocrinol Metab 2010;95(6):2536–59.
2. Araujo AB, Esche GR, Kupelian V, et al. Prevalence of symptomatic androgen deficiency in men. J Clin Endocrinol Metab 2007;92(11):4241–7.
3. Araujo AB, O'Donnell AB, Brambilla DJ, et al. Prevalence and incidence of androgen deficiency in middle-aged and older men: estimates from the Massachusetts Male Aging Study. J Clin Endocrinol Metab 2004;89(12):5920–6.
4. Wu FC, Tajar A, Beynon JM, et al. Identification of late-onset hypogonadism in middle-aged and elderly men. N Engl J Med 2010;363(2):123–35.
5. Gray A, Feldman HA, McKinlay JB, et al. Age, disease, and changing sex hormone levels in middle-aged men: results of the Massachusetts Male Aging Study. J Clin Endocrinol Metab 1991;73(5):1016–25.
6. Harman SM, Metter EJ, Tobin JD, et al. Longitudinal effects of aging on serum total and free testosterone levels in healthy men. Baltimore Longitudinal Study of Aging. J Clin Endocrinol Metab 2001;86(2):724–31.
7. Tajar A, Forti G, O'Neill TW, et al. Characteristics of secondary, primary, and compensated hypogonadism in aging men: evidence from the European Male Ageing Study. J Clin Endocrinol Metab 2010;95(4):1810–8.
8. Travison TG, Araujo AB, Kupelian V, et al. The relative contributions of aging, health, and lifestyle factors to serum testosterone decline in men. J Clin Endocrinol Metab 2007;92(2):549–55.
9. Wang C, Catlin DH, Demers LM, et al. Measurement of total serum testosterone in adult men: comparison of current laboratory methods versus liquid

chromatography-tandem mass spectrometry. J Clin Endocrinol Metab 2004; 89(2):534–43.
10. Bremner WJ, Vitiello MV, Prinz PN. Loss of circadian rhythmicity in blood testosterone levels with aging in normal men. J Clin Endocrinol Metab 1983;56(6): 1278–81.
11. Plymate SR, Tenover JS, Bremner WJ. Circadian variation in testosterone, sex hormone-binding globulin, and calculated non-sex hormone-binding globulin bound testosterone in healthy young and elderly men. J Androl 1989;10(5):366–71.
12. Brambilla DJ, Matsumoto AM, Araujo AB, et al. The effect of diurnal variation on clinical measurement of serum testosterone and other sex hormone levels in men. J Clin Endocrinol Metab 2009;94(3):907–13.
13. Brambilla DJ, O'Donnell AB, Matsumoto AM, et al. Intraindividual variation in levels of serum testosterone and other reproductive and adrenal hormones in men. Clin Endocrinol (Oxf) 2007;67(6):853–62.
14. Swerdloff RS, Wang C, Cunningham G, et al. Long-term pharmacokinetics of transdermal testosterone gel in hypogonadal men. J Clin Endocrinol Metab 2000;85(12):4500–10.
15. Anawalt BD, Hotaling JM, Walsh TJ, et al. Performance of total testosterone measurement to predict free testosterone for the biochemical evaluation of male hypogonadism. J Urol 2012;187(4):1369–73.
16. Bolona ER, Uraga MV, Haddad RM, et al. Testosterone use in men with sexual dysfunction: a systematic review and meta-analysis of randomized placebo-controlled trials. Mayo Clin Proc 2007;82(1):20–8.
17. Fernandez-Balsells MM, Murad MH, Lane M, et al. Clinical review 1: adverse effects of testosterone therapy in adult men: a systematic review and meta-analysis. J Clin Endocrinol Metab 2010;95(6):2560–75.
18. Chrisp P, Sorkin EM. Leuprorelin. A review of its pharmacology and therapeutic use in prostatic disorders. Drugs Aging 1991;1(6):487–509.
19. Fowler JE Jr, Whitmore WF Jr. The response of metastatic adenocarcinoma of the prostate to exogenous testosterone. J Urol 1981;126(3):372–5.
20. Thompson IM, Zeidman EJ, Rodriguez FR. Sudden death due to disease flare with luteinizing hormone-releasing hormone agonist therapy for carcinoma of the prostate. J Urol 1990;144(6):1479–80.
21. Basaria S, Coviello AD, Travison TG, et al. Adverse events associated with testosterone administration. N Engl J Med 2010;363(2):109–22.
22. Basaria S, Davda MN, Travison TG, et al. Risk factors associated with cardiovascular events during testosterone administration in older men with mobility limitation. J Gerontol A Biol Sci Med Sci 2013;68(2):153–60.
23. Srinivas-Shankar U, Roberts SA, Connolly MJ, et al. Effects of testosterone on muscle strength, physical function, body composition, and quality of life in intermediate-frail and frail elderly men: a randomized, double-blind, placebo-controlled study. J Clin Endocrinol Metab 2010;95(2):639–50.
24. Liu PY, Yee B, Wishart SM, et al. The short-term effects of high-dose testosterone on sleep, breathing, and function in older men. J Clin Endocrinol Metab 2003; 88(8):3605–13.
25. Sandblom RE, Matsumoto AM, Schoene RB, et al. Obstructive sleep apnea syndrome induced by testosterone administration. N Engl J Med 1983;308(9):508–10.
26. Schneider BK, Pickett CK, Zwillich CW, et al. Influence of testosterone on breathing during sleep. J Appl Physiol 1986;61(2):618–23.
27. Coviello AD, Lakshman K, Mazer NA, et al. Differences in the apparent metabolic clearance rate of testosterone in young and older men with gonadotropin

suppression receiving graded doses of testosterone. J Clin Endocrinol Metab 2006;91(11):4669–75.
28. Dobs AS, Meikle AW, Arver S, et al. Pharmacokinetics, efficacy, and safety of a permeation-enhanced testosterone transdermal system in comparison with bi-weekly injections of testosterone enanthate for the treatment of hypogonadal men. J Clin Endocrinol Metab 1999;84(10):3469–78.
29. Watts NB, Adler RA, Bilezikian JP, et al. Osteoporosis in men: an Endocrine Society clinical practice guideline. J Clin Endocrinol Metab 2012;97(6):1802–22.
30. Coviello AD, Kaplan B, Lakshman KM, et al. Effects of graded doses of testosterone on erythropoiesis in healthy young and older men. J Clin Endocrinol Metab 2008;93(3):914–9.
31. Andriole GL, Crawford ED, Grubb RL 3rd, et al. Mortality results from a randomized prostate-cancer screening trial. N Engl J Med 2009;360(13):1310–9.
32. Schroder FH, Hugosson J, Roobol MJ, et al. Screening and prostate-cancer mortality in a randomized European study. N Engl J Med 2009;360(13):1320–8.

Thyroid Disorders in Older Adults

W. Edward Visser, MD, PhD, Theo J. Visser, PhD,
Robin P. Peeters, MD, PhD*

KEYWORDS

- TSH reference range • Thyroid function tests • Nonthyroidal illness
- Hypothyroidism • Subclinical hypothyroidism • Hyperthyroidism
- Subclinical hyperthyroidism

KEY POINTS

- Changes in thyroid function tests occur in the physiology of aging.
- Application of age-specific thyroid stimulating hormone (TSH) reference ranges may avoid misclassification of elderly subjects without thyroid disease.
- Overt hypothyroidism and hyperthyroidism require immediate treatment.
- Watchful waiting is an appropriate strategy for older patients with subclinical hypothyroidism (for TSH levels up to 10 mU/L).
- After exclusion of other causes of low TSH levels such as nonthyroidal illness, treatment of subclinical hyperthyroidism may be considered in older subjects.

INTRODUCTION

The intricate relationship between aging and endocrine systems has been well recognized for decades. Important changes in endocrine signaling occur during aging and vice versa; modification of endocrine signaling may largely affect longevity. The latter is exemplified in many species in which mutations of the growth hormone/insulinlike growth factor 1 pathway prolong life span.[1]

Serum thyroid parameters are well known to change with aging.[2] It is important to recognize nonpathologic changes in thyroid function tests (TFTs) and possible confounders, in particular because features of thyroid disease in elderly patients are often less prominent. In the first part of this article, the authors focus on changes in TFTs during aging and possible confounders, with an emphasis on the serum thyroid stimulating hormone (TSH) reference range. The second part describes the features of thyroid disease in the elderly as well as the challenges and debates on diagnosis and treatment, in particular on subclinical hypothyroidism and hyperthyroidism.

Disclosure: Nothing to disclose.

Thyroid Division, Department of Internal Medicine, Erasmus Medical Center, Rotterdam, The Netherlands

* Corresponding author. Department of Internal Medicine, Erasmus Medical Centre, Room D 430, Dr Molewaterplein 50, 3015 GE, Rotterdam, The Netherlands.
E-mail address: r.peeters@erasmusmc.nl

Endocrinol Metab Clin N Am 42 (2013) 287–303
http://dx.doi.org/10.1016/j.ecl.2013.02.008 **endo.theclinics.com**

CHANGES IN TFTS

Many studies have reported changes in serum thyroid parameters with advancing age. Conflicting data may arise from differences in baseline characteristics of the populations studied such as ethnicity and genetic background, nature and prevalence of thyroid diseases, iodine status, and coexisting disease. In this section the authors discuss the changes in TSH and the iodothyronines T4, T3, and rT3 in serum as well as the prevalence and implications of thyroid autoantibodies.

Tsh

Some earlier studies indicated that serum TSH levels do not change during life and remain within the standard reference range or reported even decreased TSH levels in the elderly.[2] However, these studies were relatively small and mainly conducted in iodine-deficient areas. Later (cross-sectional) studies in the Unites States analyzed serum thyroid parameters sampled from more than 15,000 people (the National Health and Nutrition Examination Survey [NHANES] and Montefiore studies) and showed increased TSH levels with advancing age in iodine-sufficient areas,[3–5] but not in a population with borderline sufficient iodine intake[6] (see also "reference range"). The increase in TSH with age was confirmed in other large longitudinal population studies.[7,8]

Several mechanisms have been proposed to explain the changes in serum TSH levels with advancing age. Some studies have suggested that the pituitary sensitivity is changed in the elderly. However, discordant results have been found in the response of the pituitary to thyrotropin-releasing hormone or thyroid hormone (TH).[2] Therefore, it remains to be clarified if pituitary gland function changes upon aging and if the negative feedback loop between free T4 (FT4) and TSH is altered in the elderly. Also, the observations that (F)T4 levels are mostly unchanged (see later discussion) may suggest that TSH glycosylation and thus TSH bioactivity is affected.

Although the mechanism is unclear, there is increasing evidence indicating that serum TSH levels change in the elderly, up to values above the upper limit of the traditional reference range. Because TSH is regarded as the most sensitive test to detect primary thyroid disorders, it is of utmost importance to realize that changes in serum TSH levels do not necessarily reflect thyroid disease but rather may be physiologic in the elderly. The relevance for clinical practice is discussed later in this article (see section "TSH reference range").

The Iodothyronines T4, T3, and rT3

Several studies have shown that serum T4 concentrations remain unaffected during aging, although most of the studies included a limited number of participants.[2] However, the large NHANES study reported an age-dependent decrease in serum T4 concentration.[4] Cross-sectional studies mainly reported normal or slightly decreased serum FT4 levels in the elderly.[2] Two recent longitudinal studies noted unchanged and slightly increased serum FT4 levels.[7,8]

In strong contrast with conflicting data regarding serum TSH and (F)T4 levels, all studies consistently show a decline in serum T3 and FT3 levels with advancing age.[2] The consistency of this finding is striking and it is tempting to speculate about its biologic meaning. It has been postulated that decreasing T3 will lower basal metabolic rate and, consequently, lower the production of reactive oxygen species and may also reduce damage to biomolecules (eg, DNA) and slow down the aging process. Obviously, such hypotheses need to be confirmed by future (animal) studies.

Serum levels of rT3 are either normal or increased in elderly subjects.[2] In particular, serum rT3 levels may be affected by confounding factors such as illness (see later discussion).

Changes in T4, T3, and rT3 serum levels may result from changes in thyroid gland function and/or peripheral TH metabolism. An early study demonstrated that both TH synthesis and secretion decline with age, in particular in subjects older than 60 years of age.[9] This observation is underscored by the lower levothyroxine (LT4) substitution dose required in hypothyroid elderly patients compared with younger patients.[10,11]

This study also demonstrated that peripheral degradation of T4 was diminished.[9] These results suggest that T4 concentrations in the elderly are seemingly unaffected because the decrease in T4 degradation equals the decrease in thyroidal T4 secretion.[9] The age-dependent decline in serum T3 levels is likely explained by a decrease in peripheral T4 to T3 conversion, which may contribute to the decreased T4 degradation. However, an increased T3 clearance may also contribute to the declining T3 levels.

The major route of TH metabolism is its stepwise deiodination.[12] The type 1 deiodinase (D1) catalyzes the conversion of T4 to T3 and the degradation of rT3 to T2. The type 2 deiodinase (D2) "activates" TH by catalyzing the conversion of T4 to T3, whereas the type 3 deiodinase (D3) "inactivates" TH by terminating the action of its preferential substrate T3 and preventing the activation of T4. The relative contribution of the deiodinases to the changes in TH levels in aging humans has been inferred from the changes in concentrations of iodothyronines. Furthermore, genetic variation in D1 was associated with lower serum T3 levels in aging men.[13] However, direct assessment of the deiodinase activities in aging humans has not been performed. Theoretically, an increased D3 activity may also explain the decrease in serum T3 levels. Animal studies to investigate age-dependent changes in deiodinase activities are limited.[14]

The increased serum rT3 levels reported in some studies likely reflect changes in deiodinase activities. Diminished activity of D1, whose preferred substrate is rT3, may largely contribute to this observation.[14] D1 is not only known to decrease during illness and caloric restriction, but also reported to diminish in normal aging. To which extent aging per se or confounders contribute is still elusive.

In recent years, the paradigm has evolved that local TH signaling can be modified independent of serum TH levels. Because deiodinases and TH transporters govern cellular thyroid state, changes in these key players of TH regulation may affect thyroid state in a tissue-specific manner. Indeed, it has been shown that T3 uptake into the liver is reduced in aged rats, which agrees with a reduced hepatic expression of the TH transporter MCT8 as well as reduced T3-dependent D1 expression during aging.[14,15] Future studies are needed to clarify which mechanisms contribute to age-dependent changes in serum and tissue TH levels.

Thus, from the above mentioned observations the picture emerges that during aging serum T3 levels decrease, whereas TSH levels increase (at least in iodine-sufficient areas). Serum T4 levels largely remain unaffected, whereas rT3 levels tend to increase.

Thyroid Autoantibodies

It is well recognized that the prevalence of thyroid antibodies (anti-Tg, anti-TPO) increases during life, particularly in women. This increase in prevalence reaches a plateau between the sixth and eighth decade. Interestingly, in centenarians the prevalence of thyroid antibodies is much lower.[16] Also in subjects of 65 to 85 years of age, the prevalence of thyroid antibodies did not change.[8] Furthermore, thyroid antibodies were not associated with mortality or TFTs in this age range.[8] From these observations, the clinical relevance of thyroid antibodies in the elderly is not clear. Although thyroid antibodies usually indicate an increased risk for thyroid disease, this does not appear to be true in the elderly. In the NHANES study, exclusion of patients with thyroid antibodies did not alter the median TSH or its age-specific reference range.[5]

A vast amount of evidence suggest that the presence of thyroid antibodies in the elderly neither has harmful effects on morbidity and mortality nor does it predict development of thyroid disease. Therefore, the additional value of measuring thyroid antibodies in the elderly is limited.

THE OLDEST OLD

Several studies have reported on changes in TFTs in the oldest old. Mariotti and colleagues[17] reported that healthy centenarians had lower serum TSH and FT3 levels and higher serum rT3 levels, whereas FT4 levels remained normal as compared with other age groups. In a population of healthy centenarians of Ashkenazi Jewish origin, serum FT4 levels were also similar to younger controls, but serum TSH levels were increased.[18] Offspring of these centenarians also had slightly higher serum TSH levels than controls, suggesting that longevity and higher TSH levels are genetically interrelated.[19] Offspring from subjects with reported familial longevity also had lower serum FT4 and T3 and a trend for higher TSH levels, supporting the hypothesis that TH and longevity are genetically related.[20]

Two studies investigated longitudinal changes in TFTs and survival in subjects older than 80 years of age. The Leiden 85+ Study followed subjects from age 85 years through 89 years and showed that elevated serum TSH level, whether or not accompanied by low serum FT4 concentrations, was associated with decreased all-cause mortality.[21] Also within the normal range, the hazard ratios (HRs) for risk of mortality were decreased at increasing TSH and increased at increasing FT4 levels. Of interest, these HRs remained after adjustment for potential confounders such as sex, C-reactive protein levels, and number of chronic diseases. The Cardiovascular Health Study All Stars cohort noted an increase in serum TSH and FT4 and a decrease in T3 levels in individuals older than 65 years who were observed for 13 years.[8] However, in this study changes in TFTs were not associated with effects on mortality. In a large meta-analysis of more than 50,000 subjects, no effects (positive or negative) of subclinical hypothyroidism on all-cause mortality could be demonstrated.[22] However, it should be noted that all subjects in the Leiden-85+ Study were older than 85 years of age at baseline, whereas in all other cohorts the mean age was lower.

FACTORS INFLUENCING TFTS

The measurement of TFTs is influenced by many factors that are not necessarily age-related but more common in the elderly. Of particular relevance in the elderly are the changes in TFTs due to illness, in which diminished T3 and elevated rT3 levels occur in the absence of thyroid disease. These alterations in TFTs are therefore called nonthyroidal illness (NTI). Acute and chronic diseases may produce NTI.[23] In addition, caloric deprivation gives rise to similar TFT changes. Alterations in deiodinase activities (decreased D1 and increased D3 activity) may underlie the TFT changes observed in NTI[24] and caloric restriction.[25] Possibly, the changes observed in NTI and malnutrition may be part of a beneficial adaptation response, aiming to minimize further damage. Similarly, a decrease in T3 in aging may also be beneficial by reducing DNA damage and thereby slowing down the aging process (see earlier discussion).

However, this remains purely speculative and needs to be determined in future studies analyzing the role of TH in the aging process.

Because aging subjects are particularly prone to malnutrition and (as-yet-unrecognized) disease, it is of utmost importance to take the patient-specific situation into account when interpreting the obtained TFTs. This point is well illustrated in a study of elderly man in which TFTs were correlated to disease and physical function and mortality.[26] Isolated lower T3 levels were associated with better physical performance, whereas subjects with the combination of lower T3 and higher rT3 serum levels had the worst physical performance. Such interpretations explain findings in which higher serum rT3 levels are associated with shorter survival.[27]

Since drugs are more commonly prescribed in older patients, it is important to realize that some drugs may interfere with TFTs. Drugs may directly interfere with thyroid function (eg, lithium, amiodarone, glucocorticoids) or peripheral TH metabolism (eg, amiodarone, propranolol), whereas others mainly interfere with the assay (eg, furosemide, antiepileptic drugs, heparin).[28]

Thus, especially in the elderly patient, medical history, condition, and prescribed drugs should be considered when interpreting abnormal TFTs.

TSH REFERENCE RANGE

The publication of different large-population studies during the last decade has resulted in a large debate whether the standard reference range for serum TSH levels (0.4–4.5 mU/L) should be applied to the elderly.[29] Using an upper limit of 4.5 mU/L, up to 15% of subjects older than 70 years are classified having an increased TSH.[29] Because most of these individuals have normal serum FT4 values, they would be diagnosed with subclinical hypothyroidism. This assumption has been fueled by the observation that TSH does not fit a Gaussian curve, but displays a right-skewed distribution. It has been proposed that subjects with serum TSH levels within this right-skewed part of the distribution (2.5–4.5 mU/L) reflect patients with thyroid disease or at an early stage of thyroid failure.[30] Indeed, it was shown that individuals with positive thyroid antibodies and TSH levels between 2.5 and 4.5 mU/L are more prone to develop thyroid disease.[31] However, only a minority of subjects with TSH levels in this range will develop thyroid disease. In addition, median and TSH reference ranges were similar between subjects with and without thyroid antibodies.[5]

Alternatively, the possibility that the right-skewed TSH curve is a composite of several unique curves for subpopulations is an attractive explanation. Indeed, the right-skew in TSH curves disappears if a race-specific data analysis is applied.[5] Similar right-shifted curves are produced from age-specific analysis (**Fig. 1**).[3,5] These analyses suggest that the reference ranges for older people shift to the right. The 97.5 percentiles derived from these studies indicate an upper normal limit of around 7 mU/L.[3,5]

Thus, the application of an age-specific TSH reference range would largely prevent the misclassification of many elderly people having (subclinical) thyroid disease. Older subjects are likely to benefit more from adjustment of the reference range, although absolute percentages of misclassification differ amongst several studies.[32] If age-specific TSH distribution curves are applied, they should be representative for particular regions and countries, because serum TSH levels are importantly influenced by iodide state.

Thus, multiple studies have shown that subclinical hypothyroidism in the elderly is not associated with adverse outcomes. Only randomized controlled intervention trials will provide a definitive answer whether subclinical hypothyroidism in the elderly should be treated with levothyroxine substitution therapy or not.

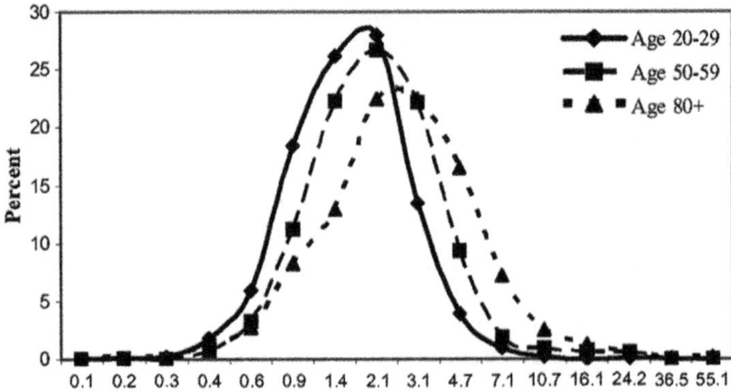

Fig. 1. TSH distribution by age groups in the NHANES III study (United States) in a disease-free population. (*Data from* Surks MI, Hollowell JG. Age-specific distribution of serum thyrotropin and antithyroid antibodies in the US population: implications for the prevalence of subclinical hypothyroidism. J Clin Endocrinol Metab 2007;92:4575–82.)

DIAGNOSIS AND TREATMENT OF (SUBCLINICAL) THYROID DISEASE

Thyroid function testing is advised for the work-up of several conditions, such as heart failure and cognitive decline, which are prevalent in older age.[33,34] When thyroid function is tested, it is important to realize that TFTs in the elderly can be confounded by factors such as the increased prevalence of chronic (nonthyroidal) illness and/or drug-induced changes (see earlier discussion).[2,28] Furthermore, clinical signs and symptoms of thyroid disease are different in older versus younger populations.[35,36]

Hypothyroidism

The frequency of overt hypothyroidism varies from 0.1% to 2%, but the prevalence may increase up to 5% in subjects older than 60 years of age.[37,38] Hypothyroidism is 5 to 8 times more common in women than men. Prevalence may be dependent on dietary and other environmental factors, especially iodine intake. Hypothyroidism has a higher prevalence in iodine-sufficient regions than in areas of mild iodine deficiency.[2] Autoimmune thyroiditis is the most frequent cause of hypothyroidism, including in the elderly, followed by iatrogenic hypothyroidism induced by treatment of thyrotoxicosis.[28,39] Iodine-induced hypothyroidism is more frequently seen in older patients than in younger patients, because of exposure to iodine overload with certain drugs (particularly amiodarone and iodinated radiographic contrast agents)[40,41] and coexistent organification defects such as Hashimoto thyroiditis or Graves disease.[42] Interestingly, amiodarone-induced hypothyroidism is more common in iodine-sufficient areas.[40,42]

It is important to realize that elderly patients with hypothyroidism may lack the classical symptoms of hypothyroidism (**Table 1**).[35] Because of the coexistence of age-related diseases and overlap between signs and symptoms of hypothyroidism (fatigue, cold intolerance, constipation, congestive heart failure, depression, etc) and the aging process, hypothyroidism in the elderly can easily be missed. For this reason, the diagnosis of hypothyroidism in the elderly can be a difficult task. As an illustration, thyroid function was determined in a population of more than 2000 elderly subjects.[43] None of the 95 subjects with increased serum TSH concentrations were suspected to be hypothyroid on the basis of a routine clinical examination.

Table 1
Comparison between young and old patients with symptoms and clinical signs of hypothyroidism

Symptoms and Clinical Signs (Percentages)	Old Patients ≥70 Y (n = 67)	Young Patients ≤55 Y (n = 54)	*P* Value[a]
Fatigue	67.7	83.4	NS[b]
Weakness	52.5	66.8	NS
Mental slowness	45.3	48.1	NS
Drowsiness	39.7	42.6	NS
Chilliness	34.9	64.8	<0.002
Dry skin	34.5	45.3	NS
Constipation	32.8	41.2	NS
Deafness	32.1	24.5	NS
Depression	28.4	51.9	NS
Hoarseness	28.1	29.4	NS
Skin infiltration	26.9	42.6	NS
Anorexia	26.6	13.2	NS
Paleness	26.6	17.8	NS
Slowed reflexes	23.8	30.8	NS
Weight gain	23.7	58.5	<0.001
Cramps	20.3	54.7	<0.001
Snoring	18.4	21.6	NS
Paresthesia	17.9	61.1	<0.001
Dizziness	14.3	33.3	NS
Weight loss	13.8	3.8	NS
Bradycardia	12.1	18.5	NS
Hair loss	11.9	27.8	NS
Buzzing	11.3	26.4	NS
Disorientation	9.0	0	NS

[a] After Bonferroni correction for multiple comparisons, a *P*<.002 was considered statistically significant.
[b] NS: not significant.
Data from Doucet J, Trivalle C, Chassagne P, et al. Does age play a role in clinical presentation of hypothyroidism? J Am Geriatr Soc 1994;42:984–6.

TH replacement therapy should be initiated in all patients with overt hypothyroidism, independent of age. It is generally advised that elderly hypothyroid patients are given a lower starting dose than younger adults. TH increases myocardial oxygen demand, and may thereby induce angina pectoris, myocardial infarction, or cardiac arrhythmias in older patients.[28,34] For this reason, initiation of LT4 treatment in elderly hypothyroid patients should be started at a low dose, especially in patients with (an increased risk of) coronary heart disease. In a prospective study, in which hypothyroid patients were randomly assigned to a full starting dose or to 25 μg LT4 per day with dose adjustments every 4 weeks, symptoms of hypothyroidism improved at a similar rate in both groups, although serum TSH and FT4 normalized more rapidly in the full-dose group. These data suggest no clinical benefit of a higher starting dose of LT4.[44] An additional argument for starting with a low LT4 dose in elderly patients is the observation that elderly patients need lower doses of LT4 to suppress serum TSH levels. Close monitoring is necessary to avoid overtreatment, because unintended TSH suppression therapy is a very frequent cause of subclinical hyperthyroidism (see also the section on subclinical hyperthyroidism).[10,45–47]

Subclinical Hypothyroidism

Subclinical hypothyroidism is defined as an elevated TSH in combination with an FT4 within the reference range, and it is generally considered to represent early, mild thyroid failure.[48,49] Most patients with subclinical hypothyroidism have thyroid autoantibodies, suggestive of Hashimoto thyroiditis.[4,48] Patients treated for overt hypothyroidism may have subclinical hypothyroidism due to inadequate substitution therapy.[4,45,47]

Most patients with subclinical hypothyroidism have a mildly elevated TSH level (above the reference range, but below 10 mU/L).[45] The frequency of subclinical hypothyroidism varies from 4% to 10% in different populations.[4,38,45,50] This percentage is more prevalent in iodine-sufficient countries,[51] and the incidence increases with age when nonage adjusted TSH reference ranges are used (see earlier discussion). Subclinical hypothyroidism may be present in up to 20% of elderly women and in 8% of elderly men. Of subjects with subclinical hypothyroidism older than 55 years, approximately a few percent per year progress to overt hypothyroidism.[28,52] However, it should be noticed that TSH levels may also normalize in almost 50% of patients.[53] For this reason, serum TSH measurements should always be redetermined after 3 to 6 months, to rule out a temporary increase in TSH.[48,54] The most powerful predictor for progression to overt hypothyroidism is magnitude of TSH elevation, but the presence of thyroid antibodies, clinical symptoms of hypothyroidism, goiter, and/or a low normal FT4 are also related to an increased risk of progression.[38,55–57] These predictors might be different in elderly subjects, because thyroid antibodies seem to have less effect in this age group.[2]

Subclinical hypothyroidism may be associated with similar symptoms as overt hypothyroidism, but in the elderly it may very well be asymptomatic. In subjects older than 65 years, subclinical hypothyroidism was not associated with cognitive function or depression in 2 large studies,[58,59] and in subjects older than 70 years it was even associated with a better preservation of physical function compared with euthyroid controls.[60]

In addition to symptoms, subclinical hypothyroidism has also been associated with a wide variety of cardiovascular risk factors and cardiovascular mortality (see Biondi & Cooper[54] for a detailed overview of the literature), as well as an increased risk of hip fractures.[61] A recent participant-based meta-analysis demonstrated an increased risk of cardiovascular events and cardiovascular mortality, but not all-cause mortality, in subjects with an elevated TSH, especially in those with a TSH level greater than 10 mU/L (**Fig. 2**).[22] Various studies have assessed the effects of treatment on signs and symptoms. Although it has been shown that LT4 treatment improves systolic and diastolic function, lipid profile, endothelial function, and carotid intima-media thickness (see Refs.[48,54,62] for reviews), no randomized studies on the effect of treatment of subclinical hypothyroidism on cardiovascular events or mortality are yet available. However, this topic has been addressed indirectly by 2 cohort studies, in which patients with subclinical hypothyroidism who received LT4 treatment were compared with patients who were not treated. Patients who received LT4 therapy had a significantly lower risk of heart failure[63] and lower all-cause mortality.[64] The issue of treatment in relation to age was not addressed specifically in these studies, but it was in a study of data from general practitioners in the United Kingdom in which lower rates of ischemic heart disease were found in LT4-treated younger patients, but not in LT4-treated older patients.[65] In very old subjects (ie, aged 80 years), the

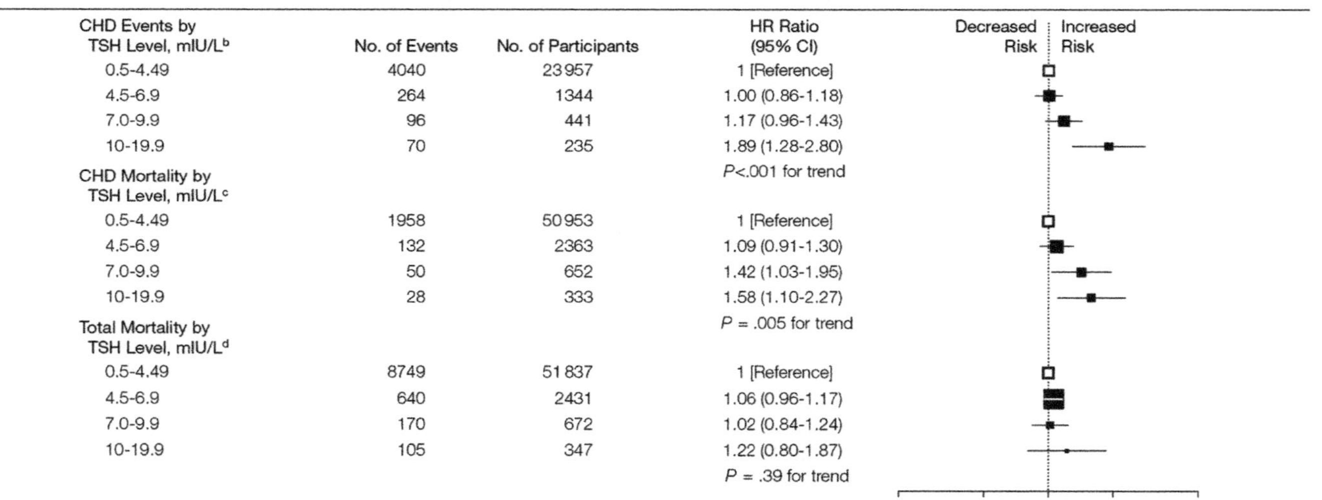

Hazard Ratios (HRs) for Coronary Heart Disease (CHD) Events, CHD Mortality, and Total Mortality According to Elevated Thyroid-Stimulating Hormone (TSH) Categories and Subclinical Hypothyroidism Stratified by Age vs Euthyroidism[a]

	No. of Events	No. of Participants	HR Ratio (95% CI)
CHD Events by TSH Level, mIU/L[b]			
0.5-4.49	4040	23957	1 [Reference]
4.5-6.9	264	1344	1.00 (0.86-1.18)
7.0-9.9	96	441	1.17 (0.96-1.43)
10-19.9	70	235	1.89 (1.28-2.80)
			P<.001 for trend
CHD Mortality by TSH Level, mIU/L[c]			
0.5-4.49	1958	50953	1 [Reference]
4.5-6.9	132	2363	1.09 (0.91-1.30)
7.0-9.9	50	652	1.42 (1.03-1.95)
10-19.9	28	333	1.58 (1.10-2.27)
			P = .005 for trend
Total Mortality by TSH Level, mIU/L[d]			
0.5-4.49	8749	51837	1 [Reference]
4.5-6.9	640	2431	1.06 (0.96-1.17)
7.0-9.9	170	672	1.02 (0.84-1.24)
10-19.9	105	347	1.22 (0.80-1.87)
			P = .39 for trend

Fig. 2. HRs for coronary heart disease (CHD) events, CHD mortality, and total mortality according to elevated TSH categories. (*Data from* Rodondi N, den Elzen WP, Bauer DC, et al. Subclinical hypothyroidism and the risk of coronary heart disease and mortality. JAMA 2010;304:1365–74.)

consequences of LT4 therapy may be different than in younger subjects, because observational studies in older subjects (older than 73 and 85 years, respectively) have shown that high TSH and/or low FT4 levels are associated with a lower mortality rate[8,21,26] (see earlier discussion). However, results from studies in these selected populations may also be because of selection bias and randomized clinical trials are urgently needed.[66–68]

In general, treatment is recommended for patients who have a TSH level greater than 10 mU/L. For patients with a mildly elevated TSH, the decision to treat or not to treat is based on clinical judgment and expert opinion, until the results of large scale randomized clinical trials are available.

Hyperthyroidism

The prevalence of hyperthyroidism is increased in the elderly, with frequencies varying from 0.5% to 3% in populations older than 60 years of age.[2,4,39,69] Whereas toxic (multinodular) goiter is the most frequent cause of hyperthyroidism in areas with a low iodine intake, Graves disease is a more common cause of hyperthyroidism in elderly living in areas with a relatively high iodine intake such as the United States and Northern Europe.[2,70,71] In aged patients, hyperthyroidism may also be precipitated by excess iodine intake from drugs or radiographic contrast agents,[28,41] especially in patients with underlying thyroid disease and functional autonomy.

Similar to hypothyroidism, elderly patients with hyperthyroidism usually display fewer signs and symptoms of hyperthyroidism than younger patients (**Table 2**).[2,36] They often lack a tremor, nervousness, increased appetite, heat intolerance, ocular signs, and nervousness. However, the frequency of atrial fibrillation and unexplained weight loss is higher in the elderly.[72,73] About 15% of elderly individuals with atrial fibrillation have elevated T4 levels or a history of thyrotoxicosis.[36,74,75] Hyperthyroidism in the elderly may even present as depression or mania.[76]

Administration of radioactive iodine is a good choice in most cases of hyperthyroidism in the elderly, resulting in a definitive cure and avoidance of the risks of surgery.[28] Alternatively, long-term thionamide treatment may be considered in the elderly with Graves disease,[34] but this may not be practical because of difficulties in patients' compliance and side effects.[2] Beta-blockers should be administered to elderly patients with hyperthyroidism, also in the initial phase after radioiodine administration, to reduce the heart rate and the risk of tachyarrhythmias. A potential concern is post-radioiodine exacerbation of hyperthyroidism due to radiation-related thyroiditis. The precise frequency of this complication in the elderly is unknown, but may be roughly around 10%.[2] Thus, hyperthyroidism in the elderly warrants treatment, preferably with 131-I.

Subclinical Hyperthyroidism

Subclinical hyperthyroidism is defined as a low serum TSH, combined with an FT4 and FT3 in the reference range.[49] The prevalence of subclinical hyperthyroidism is relatively low compared with subclinical hypothyroidism and varies from 1% to 2.5% in iodine-sufficient populations[4,77,78] and up to 9% in iodine-deficient populations.[79] Its prevalence increases in older populations, especially in women.[28] Before making the diagnosis of subclinical hyperthyroidism, other causes of a low TSH such as nonthyroidal illness, fasting, and the administration of drugs (eg, glucocorticoids) should be excluded (see earlier discussion). Furthermore, a second measurement is necessary because low serum TSH levels are often transitory.[80,81]

Subclinical hyperthyroidism may be caused by similar mechanisms as overt hyperthyroidism but it may also result from excessive LT4 substitution therapy.[48,75]

Table 2
Comparison between young and old patients with symptoms and clinical signs of hyperthyroidism

Symptoms and Clinical Signs	Percentage of Old Patients ≥70 Y (n = 34)	Percentage of Young Patients ≤50 Y (n = 50)	*P* Value[a]
Tachycardia	71	96	.01
Fatigue	56	84	.01
Weight loss	50	51	.87
Tremor	44	84	<.001
Dyspnea	41	56	.20
Apathy	41	25	.20
Anorexia	32	4	<.001
Nervousness	31	84	<.001
Hyperactive reflexes	28	96	<.001
Weakness	27	61	.01
Depression	24	22	87
Increased sweating	24	95	<.001
Polydipsia	21	67	<.001
Diarrhea	18	43	.02
Confusion	16	0	.01
Muscular atrophy	16	10	.52
Heat intolerance	15	92	<.001
Constipation	15	0	.01
Increased appetite	0	57	<.001

[a] After Bonferroni correction for multiple comparisons, a *P*<.002 was considered statistically significant.

Data from Trivalle C, Doucet J, Chassagne P, et al. Differences in the signs and symptoms of hyperthyroidism in older and younger patients. J Am Geriatr Soc 1996;44:50–3.

Whereas Graves disease is the most common cause of endogenous subclinical hyperthyroidism in young patients, toxic multinodular goiter and toxic adenomas may be more common causes in elderly patients. In the elderly, exogenous subclinical hyperthyroidism is more common than endogenous subclinical hyperthyroidism and can be intentional (ie, TSH suppressive therapy in patients with thyroid cancer) as well as unintentional in case of overtreatment of hypothyroid patients. It should be realized that 20% to 40% of patients older than 65 years of age who are on LT4 treatment have a low serum TSH.[45–47] Older patients are especially prone to exogenous subclinical hyperthyroidism, because LT4 requirements decrease with age.[10] Whether or not an altered sensitivity of the pituitary to the negative feedback of T4 plays a role as well remains to be determined.[2]

Approximately 1% to 5% of patients older than 60 years of age with subclinical hyperthyroidism progress to overt hyperthyroidism.[81–84] Progression to overt hyperthyroidism occurs more often in patients with a TSH less than 0.1 mU/L than in patients with a TSH between 0.1 and 0.4 mU/L and in patients with Graves disease than in patients with toxic multinodular goiter.[54] In addition to progression to overt hyperthyroidism, subclinical hyperthyroidism is also related to an increased risk of atrial fibrillation, cardiac dysfunction, cardiovascular and overall mortality, decreased bone mineral density, and decreased quality of life and cognition[61,72,73,85,86] (see[48,54] for 2 excellent reviews).

There is a lack of prospective, randomized controlled trials investigating the benefits of treatment of subclinical hyperthyroidism. The choice between treatment and a wait-and-see policy depends on the level of TSH (<0.1 mU/L vs 0.1–0.4 mU/L), clinical risk factors (atrial fibrillation, osteoporosis, etc), and the cause of subclinical hyperthyroidism. However, it is generally accepted that treatment of subclinical hyperthyroidism should be initiated more readily in older subjects than in younger subjects.[33,48] In patients with toxic multinodular goiter or toxic adenoma, radioactive iodine is the preferred treatment of choice because it is definitive and remission is very unlikely to occur. In patients with subclinical hyperthyroidism due to Graves disease, medical therapy can be considered as well. If it is decided not to treat the subclinical hyperthyroidism in elderly patients, provision of a beta-blocker should be considered, as well as calcium supplementation and treatment with a bisphosphonate in patients with a low bone mineral density or at risk for osteoporosis.[33,48]

SUMMARY

Significant changes in thyroid parameters are observed during aging. Most of these changes naturally occur during the aging process and may be regarded as physiologic. The most important consequence is that the traditional TSH reference range may not be applicable for elderly patients and this implies that an age-specific TSH reference range is desired to avoid misclassification of patients. The value of additive testing for thyroid antibodies is much less in the elderly. Furthermore, confounders such as illness and malnutrition, which are more common in the elderly, may disturb the interpretation of TFTs.

Diagnosing thyroid disease in elderly patients may be challenging, because clinical features of abnormal thyroid function are less pronounced. Whereas overt hypothyroidism requires prompt treatment, this is less clear for subclinical hypothyroidism. In subclinical hypothyroidism with TSH levels up to 10 mU/L, watchful waiting can be an appropriate strategy. Also overt hyperthyroidism needs immediate treatment in which I-131 therapy appears a logical choice. Depending on TSH levels and clinical symptoms, subclinical hyperthyroidism does not necessarily warrant immediate treatment. However, treatment is more strongly indicated in older patients than in younger patients. Randomized controlled trials should provide the definitive answer whether or not to treat elderly patients with subclinical thyroid disease.

Because life expectancy in western populations is still increasing, the topics discussed in this article will remain of great importance. Therefore, future studies should be dedicated to investigating the mechanisms underlying physiologic changes in thyroid function and metabolism as well as optimal treatment strategies for thyroid diseases in the elderly.

REFERENCES

1. Russell SJ, Kahn CR. Endocrine regulation of ageing. Nat Rev Mol Cell Biol 2007;8:681–91.
2. Mariotti S, Franceschi C, Cossarizza A, et al. The aging thyroid. Endocr Rev 1995;16:686–715.
3. Boucai L, Surks MI. Reference limits of serum TSH and free T4 are significantly influenced by race and age in an urban outpatient medical practice. Clin Endocrinol (Oxf) 2009;70:788–93.
4. Hollowell JG, Staehling NW, Flanders WD, et al. Serum TSH, T(4), and thyroid antibodies in the United States population (1988 to 1994): National Health and

Nutrition Examination Survey (NHANES III). J Clin Endocrinol Metab 2002;87: 489–99.

5. Surks MI, Hollowell JG. Age-specific distribution of serum thyrotropin and antithyroid antibodies in the US population: implications for the prevalence of subclinical hypothyroidism. J Clin Endocrinol Metab 2007;92:4575–82.
6. Hoogendoorn EH, Hermus AR, de Vegt F, et al. Thyroid function and prevalence of anti-thyroperoxidase antibodies in a population with borderline sufficient iodine intake: influences of age and sex. Clin Chem 2006;52:104–11.
7. Bremner AP, Feddema P, Leedman PJ, et al. Age-related changes in thyroid function: a longitudinal study of a community-based cohort. J Clin Endocrinol Metab 2012;97:1554–62.
8. Waring AC, Arnold AM, Newman AB, et al. Longitudinal changes in thyroid function in the oldest old and survival: the cardiovascular health study all-stars study. J Clin Endocrinol Metab 2012;97:3944–50.
9. Gregerman RI, Gaffney GW, Shock NW, et al. Thyroxine turnover in euthyroid man with special reference to changes with age. J Clin Invest 1962;41:2065–74.
10. Rosenbaum RL, Barzel US. Levothyroxine replacement dose for primary hypothyroidism decreases with age. Ann Intern Med 1982;96:53–5.
11. Sawin CT, Herman T, Molitch ME, et al. Aging and the thyroid. Decreased requirement for thyroid hormone in older hypothyroid patients. Am J Med 1983;75: 206–9.
12. Bianco AC, Salvatore D, Gereben B, et al. Biochemistry, cellular and molecular biology, and physiological roles of the iodothyronine selenodeiodinases. Endocr Rev 2002;23:38–89.
13. Peeters RP, van den Beld AW, van Toor H, et al. A polymorphism in type I deiodinase is associated with circulating free insulin-like growth factor I levels and body composition in humans. J Clin Endocrinol Metab 2005;90: 256–63.
14. Silvestri E, Lombardi A, de Lange P, et al. Age-related changes in renal and hepatic cellular mechanisms associated with variations in rat serum thyroid hormone levels. Am J Physiol Endocrinol Metab 2008;294:E1160–8.
15. Mooradian AD. The hepatic transcellular transport of 3,5,3'-triiodothyronine is reduced in aged rats. Biochim Biophys Acta 1990;1054:1–7.
16. Mariotti S, Sansoni P, Barbesino G, et al. Thyroid and other organ-specific autoantibodies in healthy centenarians. Lancet 1992;339:1506–8.
17. Mariotti S, Barbesino G, Caturegli P, et al. Complex alteration of thyroid function in healthy centenarians. J Clin Endocrinol Metab 1993;77:1130–4.
18. Atzmon G, Barzilai N, Hollowell JG, et al. Extreme longevity is associated with increased serum thyrotropin. J Clin Endocrinol Metab 2009;94:1251–4.
19. Atzmon G, Barzilai N, Surks MI, et al. Genetic predisposition to elevated serum thyrotropin is associated with exceptional longevity. J Clin Endocrinol Metab 2009;94:4768–75.
20. Rozing MP, Westendorp RG, de Craen AJ, et al. Low serum free triiodothyronine levels mark familial longevity: the Leiden Longevity Study. J Gerontol A Biol Sci Med Sci 2010;65:365–8.
21. Gussekloo J, van Exel E, de Craen AJ, et al. Thyroid status, disability and cognitive function, and survival in old age. JAMA 2004;292:2591–9.
22. Rodondi N, den Elzen WP, Bauer DC, et al. Subclinical hypothyroidism and the risk of coronary heart disease and mortality. JAMA 2010;304:1365–74.
23. Peeters RP, Debaveye Y, Fliers E, et al. Changes within the thyroid axis during critical illness. Crit Care Clin 2006;22:41–55, vi.

24. Peeters RP, Wouters PJ, van Toor H, et al. Serum 3,3',5'-triiodothyronine (rT3) and 3,5,3'-triiodothyronine/rT3 are prognostic markers in critically ill patients and are associated with postmortem tissue deiodinase activities. J Clin Endocrinol Metab 2005;90:4559–65.
25. Araujo RL, Andrade BM, da Silva ML, et al. Tissue-specific deiodinase regulation during food restriction and low replacement dose of leptin in rats. Am J Physiol Endocrinol Metab 2009;296:E1157–63.
26. van den Beld AW, Visser TJ, Feelders RA, et al. Thyroid hormone concentrations, disease, physical function, and mortality in elderly men. J Clin Endocrinol Metab 2005;90:6403–9.
27. Forestier E, Vinzio S, Sapin R, et al. Increased reverse triiodothyronine is associated with shorter survival in independently-living elderly: the Alsanut study. Eur J Endocrinol 2009;160:207–14.
28. Peeters RP. Thyroid hormones and aging. Hormones (Athens) 2008;7:28–35.
29. Surks MI, Boucai L. Age- and race-based serum thyrotropin reference limits. J Clin Endocrinol Metab 2010;95:496–502.
30. Baloch Z, Carayon P, Conte-Devolx B, et al. Laboratory medicine practice guidelines. Laboratory support for the diagnosis and monitoring of thyroid disease. Thyroid 2003;13:3–126.
31. Surks MI, Goswami G, Daniels GH. The thyrotropin reference range should remain unchanged. J Clin Endocrinol Metab 2005;90:5489–96.
32. Kahapola-Arachchige KM, Hadlow N, Wardrop R, et al. Age-specific TSH reference ranges have minimal impact on the diagnosis of thyroid dysfunction. Clin Endocrinol (Oxf) 2012;77:773–9.
33. Bahn RS, Burch HB, Cooper DS, et al. Hyperthyroidism and other causes of thyrotoxicosis: management guidelines of the American Thyroid Association and American Association of Clinical Endocrinologists. Thyroid 2011;21:593–646.
34. Garber JR, Cobin RH, Gharib H, et al. Clinical practice guidelines for hypothyroidism in adults: cosponsored by the american association of clinical endocrinologists and the american thyroid association. Thyroid 2012;18(6):988–1028.
35. Doucet J, Trivalle C, Chassagne P, et al. Does age play a role in clinical presentation of hypothyroidism? J Am Geriatr Soc 1994;42:984–6.
36. Trivalle C, Doucet J, Chassagne P, et al. Differences in the signs and symptoms of hyperthyroidism in older and younger patients. J Am Geriatr Soc 1996;44:50–3.
37. Almandoz JP, Gharib H. Hypothyroidism: etiology, diagnosis, and management. Med Clin North Am 2012;96:203–21.
38. Vanderpump MP, Tunbridge WM, French JM, et al. The incidence of thyroid disorders in the community: a twenty-year follow-up of the Whickham Survey. Clin Endocrinol (Oxf) 1995;43:55–68.
39. Diez JJ. Hypothyroidism in patients older than 55 years: an analysis of the etiology and assessment of the effectiveness of therapy. J Gerontol A Biol Sci Med Sci 2002;57:M315–20.
40. Eskes SA, Wiersinga WM. Amiodarone and thyroid. Best Pract Res Clin Endocrinol Metab 2009;23:735–51.
41. Rhee CM, Bhan I, Alexander EK, et al. Association between iodinated contrast media exposure and incident hyperthyroidism and hypothyroidism. Arch Intern Med 2012;172:153–9.
42. Martino E, Aghini-Lombardi F, Bartalena L, et al. Enhanced susceptibility to amiodarone-induced hypothyroidism in patients with thyroid autoimmune disease. Arch Intern Med 1994;154:2722–6.

43. Sawin CT, Castelli WP, Hershman JM, et al. The aging thyroid. Thyroid deficiency in the Framingham Study. Arch Intern Med 1985;145:1386–8.
44. Roos A, Linn-Rasker SP, van Domburg RT, et al. The starting dose of levothyroxine in primary hypothyroidism treatment: a prospective, randomized, double-blind trial. Arch Intern Med 2005;165:1714–20.
45. Canaris GJ, Manowitz NR, Mayor G, et al. The Colorado thyroid disease prevalence study. Arch Intern Med 2000;160:526–34.
46. Parle JV, Franklyn JA, Cross KW, et al. Thyroxine prescription in the community: serum thyroid stimulating hormone level assays as an indicator of undertreatment or overtreatment. Br J Gen Pract 1993;43:107–9.
47. Somwaru LL, Arnold AM, Joshi N, et al. High frequency of and factors associated with thyroid hormone over-replacement and under-replacement in men and women aged 65 and over. J Clin Endocrinol Metab 2009;94:1342–5.
48. Cooper DS, Biondi B. Subclinical thyroid disease. Lancet 2012;379:1142–54.
49. Surks MI, Ortiz E, Daniels GH, et al. Subclinical thyroid disease: scientific review and guidelines for diagnosis and management. JAMA 2004;291: 228–38.
50. Bagchi N, Brown TR, Parish RF. Thyroid dysfunction in adults over age 55 years. A study in an urban US community. Arch Intern Med 1990;150:785–7.
51. Teng W, Shan Z, Teng X, et al. Effect of iodine intake on thyroid diseases in China. N Engl J Med 2006;354:2783–93.
52. Biondi B. Natural history, diagnosis and management of subclinical thyroid dysfunction. Best Pract Res Clin Endocrinol Metab 2012;26:431–46.
53. Somwaru LL, Rariy CM, Arnold AM, et al. The natural history of subclinical hypothyroidism in the elderly: the cardiovascular health study. J Clin Endocrinol Metab 2012;97:1962–9.
54. Biondi B, Cooper DS. The clinical significance of subclinical thyroid dysfunction. Endocr Rev 2008;29:76–131.
55. Diez JJ, Iglesias P. Spontaneous subclinical hypothyroidism in patients older than 55 years: an analysis of natural course and risk factors for the development of overt thyroid failure. J Clin Endocrinol Metab 2004;89:4890–7.
56. Walsh JP, Bremner AP, Feddema P, et al. Thyrotropin and thyroid antibodies as predictors of hypothyroidism: a 13-year, longitudinal study of a community-based cohort using current immunoassay techniques. J Clin Endocrinol Metab 2010;95:1095–104.
57. Li Y, Teng D, Shan Z, et al. Antithyroperoxidase and antithyroglobulin antibodies in a five-year follow-up survey of populations with different iodine intakes. J Clin Endocrinol Metab 2008;93:1751–7.
58. de Jongh RT, Lips P, van Schoor NM, et al. Endogenous subclinical thyroid disorders, physical and cognitive function, depression, and mortality in older individuals. Eur J Endocrinol 2011;165:545–54.
59. Roberts LM, Pattison H, Roalfe A, et al. Is subclinical thyroid dysfunction in the elderly associated with depression or cognitive dysfunction? Ann Intern Med 2006;145:573–81.
60. Simonsick EM, Newman AB, Ferrucci L, et al. Subclinical hypothyroidism and functional mobility in older adults. Arch Intern Med 2009;169:2011–7.
61. Lee JS, Buzkova P, Fink HA, et al. Subclinical thyroid dysfunction and incident hip fracture in older adults. Arch Intern Med 2010;170:1876–83.
62. Biondi B, Palmieri EA, Fazio S, et al. Endogenous subclinical hyperthyroidism affects quality of life and cardiac morphology and function in young and middle-aged patients. J Clin Endocrinol Metab 2000;85:4701–5.

63. Rodondi N, Bauer DC, Cappola AR, et al. Subclinical thyroid dysfunction, cardiac function, and the risk of heart failure. The Cardiovascular Health study. J Am Coll Cardiol 2008;52:1152–9.
64. Razvi S, Weaver JU, Vanderpump MP, et al. The incidence of ischemic heart disease and mortality in people with subclinical hypothyroidism: reanalysis of the Whickham Survey cohort. J Clin Endocrinol Metab 2010;95:1734–40.
65. Razvi S, Weaver JU, Butler TJ, et al. Levothyroxine treatment of subclinical hypothyroidism, fatal and nonfatal cardiovascular events, and mortality. Arch Intern Med 2012;172:811–7.
66. Goichot B, Vinzio S. Subclinical thyroid disorders. Lancet 2012;380:335 [author reply: 336–7].
67. Mooijaart SP. Subclinical thyroid disorders. Lancet 2012;380:335 [author reply: 336–7].
68. Quinn TJ, Gussekloo J, Kearney P, et al. Subclinical thyroid disorders. Lancet 2012;380:335–6 [author reply: 336–7].
69. Tunbridge WM, Evered DC, Hall R, et al. The spectrum of thyroid disease in a community: the Whickham survey. Clin Endocrinol (Oxf) 1977;7:481–93.
70. Diez JJ. Hyperthyroidism in patients older than 55 years: an analysis of the etiology and management. Gerontology 2003;49:316–23.
71. Laurberg P, Pedersen KM, Vestergaard H, et al. High incidence of multinodular toxic goitre in the elderly population in a low iodine intake area vs. high incidence of Graves' disease in the young in a high iodine intake area: comparative surveys of thyrotoxicosis epidemiology in East-Jutland Denmark and Iceland. J Intern Med 1991;229:415–20.
72. Gammage MD, Parle JV, Holder RL, et al. Association between serum free thyroxine concentration and atrial fibrillation. Arch Intern Med 2007;167:928–34.
73. Heeringa J, Hoogendoorn EH, van der Deure WM, et al. High-normal thyroid function and risk of atrial fibrillation: the Rotterdam study. Arch Intern Med 2008;168:2219–24.
74. Cobler JL, Williams ME, Greenland P. Thyrotoxicosis in institutionalized elderly patients with atrial fibrillation. Arch Intern Med 1984;144:1758–60.
75. Franklyn JA, Boelaert K. Thyrotoxicosis. Lancet 2012;379:1155–66.
76. Mokshagundam S, Barzel US. Thyroid disease in the elderly. J Am Geriatr Soc 1993;41:1361–9.
77. Cappola AR, Fried LP, Arnold AM, et al. Thyroid status, cardiovascular risk, and mortality in older adults. JAMA 2006;295:1033–41.
78. Vadiveloo T, Donnan PT, Cochrane L, et al. The Thyroid Epidemiology, Audit, and Research Study (TEARS): the natural history of endogenous subclinical hyperthyroidism. J Clin Endocrinol Metab 2011;96:E1–8.
79. Laurberg P, Pedersen KM, Hreidarsson A, et al. Iodine intake and the pattern of thyroid disorders: a comparative epidemiological study of thyroid abnormalities in the elderly in Iceland and in Jutland, Denmark. J Clin Endocrinol Metab 1998;83:765–9.
80. Meyerovitch J, Rotman-Pikielny P, Sherf M, et al. Serum thyrotropin measurements in the community: five-year follow-up in a large network of primary care physicians. Arch Intern Med 2007;167:1533–8.
81. Parle JV, Franklyn JA, Cross KW, et al. Prevalence and follow-up of abnormal thyrotrophin (TSH) concentrations in the elderly in the United Kingdom. Clin Endocrinol (Oxf) 1991;34:77–83.

32. Sawin CT, Geller A, Kaplan MM, et al. Low serum thyrotropin (thyroid-stimulating hormone) in older persons without hyperthyroidism. Arch Intern Med 1991;151:165–8.
33. Sawin CT, Geller A, Wolf PA, et al. Low serum thyrotropin concentrations as a risk factor for atrial fibrillation in older persons. N Engl J Med 1994;331:1249–52.
34. Sundbeck G, Eden S, Jagenburg R, et al. Thyroid dysfunction in 85-year-old men and women. Influence of non-thyroidal illness and drug treatment. Acta Endocrinol (Copenh) 1991;125:475–86.
35. Ceresini G, Ceda GP, Lauretani F, et al. Mild thyroid hormone excess is associated with a decreased physical function in elderly men. Aging Male 2011;14:213–9.
36. Collet TH, Gussekloo J, Bauer DC, et al. Subclinical hyperthyroidism and the risk of coronary heart disease and mortality. Arch Intern Med 2012;172:799–809.

Diagnosis and Treatment of Osteoporosis in Older Adults

Dima L. Diab, MD[a,*], Nelson B. Watts, MD[b]

KEYWORDS

• Osteoporosis • Fractures • Older adults • Elderly • Frailty • Diagnosis • Treatment • Fall prevention

KEY POINTS

- Osteoporosis is predominantly a condition of the elderly.
- The diagnosis of osteoporosis is established by measurement of bone mineral density by dual-energy x-ray absorptiometry of the spine, hip, and/or forearm (T-score of −2.5 or lower), or by the presence of a low-trauma or fragility fracture.
- Several US Food and Drug Administration-approved pharmacologic treatments have been shown to significantly reduce the risk of fracture in older adults.
- Nonskeletal risk factors leading to falls become increasingly important with older age and should be addressed.

INTRODUCTION

Osteoporosis is defined as a generalized skeletal disorder characterized by compromised bone strength predisposing to an increased risk of fractures. Bone strength reflects the integration of 2 main features: bone density and bone quality.[1] Based on the US Surgeon General's report on bone health and osteoporosis published in 2004, osteoporosis affects 8 million women and 2 million men, and 34 million people have low bone mass.[2] With an increasingly aged population, these numbers are likely to steadily increase in the future, with osteoporosis affecting an estimated 14 million people and low bone mass affecting an estimated 48 million people by the year 2020. Based on data from the same report, the annual incidence of osteoporotic fractures is greater than 2 million, and this is expected to rise to more than 3 million by the year 2020.

[a] Division of Endocrinology/Metabolism, Department of Internal Medicine, Cincinnati VA Medical Center, University of Cincinnati Bone Health and Osteoporosis Center, 260 Stetson Street, Suite 4200, Cincinnati, OH 45219, USA; [b] Mercy Health Osteoporosis and Bone Health Services, 4760 East Galbraith Road, Suite 212, Cincinnati, OH 45236, USA

* Corresponding author.

E-mail address: diabd@ucmail.uc.edu

Endocrinol Metab Clin N Am 42 (2013) 305–317

http://dx.doi.org/10.1016/j.ecl.2013.02.007 endo.theclinics.com

0889-8529/13/$ – see front matter

EPIDEMIOLOGY OF OSTEOPOROSIS IN OLDER ADULTS

Osteoporosis is predominantly a condition of the elderly.[3] Both men and women lose bone mass with advancing age,[4] and the prevalence of osteoporosis increases in older adults.[5] Furthermore, the age profile varies for the different fractures, with the incidence of vertebral and hip fractures increasing steeply with age.[6,7] The incidence of hip fractures, which are regarded as the most devastating of the osteoporotic fractures because of their association with significant morbidity and mortality, increases exponentially with age until about the age of 84, after which the increase is slower (**Fig. 1**). This increase is more rapid than would be expected from age-related decline in bone mass,[8] mainly because nonskeletal risk factors leading to falls become increasingly important with older age.[9] Moreover, osteoporosis is more common in nursing home residents compared with the general population but is undertreated,[10,11] leading to much higher fracture rates and increased health care use in nursing home residents than in age-matched community dwellers.[12]

DIAGNOSIS OF OSTEOPOROSIS IN OLDER ADULTS

The diagnosis of osteoporosis is established by measurement of bone mineral density (BMD) by dual-energy x-ray absorptiometry (DXA) of the spine, hip, and/or forearm (T-score of −2.5 or lower), although a clinical diagnosis can be made in individuals who sustain a low-trauma or fragility fracture (**Table 1**). In agreement with the US Preventive Service Task Force recommendations for postmenopausal women,[13] the National Osteoporosis Foundation (NOF) recommends BMD testing for all women 65 years of age and older. NOF also recommends testing men 70 years of age and older. Testing should be done sooner (starting age 50) in subjects with clinical risk factors for fracture such as low body weight, history of prior fracture, family history of osteoporosis, smoking, excessive alcohol intake, or long-term use of high-risk medications such as glucocorticoids.[14]

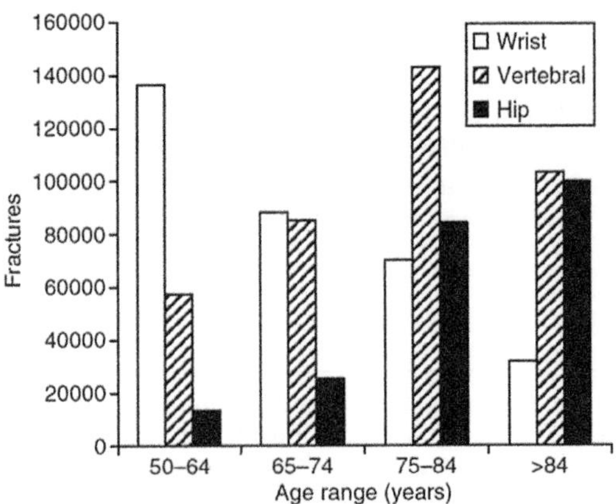

Fig. 1. Total incident fractures by skeletal site in the year 2005 in the United States. (*Data from* Burge R, Dawson-Hughes B, Solomon DH, et al. Incidence and economic burden of osteoporosis-related fractures in the United States, 2005–2025. J Bone Miner Res 2007;22:465; and Rizzoli R, Bruyere O, Cannata-Andia JB, et al. Management of osteoporosis in the elderly. Curr Med Res Opin 2009;25:2373.)

Table 1
WHO diagnostic classification of osteoporosis

Category	T-score[a]
Normal	−1.0 and above
Low bone mass (osteopenia)	Between −1.0 and −2.5
Osteoporosis	−2.5 and below

The T-score compares an individual's BMD with the mean value for young normal individuals and expresses the difference as a standard deviation score.

TREATMENT OF OSTEOPOROSIS IN OLDER ADULTS

Pharmacologic Management

Based on the NOF guidelines,[14] health care providers should consider treating patients based on the following

- T-score ≤ -2.5 at the lumbar spine, femoral neck, total hip or one-third distal radius (after appropriate evaluation to exclude secondary causes)
- A hip or vertebral (clinical or morphometric) fracture
- Low bone mass (T-score between −1.0 and −2.5) and a 10-year probability of a hip fracture $\geq$3% or a 10-year probability of a major osteoporosis-related fracture $\geq$20% based on the US-adapted World Health Organization (WHO) algorithm (ie, using the Fracture Risk Assessment Model (FRAX) Web-based tool, **Box 1**)
- Clinician's judgment and/or patient preferences may indicate treatment for people with 10-year fracture probabilities below these levels

The current US Food and Drug Administration (FDA)-approved indications for bone-active agents and their evidence for fracture reduction are shown in **Tables 2** and **3**, respectively. The efficacy of these agents has been established in several large randomized clinical trials, and the mean age of subjects in these pivotal clinical trials with fracture end points ranges between 68 and 83 years of age (**Table 4**).

Box 1
Clinical risk factors for fracture included in the WHO FRAX

Current age

Gender

Low body mass index (kg/m^2)

A prior osteoporotic fracture (including morphometric vertebral fracture)

Parental history of hip fracture

Oral glucocorticoids $\geq$5 mg/d of prednisone for $\geq$3 mo (ever)

Current smoking

Alcohol intake (3 or more drinks per day)

Rheumatoid arthritis

Secondary osteoporosis

Femoral neck BMD

Table 2
FDA-approved indications for bone-active agents

Drug	Postmenopausal Osteoporosis		Glucocorticoid-Induced Osteoporosis		
	Prevention	Treatment	Prevention	Treatment	Men
Estrogen	✔				
Calcitonin (Miacalcin, Fortical)		✔			
Raloxifene (Evista)	✔	✔			
Ibandronate (Boniva)	✔	✔			
Alendronate (Fosamax)	✔	✔		✔	✔
Risedronate (Actonel)	✔	✔	✔	✔	✔
Risedronate (Atelvia)		✔			
Zoledronate (Reclast)	✔	✔	✔	✔	✔
Denosumab (Prolia)		✔			✔
Teriparatide (Forteo)		✔		✔	✔

Raloxifene

Selective estrogen modulators (SERMs) are compounds that can bind to estrogen receptors and cause estrogen or antiestrogenic responses in different tissues. Raloxifene was the first SERM approved for the treatment of osteoporosis. In the Multiple Outcomes of Raloxifene Evaluation (MORE) trial (mean age 69 years),[15] the risk of vertebral fracture was reduced in both study groups receiving raloxifene (30% Relative Risk Reduction [RRR] for 60 mg/d group, 50% RRR for 120 mg/d group). Women receiving raloxifene had an increased risk of thromboembolism. A study examining the effect of raloxifene in elderly women living in long-term care facilities showed that raloxifene reduces bone turnover in these women to a level comparable to what is seen in younger postmenopausal women.[16]

Calcitonin

Calcitonin acts directly on osteoclasts, inhibiting bone resorption. The Prevent Recurrence of Osteoporotic Fractures (PROOF) study in postmenopausal women with osteoporosis (mean age 69 years) showed that 200 IU salmon calcitonin nasal spray per

Table 3
Evidence for fracture reduction for FDA-approved bone-active agents

Drug	Vertebral Fracture	Nonvertebral Fracture	Hip Fracture
Calcitonin (Miacalcin, Fortical)	✔	No effect demonstrated	No effect demonstrated
Raloxifene (Evista)	✔	No effect demonstrated	No effect demonstrated
Ibandronate (Boniva)	✔	No effect demonstrated	No effect demonstrated
Alendronate (Fosamax)	✔	★	✔
Risedronate (Actonel, Atelvia)	✔	✔	★
Zoledronic acid (Reclast)	✔	✔	✔
Denosumab (Prolia)	✔	✔	✔
Teriparatide (Forteo)	✔	✔	No effect demonstrated

★ Evidence for effect but not an FDA-approved indication.

Table 4
Mean age of subjects in pivotal clinical trials with fracture end-points

Trial	Intervention	Population Mean Age
VERT-NA[75]	Risedronate	68
FIT-2[76]	Alendronate	69
PROOF[17]	Calcitonin	69
TPTD[32]	Teriparatide	69
MORE[15]	Raloxifene	69
FIT-1[18]	Alendronate	71
VERT-MN[77]	Risedronate	71
FREEDOM[78]	Denosumab	72
HIP Group 1[21]	Risedronate	74
HORIZON RFT[24]	Zoledronic acid	75
HIP Group 2[21]	Risedronate	83

day decreased the risk of new vertebral fractures by 33% to 36% at the end of 5 years.[17] It is important to note that the discontinuation rate at the end of the study was 59%.

Bisphosphonates

Bisphosphonates reduce osteoclastic bone resorption by entering the osteoclast and causing loss or resorptive function as well as accelerating osteoclast apoptosis. Alendronate was the first bisphosphonate approved by the FDA (1995) for the treatment of osteoporosis. A post-hoc analysis of the Fracture Intervention Trial (FIT)[18] revealed that the relative risk reductions for all fractures with alendronate treatment were constant across age groups, without evidence of a decline at older ages, and the absolute risk reduction increased with age because of the age-related increase in fracture risk in the placebo group.[19] Furthermore, in a study of elderly female residents of long-term care facilities, alendronate increased BMD at both the spine and hip compared with placebo.[20]

Similarly, the Hip Intervention Program (HIP) study revealed that risedronate increased BMD at the femoral neck and trochanter in elderly women.[21] The incidence of hip fracture among those assigned to risedronate was 1.9%, compared with 3.2% among those assigned to placebo (RRR 40%, P = .009). However, in the group of women 80 years of age and older who were selected primarily on the basis of nonskeletal risk factors, risedronate had no significant reduction in fracture rates. A post-hoc analysis of the 2 Vertebral Efficacy With Risedronate Therapy (VERT) trials (VERT-MN and VERT-NA) showed that 1 year of treatment with risedronate 5 mg/d reduced vertebral fracture risk in high-risk subjects, including postmenopausal women at least 70 years of age, compared with placebo (RRR 62%. P<.001).[22] A pooled analysis of women with osteoporosis aged 80 and older from 3 risedronate trials (HIP study and the 2 VERT trials) revealed that risedronate decreased the incidence of vertebral fractures by 81% at 1 year and 44% at 3 years, but had no effect on nonvertebral fractures.[23]

In the Health Outcomes and Reduced Incidence with Zoledronic acid Once Yearly (HORIZON) Recurrent Fracture Trial (RFT), once-yearly zoledronic acid reduced the rates of clinical fractures in patients with recent hip fracture by 35% (P = .001), with a 28% reduction in all-cause mortality at 2 years.[24] The mean age of patients in this study was 74.5 years, with 14% of subjects over 85 years of age. The increases in BMD in men were of a similar magnitude to those observed in women in the same study.[25] A post-hoc subgroup analysis of the HORIZON Pivotal Fracture Trial (PFT) and RFT revealed that once-yearly zoledronic acid was associated with a significant reduction in the risk of new clinical fractures (vertebral and nonvertebral) in elderly postmenopausal women with osteoporosis. The incidence of hip fracture was lower with zoledronic acid but did not reach statistical significance.[26]

Therefore, a high level of evidence suggests that bisphosphonates are at least as effective in older patients as in younger patients, with similar safety profiles.[27] Furthermore, cost-effectiveness analyses suggest that treatment with an oral bisphosphonate for 5 years is cost-effective for all women, regardless of quartile of life expectancy.[28]

Denosumab

Denosumab is a fully human monoclonal antibody to the receptor activator of nuclear factor kappa-B ligand (RANKL), an osteoclast-differentiating factor. It inhibits osteoclast formation, thus decreasing bone resorption. Although not formally evaluated in the elderly, 5 years of denosumab exposure in postmenopausal women with osteoporosis in the Fracture Reduction Evaluation of Denosumab in Osteoporosis Every 6 Months (FREEDOM) Extension trial (mean age 75 years) was associated with a progressive increase in bonedensity and sustained but not progressive decrease in bone turnover, with low fracture rates and a favorable risk/benefit profile.[29] A post-hoc analysis of the FREEDOM trial revealed that 3 years of treatment with denosumab significantly reduced the risk of hip fractures in subjects aged 75 years or older (2.3% placebo vs 0.9% denosumab; $P<.01$). Furthermore, no significant differences were noted in the safety profile between placebo-treated and denosumab-treated subjects in the various higher-risk and lower-risk subgroups, including subjects who were 75 years of age or older.[30] Similarly, a recent subgroup analysis of the same trial showed that the effect of denosumab treatment on reduction in risk of vertebral and nonvertebral fractures was similar in subjects older or younger than 75 years of age.[31]

Teriparatide

In contrast to the other available antiresorptive therapies for osteoporosis, teriparatide is an anabolic agent that stimulates bone remodeling, preferentially increasing bone formation over resorption. A subgroup analysis of data from the Fracture Prevention Trial (FPT)[32] showed that teriparatide treatment was associated with a significant reduction in the risk of new vertebral fracture (RRR 65%, $P<.05$) in postmenopausal women aged 75 years and older but no significant reduction in nonvertebral fractures.[33]

In summary, several pharmacologic treatments have been shown to significantly reduce the risk of fracture. It is important to note that therapy needs to be individualized based on risk/benefit assessments, taking into account the presence of comorbid medical conditions that are prevalent in the elderly.[34]

Nonadherence to treatment

Poor adherence appears to be a major limiting factor in clinical practice, with advancing age predicting a greater risk of noncompliance.[35] Other factors associated with nonadherence include adverse effects, pain, being unsure about BMD test results, patient health beliefs, and inadequate patient education.[36,37] Another challenge is following the specific administration requirements of oral bisphosphonates (fasting, with a full glass of water, remaining upright, and not eating for at least 30 minutes). Strategies to increase adherence include reducing administration frequency if possible, monitoring patients with bone markers and BMD testing, providing adequate instructions, practitioner feedback and support, and educational materials and sessions. More studies are needed to assess strategies aimed at increasing adherence to osteoporosis therapies.

Nonpharmacologic Management

Nonpharmacologic management aimed at decreasing fracture risk becomes increasingly important in older patients. Schott and colleagues[38] showed that women aged 75 to 79 with osteoporosis are 4.4 times more likely to fracture than those without, while women aged 85 and older with osteoporosis are only 60% more likely to fracture than those without, suggesting the nonskeletal risk factors play a bigger role in determining fracture risk in the elderly compared with younger patients.

Fall risk reduction

Poor vision, poor hearing, poor balance, and muscle weakness become critical determinants of fall risk, hence fracture risk, in older patients.[39] Furthermore, neuromuscular and visual impairments are significant independent predictors of the risk of hip fracture in elderly women, and their combined assessment with BMD measurements improves the prediction of hip fractures.[40–42] Effective fall prevention interventions in the elderly include home safety evaluation for high-risk or visually impaired patients, withdrawal of psychoactive medications, cataract surgery, exercise interventions (such as Tai Chi), and vitamin D repletion in those with low vitamin D levels.[43,44] Using proper footwear and avoiding stairs if possible are also important measures in reducing fall risk.

Physical exercise programs should emphasize improving muscle strength and balance. Exercise programs that included balance training, such as Tai Chi, were more effective at reducing falls than others.[45] A review and meta-analysis confirmed this finding and also showed that programs with a high dose of exercise and those that did not involve walking reduced fall rates more than programs with a low dose of exercise and those involving walking. Specifically, the greatest relative effects of exercise on fall rates (relative risk [RR] = 0.58, 95% confidence interval [CI] = 0.48–0.69) were seen in programs that included a combination of a higher total dose of exercise (>50 hours over the trial period) and challenging balance exercises (exercises conducted while standing in which people aimed to stand with their feet closer together or on 1 leg, minimize use of their hands to assist, and practice controlled movements of the center of mass) and did not include a walking program.[46] The negative effect of walking may in part be due to time taken away from balance training.

Vitamin D deficiency is common in the elderly, and supplementation is essential for the maintenance of bone and muscle strength.[47–49] Risk factors for vitamin D deficiency include low exposure to sunlight among others,[50] and age decreases the capacity of human skin to produce vitamin D3.[51] Vitamin D replacement therapy has been shown to reduce body sway and decrease fall risk in older individuals,[52–55] as well as decrease fracture risk in men and women aged 65 years and over living in the community.[56] A meta-analysis of double-blind studies of vitamin D supplementation showed that oral vitamin D supplementation between 700 to 800 IU/d reduced the risk of hip and any nonvertebral fractures in ambulatory or institutionalized elderly persons.[57] Similarly, a recent pooled analysis of 11 double-blind, randomized, controlled trials of oral vitamin D supplementation in persons 65 years of age or older revealed that high-dose vitamin D supplementation (≥800 IU daily) was somewhat favorable in the prevention of hip fracture and any nonvertebral fracture in persons 65 years of age or older.[58] Vitamin D status is assessed by measurement of its major circulating metabolite, 25-hydroxy vitamin D,[59] with the minimum desirable 30 ng/dL.[60,61] Many patients require supplements of vitamin D, 2000 IU daily or more, to achieve this level. Adequate calcium intake is another important component in the prevention and treatment of osteoporosis in the elderly. One of the earliest trials assessing the effectiveness of calcium and vitamin D in elderly women (mean age 84 years) revealed a reduction in the number of hip and all nonvertebral fractures after daily supplementation for 18 months.[62] Randomized double-blind placebo-controlled trials in elderly women have shown that calcium supplementation decreases bone loss and reduces bone turnover.[63,64] A recent study examined the health benefits and risks of calcium and vitamin D supplementation using data from the Women's Health Initiative, with emphasis on fractures, cardiovascular disease, cancer, and total mortality.[65] This showed a substantial reduction in hip fracture risk (hazard ratio [HR] 0.65; 95% CI, 0.44–0.98) but no significant effect on other outcomes. The recommended total calcium intake for men and women age 70 and older is 1200 mg daily, with the preferred source being dietary[66,67]; supplementation is recommended if this cannot be obtained through diet alone.

Hip protectors and other assistive devices

Hip protectors may reduce the risk of hip fractures, but poor adherence is a key problem contributing to the continuing uncertainty on their effectiveness.[68–71] However, a study in nursing home residents (mean age 85 years) did not detect a protective effect on the risk of hip fracture despite good adherence to the study protocol (overall adherence 74%).[72] There are several different styles of hip protectors, and it remains unknown if findings from different studies performed to date apply to all types of hip protectors. Patients may benefit from balance, gait, and transfer training, as well as the use of assistive devices such as canes, walkers, bed handlers, bath rails, shower chairs, reachers, and transfer aids.

Psychosocial support

Both the functional limitation and the pain associated with osteoporotic fractures often lead to the serious social consequences of role loss and isolation. There are 3 stages of psychosocial impairment associated with osteoporosis-related complications[73]:

1. Primary: reduced capacity to fulfill social roles and to perform activities of daily living
2. Secondary: diminished self-esteem and reduced social involvement outside the family, leading to loneliness, isolation, and depression
3. Tertiary: overall quality of life is substantially reduced due extremely limited social interactions and depression

Despite the substantial psychosocial impact of osteoporosis, little research has evolved in this area.[74]Psychosocial consequences of osteoporosis must be identified and addressed to improve quality of life and compliance with medical recommendations.

SUMMARY

The incidence of osteoporotic fracture increases with advancing age. The risk of fractures in the elderly is determined by skeletal risk factors (BMD) and nonskeletal risk factors (frailty, poor balance, and hazards in the home environment). There are numerous opportunities for intervention to decrease fracture risk. The management of osteoporosis in older people involves improving bone health via calcium and vitamin D supplements as well as fall prevention strategies. Although these measures are important in the management of all patients, most elderly patients will likely require pharmacologic therapy to adequately reduce their fracture risk. Pharmacologic treatment options that are FDA-approved for osteoporosis include SERMs, calcitonin, bisphosphonates, denosumab, and teriparatide. Pharmacologic therapy must be individualized and must be paralleled with the treatment of potentially modifiable risk factors and improved household safety, which are important adjuncts to pharmacologic therapy.

REFERENCES

1. Osteoporosis prevention, diagnosis, and therapy. NIH Consensus Statement 2000;17:1.
2. Bone health and osteoporosis: a report of the Surgeon General. Available at: http://www.surgeongeneral.gov/library/reports/bonehealth/full_report.pdf. Accessed November 30, 2012.
3. Melton LJ 3rd. How many women have osteoporosis now? J Bone Miner Res 1995;10:175.
4. Burger H, de Laet CE, van Daele PL, et al. Risk factors for increased bone loss in an elderly population: the Rotterdam Study. Am J Epidemiol 1998;147:871.
5. Schuit SC, van der Klift M, Weel AE, et al. Fracture incidence and association with bone mineral density in elderly men and women: the Rotterdam Study. Bone 2004;34:195.
6. Burge R, Dawson-Hughes B, Solomon DH, et al. Incidence and economic burden of osteoporosis-related fractures in the United States, 2005-2025. J Bone Miner Res 2007;22:465.
7. Rizzoli R, Bruyere O, Cannata-Andia JB, et al. Management of osteoporosis in the elderly. Curr Med Res Opin 2009;25:2373.
8. Kanis JA, Johnell O, Oden A, et al. Ten year probabilities of osteoporotic fractures according to BMD and diagnostic thresholds. Osteoporos Int 2001;12:989.
9. Birge SJ. Osteoporotic fractures: a brain or bone disease? Curr Osteoporos Rep 2008;6:57.
10. Zimmerman SI, Girman CJ, Buie VC, et al. The prevalence of osteoporosis in nursing home residents. Osteoporos Int 1999;9:151.
11. Rojas-Fernandez CH, Lapane KL, MacKnight C, et al. Undertreatment of osteoporosis in residents of nursing homes: population-based study with use of the Systematic Assessment of Geriatric Drug Use via Epidemiology (SAGE) database. Endocr Pract 2002;8:335.
12. Zimmerman S, Chandler JM, Hawkes W, et al. Effect of fracture on the health care use of nursing home residents. Arch Intern Med 2002;162:1502.
13. US Preventive Services Task Force. Screening for osteoporosis: US Preventive Services Task Force recommendation statement. Ann Intern Med 2011;154:356.
14. National Osteoporosis Foundation. Clinician's guide to prevention and treatment of osteoporosis. Available at: http://www.nof.org/files/nof/public/content/file/344/upload/159.pdf. Accessed November 30, 2012.
15. Ettinger B, Black DM, Mitlak BH, et al. Reduction of vertebral fracture risk in postmenopausal women with osteoporosis treated with raloxifene: results from a 3-year randomized clinical trial. Multiple Outcomes of Raloxifene Evaluation (MORE) Investigators. JAMA 1999;282:637.
16. Hansdottir H, Franzson L, Prestwood K, et al. The effect of raloxifene on markers of bone turnover in older women living in long-term care facilities. J Am Geriatr Soc 2004;52:779.
17. Chesnut CH 3rd, Silverman S, Andriano K, et al. A randomized trial of nasal spray salmon calcitonin in postmenopausal women with established osteoporosis: the prevent recurrence of osteoporotic fractures study. PROOF Study Group. Am J Med 2000;109:267.

18. Black DM, Cummings SR, Karpf DB, et al. Randomised trial of effect of alendronate on risk of fracture in women with existing vertebral fractures. Fracture Intervention Trial Research Group. Lancet 1996;348:1535.
19. Hochberg MC, Thompson DE, Black DM, et al. Effect of alendronate on the age-specific incidence of symptomatic osteoporotic fractures. J Bone Miner Res 2005;20:971.
20. Greenspan SL, Schneider DL, McClung MR, et al. Alendronate improves bone mineral density in elderly women with osteoporosis residing in long-term care facilities. A randomized, double-blind, placebo-controlled trial. Ann Intern Med 2002;136:742.
21. McClung MR, Geusens P, Miller PD, et al. Effect of risedronate on the risk of hip fracture in elderly women. Hip Intervention Program Study Group. N Engl J Med 2001;344:333.
22. Watts NB, Josse RG, Hamdy RC, et al. Risedronate prevents new vertebral fractures in postmenopausal women at high risk. J Clin Endocrinol Metab 2003;88: 542.
23. Boonen S, McClung MR, Eastell R, et al. Safety and efficacy of risedronate in reducing fracture risk in osteoporotic women aged 80 and older: implications for the use of antiresorptive agents in the old and oldest old. J Am Geriatr Soc 2004;52:1832.
24. Lyles KW, Colon-Emeric CS, Magaziner JS, et al. Zoledronic acid and clinical fractures and mortality after hip fracture. N Engl J Med 2007;357:1799.
25. Boonen S, Orwoll E, Magaziner J, et al. Once-yearly zoledronic acid in older men compared with women with recent hip fracture. J Am Geriatr Soc 2011;59:2084.
26. Boonen S, Black DM, Colon-Emeric CS, et al. Efficacy and safety of a once-yearly intravenous zoledronic acid 5 mg for fracture prevention in elderly postmenopausal women with osteoporosis aged 75 and older. J Am Geriatr Soc 2010;58:292.
27. Crandall CJ, Newberry SJ, Diamant A, et al. Treatment to prevent fractures in men and women with low bone density or osteoporosis: update of a 2007 report. In: AHRQ comparative effectiveness reviews. Rockville (MD): 2012. Available at: http://www.ncbi.nlm.nih.gov/books/NBK92566/. Accessed November 30, 2012.
28. Pham AN, Datta SK, Weber TJ, et al. Cost-effectiveness of oral bisphosphonates for osteoporosis at different ages and levels of life expectancy. J Am Geriatr Soc 2011;59:1642.
29. Papapoulos S, Chapurlat R, Libanati C, et al. Five years of denosumab exposure in women with postmenopausal osteoporosis: results from the first two years of the FREEDOM extension. J Bone Miner Res 2012;27:694.
30. Boonen S, Adachi JD, Man Z, et al. Treatment with denosumab reduces the incidence of new vertebral and hip fractures in postmenopausal women at high risk. J Clin Endocrinol Metab 2011;96:1727.
31. McClung M, Boonen S, Torring O, et al. Effect of denosumab treatment on the risk of fractures in subgroups of women with postmenopausal osteoporosis. J Bone Miner Res 2012;27:211.
32. Neer RM, Arnaud CD, Zanchetta JR, et al. Effect of parathyroid hormone (1–34) on fractures and bone mineral density in postmenopausal women with osteoporosis. N Engl J Med 2001;344:1434.
33. Boonen S, Marin F, Mellstrom D, et al. Safety and efficacy of teriparatide in elderly women with established osteoporosis: bone anabolic therapy from a geriatric perspective. J Am Geriatr Soc 2006;54:782.
34. Curtis JR, Safford MM. Management of osteoporosis among the elderly with other chronic medical conditions. Drugs Aging 2012;29:549.

35. Penning-van Beest FJ, Erkens JA, Olson M, et al. Determinants of non-compliance with bisphosphonates in women with postmenopausal osteoporosis. Curr Med Res Opin 2008;24:1337.
36. Papaioannou A, Kennedy CC, Dolovich L, et al. Patient adherence to osteoporosis medications: problems, consequences and management strategies. Drugs Aging 2007;24:37.
37. Gold DT, Silverman S. Review of adherence to medications for the treatment of osteoporosis. Curr Osteoporos Rep 2006;4:21.
38. Schott AM, Cormier C, Hans D, et al. How hip and whole-body bone mineral density predict hip fracture in elderly women: the EPIDOS Prospective Study. Osteoporos Int 1998;8:247.
39. Cummings SR, Nevitt MC, Browner WS, et al. Risk factors for hip fracture in white women. Study of Osteoporotic Fractures Research Group. N Engl J Med 1995; 332:767.
40. Dargent-Molina P, Favier F, Grandjean H, et al. Fall-related factors and risk of hip fracture: the EPIDOS prospective study. Lancet 1996;348:145.
41. Girman CJ, Chandler JM, Zimmerman SI, et al. Prediction of fracture in nursing home residents. J Am Geriatr Soc 2002;50:1341.
42. Grundstrom AC, Guse CE, Layde PM. Risk factors for falls and fall-related injuries in adults 85 years of age and older. Arch Gerontol Geriatr 2012;54:421.
43. Gillespie LD, Robertson MC, Gillespie WJ, et al. Interventions for preventing falls in older people living in the community. Cochrane Database Syst Rev 2012;(9):CD007146.
44. Waldron N, Hill AM, Barker A. Falls prevention in older adults—assessment and management. Aust Fam Physician 2012;41:930.
45. Li F, Harmer P, Fisher KJ, et al. Tai Chi and fall reductions in older adults: a randomized controlled trial. J Gerontol A Biol Sci Med Sci 2005;60:187.
46. Sherrington C, Whitney JC, Lord SR, et al. Effective exercise for the prevention of falls: a systematic review and meta-analysis. J Am Geriatr Soc 2008;56:2234.
47. Holick MF. The role of vitamin D for bone health and fracture prevention. Curr Osteoporos Rep 2006;4:96.
48. Visser M, Deeg DJ, Lips P. Low vitamin D and high parathyroid hormone levels as determinants of loss of muscle strength and muscle mass (sarcopenia): the Longitudinal Aging Study Amsterdam. J Clin Endocrinol Metab 2003;88:5766.
49. Bischoff-Ferrari HA, Staehelin HB. Importance of vitamin D and calcium at older age. Int J Vitam Nutr Res 2008;78:286.
50. Holick MF. High prevalence of vitamin D inadequacy and implications for health. Mayo Clin Proc 2006;81:353.
51. MacLaughlin J, Holick MF. Aging decreases the capacity of human skin to produce vitamin D3. J Clin Invest 1985;76:1536.
52. Bischoff HA, Stahelin HB, Dick W, et al. Effects of vitamin D and calcium supplementation on falls: a randomized controlled trial. J Bone Miner Res 2003;18:343.
53. Bischoff-Ferrari HA, Dawson-Hughes B, Willett WC, et al. Effect of Vitamin D on falls: a meta-analysis. JAMA 2004;291:1999.
54. Pfeifer M, Begerow B, Minne HW, et al. Effects of a short-term vitamin D and calcium supplementation on body sway and secondary hyperparathyroidism in elderly women. J Bone Miner Res 2000;15:1113.
55. Pfeifer M, Begerow B, Minne HW, et al. Effects of a long-term vitamin D and calcium supplementation on falls and parameters of muscle function in community-dwelling older individuals. Osteoporos Int 2009;20:315.

56. Trivedi DP, Doll R, Khaw KT. Effect of four monthly oral vitamin D3 (cholecalciferol) supplementation on fractures and mortality in men and women living in the community: randomised double blind controlled trial. BMJ 2003;326:469.
57. Bischoff-Ferrari HA, Willett WC, Wong JB, et al. Fracture prevention with vitamin D supplementation: a meta-analysis of randomized controlled trials. JAMA 2005; 293:2257.
58. Bischoff-Ferrari HA, Willett WC, Orav EJ, et al. A pooled analysis of vitamin D dose requirements for fracture prevention. N Engl J Med 2012;367:40.
59. Holick MF, Binkley NC, Bischoff-Ferrari HA, et al. Evaluation, treatment, and prevention of vitamin D deficiency: an Endocrine Society clinical practice guideline. J Clin Endocrinol Metab 2011;96:1911.
60. Bischoff-Ferrari HA. Optimal serum 25-hydroxyvitamin D levels for multiple health outcomes. Adv Exp Med Biol 2008;624:55.
61. Holick MF, Binkley NC, Bischoff-Ferrari HA, et al. Guidelines for preventing and treating vitamin D deficiency and insufficiency revisited. J Clin Endocrinol Metab 2012;97:1153.
62. Chapuy MC, Arlot ME, Duboeuf F, et al. Vitamin D3 and calcium to prevent hip fractures in the elderly women. N Engl J Med 1992;327:1637.
63. Riggs BL, O'Fallon WM, Muhs J, et al. Long-term effects of calcium supplementation on serum parathyroid hormone level, bone turnover, and bone loss in elderly women. J Bone Miner Res 1998;13:168.
64. Storm D, Eslin R, Porter ES, et al. Calcium supplementation prevents seasonal bone loss and changes in biochemical markers of bone turnover in elderly New England women: a randomized placebo-controlled trial. J Clin Endocrinol Metab 1998;83:3817.
65. Prentice RL, Pettinger MB, Jackson RD, et al. Health risks and benefits from calcium and vitamin D supplementation: women's health initiative clinical trial and cohort study. Osteoporos Int 2012;24(2):567–80.
66. Verbrugge FH, Gielen E, Milisen K, et al. Who should receive calcium and vitamin D supplementation? Age Ageing 2012;41:576.
67. Tang BM, Eslick GD, Nowson C, et al. Use of calcium or calcium in combination with vitamin D supplementation to prevent fractures and bone loss in people aged 50 years and older: a meta-analysis. Lancet 2007;370:657.
68. Gillespie WJ, Gillespie LD, Parker MJ. Hip protectors for preventing hip fractures in older people. Cochrane Database Syst Rev 2010;(6):CD001255.
69. Kannus P, Parkkari J. Hip protectors for preventing hip fracture. JAMA 2007;298:454.
70. Kannus P, Parkkari J, Niemi S, et al. Prevention of hip fracture in elderly people with use of a hip protector. N Engl J Med 2000;343:1506.
71. Kannus P, Sievanen H, Palvanen M, et al. Prevention of falls and consequent injuries in elderly people. Lancet 2005;366:1885.
72. Kiel DP, Magaziner J, Zimmerman S, et al. Efficacy of a hip protector to prevent hip fracture in nursing home residents: the HIP PRO randomized controlled trial. JAMA 2007;298:413.
73. Gold DT, Shipp KM, Lyles KW. Managing patients with complications of osteoporosis. Endocrinol Metab Clin North Am 1998;27:485.
74. Gold DT. Osteoporosis and quality of life psychosocial outcomes and interventions for individual patients. Clin Geriatr Med 2003;19:271.
75. Harris ST, Watts NB, Genant HK, et al. Effects of risedronate treatment on vertebral and nonvertebral fractures in women with postmenopausal osteoporosis: a randomized controlled trial. Vertebral Efficacy With Risedronate Therapy (VERT) Study Group. JAMA 1999;282:1344.

76. Cummings SR, Black DM, Thompson DE, et al. Effect of alendronate on risk of fracture in women with low bone density but without vertebral fractures: results from the Fracture Intervention Trial. JAMA 1998;280:2077.
77. Reginster J, Minne HW, Sorensen OH, et al. Randomized trial of the effects of risedronate on vertebral fractures in women with established postmenopausal osteoporosis. Vertebral Efficacy with Risedronate Therapy (VERT) Study Group. Osteoporos Int 2000;11:83.
78. Cummings SR, San Martin J, McClung MR, et al. Denosumab for prevention of fractures in postmenopausal women with osteoporosis. N Engl J Med 2009;361:756.

Vitamin D and Aging

J. Christopher Gallagher, MD, MRCP

KEYWORDS

• Vitamin D metabolism • Aging • Vitamin D insufficiency • Vitamin D treatment

KEY POINTS

- There are age-related changes that affect vitamin D metabolism and increase the requirement for vitamin D in the elderly.
- The optimal total calcium intake is unclear. Increasing calcium from dietary sources may be preferred to supplements, and requires increasing the intake of dairy products and calcium-fortified foods.
- Evidence suggests that vitamin D and calcium nutrition can be improved in the elderly by increasing the vitamin D intake to 800 IU daily together with calcium 1000 mg daily. This combination is a simple, inexpensive strategy that can reduce fractures in independent living by ~12 percent and in institutionalized individuals by 30%.

Aging affects the formation of 1,25-dihydroxyvitamin D (1,25[OH]$_2$D; calcitriol), the active form of vitamin D. Production of 1,25(OH)$_2$D is reduced by 50% as a result of an age-related decline in renal function, although serum 1,25(OH)$_2$D levels are maintained in part by secondary hyperparathyroidism. Aging also causes a decrease in calcium absorption that precedes the decrease in 1,25(OH)$_2$D by 10 to 15 years. Because 1,25(OH)$_2$D is dependent on an adequate supply of the substrate vitamin D, the development of vitamin D deficiency leads to further reduction in the formation of 1,25(OH)$_2$D. Measurement of the metabolite 25OHD provides the most widely used assessment of vitamin D deficiency. A serum 25OHD level lower than 10 ng/mL (25 nmol/L) represents vitamin D deficiency and leads to a reduction in serum 1,25(OH)$_2$D. Vitamin D deficiency, is uncommon in North America, probably because of supplementation of dairy products and other foods with vitamin D. Sunlight exposure increases serum 25OHD levels by about 10 ng/mL during the months of April through September, resulting in low serum 25OHD for about 3 to 4 months in winter, with 2 additional months of low levels in more northern latitudes, such as Canada, and 2 fewer months in the southern states. Vitamin D supplementation in the winter can

Disclosures: None.
Funding: National Institute on Aging (RO1-AG28168).
Conflict of Interest: None.
Endocrine Department, Creighton University Medical School, 601 North 30th Street, Omaha, NE 68131, USA
E-mail address: jcg@creighton.edu

Endocrinol Metab Clin N Am 42 (2013) 319–332
http://dx.doi.org/10.1016/j.ecl.2013.02.004 endo.theclinics.com
0889-8529/13/$ – see front matter

prevent vitamin D deficiency. Vitamin D insufficiency has been defined by the Institute of Medicine as a serum 25OHD level lower than 20 ng/mL (and >10 ng/mL). A serum 25OHD level lower than 20 ng/mL is associated with an increased fracture rate and increased rate of bone loss and treatment. Although other diseases have been associated with low serum 25OHD levels, the evidence for a causative role has not yet been established. Treatment of elderly people with vitamin D 800 IU daily will increase serum 25OHD levels to higher than 20 ng/mL and reduce fractures; this is particularly important in institutionalized people.

VITAMIN D METABOLISM

Vitamin D is derived from diet and sunlight and is not biologically active. Vitamin D must be sequentially converted into 25-hydroxyvitamin D (25OHD) in the liver by the enzyme CYP2R1 and then into 1,25-dihydroxyvitamin D (1,25[OH]$_2$D) in the kidney by the CYP27B1 enzyme (1α hydroxylase) (**Fig. 1**). Both 1,25(OH)$_2$D and 25OHD are carried in the circulation by vitamin D–binding protein (DBP).

The active hormonal form of vitamin D is 1,25(OH)$_2$D, which binds to the vitamin D receptor (VDR) together with the retinoid X receptor to activate specific genes in target organs.[1] VDR is present in many tissues besides bone, and certain cells, such as immune and osteoprogenitor cells, also contain the 1α hydroxylase enzyme as part of an intracrine and paracrine system. The regulation of the 1α hydroxylase enzyme is tightly maintained so as to keep serum 1,25(OH)$_2$D levels constant. Production of 1,25(OH)$_2$D is upregulated by parathyroid hormone (PTH) and low serum phosphorus and inhibited by fibroblast growth factor (FGF-23), which also regulates serum phosphorus levels. The enzyme CYP24 hydroxylase converts 25OHD to the nonactive metabolite 24,25(OH)$_2$D in the kidney, thereby limiting the production of 1,25(OH)$_2$D. Local formation of 24,25(OH)$_2$D is also induced in many target tissues through negative feedback by 1,25(OH)$_2$D.

1,25(OH)$_2$D is essential for the efficient absorption of dietary calcium and phosphorus and for mineralization of bone. Recently, 1,25(OH)$_2$D has been recognized

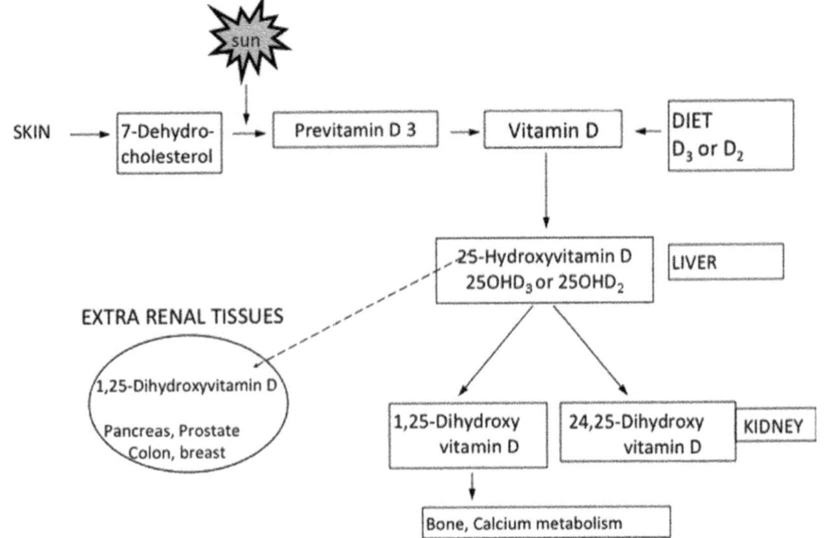

Fig. 1. Vitamin D metabolism.

to have a multitude of other biologic functions. Studies suggest that it is unlikely that serum 25OHD has an independent physiologic function that is not fulfilled by $1,25(OH)_2D$.

EFFECT OF AGE ON VITAMIN D AND CALCIUM METABOLISM

The following are effects of age on vitamin D and calcium metabolism:

- Decreased calcium absorption
- Intestinal resistance of calcium absorption to circulating $1,25(OH)_2D$
- Decreased VDR
- Decreased renal production of $1,25(OH)_2D$ by the aging kidney
- Decreased skin production of vitamin D
- Substrate deficiency of vitamin D

Decreased Calcium Absorption

Malabsorption of calcium occurs as part of aging and starts at approximately age 65 to 70 years.[2,3] As a result, it leads to negative calcium balance, secondary hyperparathyroidism, increased bone loss, and osteoporosis. Because of malabsorption of calcium, there is a decreased ability to adapt to a low-calcium diet by increasing fractional calcium absorption.[4] Although several independent dietary factors affect calcium absorption, such as protein intake, sodium intake, or glucose, the main regulator is $1,25(OH)_2D$ acting through the VDR and synthesizing genes and proteins involved in calcium transport.[5] Deletion of the VDR results in malabsorption of calcium.[6] Calcium absorption occurs by both an active saturable system and a passive diffusion transport system. Active transport of calcium occurs through transcellular and paracellular pathways in the duodenum and jejunum, whereas passive paracellular absorption is the main process of calcium absorption throughout the intestine.[7] At the molecular level, the calcium-binding protein calbindin-D_{9k} and an epithelial calcium channel transient receptor potential vanilloid type 6 (TRPV6) were initially thought to mediate the diffusion of calcium across the gut.[7–9] However, in TRPV6/Calbindin-D_{9k} double knockout mice, calcium absorption still responds to $1,25(OH)_2D$ administration, challenging this mechanism.[10] The tight junction proteins Claudins-2 and Claudins-12 facilitate paracellular calcium transport and are upregulated by $1,25(OH)_2D$ via the VDR receptor.[11] In summary, part of the change in calcium absorption with aging may be because of abnormalities in the transport proteins that are regulated by $1,25(OH)_2D$.

Intestinal Resistance of Calcium Absorption to Circulating $1,25(OH)_2D$

In young healthy people, there is a positive correlation between calcium absorption and serum $1,25(OH)_2D$, but in older people and patients with osteoporosis, the calcium absorption response is lower relative to serum $1,25(OH)_2D$ than in young people (**Fig. 2**), suggesting intestinal resistance to endogenous circulating $1,25(OH)_2D$.[12,13] However, administration of a small oral dose of calcitriol 0.25 μg twice daily to elderly people completely normalizes malabsorption of calcium, suggesting that calcitriol may have a first-pass effect on intestinal transport.[14]

Decreased VDR

Aging may affect the intestinal concentration of VDR to cause a decrease in calcium absorption, as demonstrated in aging rats.[15] There have been 2 studies of intestinal VDR performed on biopsies in humans. A small study of 9 subjects older than 65 years

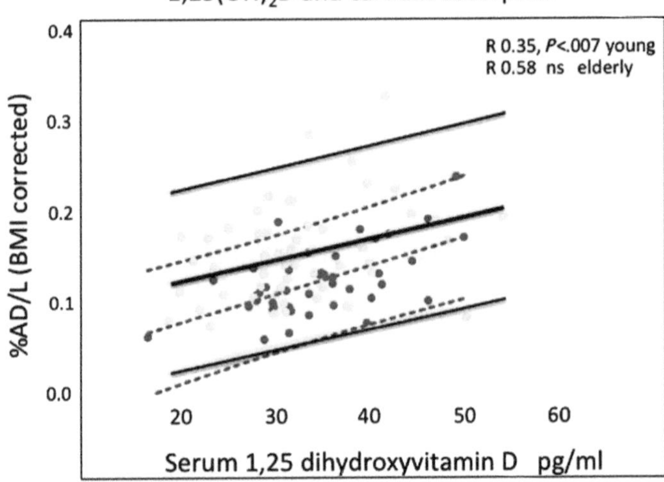

Fig. 2. Calcium absorption is lower in elderly (*red*) compared with young (*yellow*) women for any given serum 1,25 dihydroxyvitamin D level. (*Data from* Kinyamu HK, Gallagher JC, Prahl JM, et al. Association between intestinal vitamin D receptor, calcium absorption, and serum $1,25(OH)_2D$ in normal young and elderly women. J Bone Miner Res 1996;11:1400–5.)

showed a decrease in intestinal VDR concentration with age but no change in serum $1,25(OH)_2D$.[16] In a similar study of 41 women older than 65, 10 of whom were older than 75, there was no difference in intestinal VDR concentration compared with 59 women younger than 35.[17]

Decreased Renal Production of $1,25(OH)_2D$ by the Aging Kidney

As renal function declines with age, there is a decrease in the activity of the renal enzyme 1α hydroxylase that converts 25OHD into $1,25(OH)_2D$. Serum $1,25(OH)_2D$ levels are inversely related to serum creatinine and glomerular function rate (GFR) and a GFR of 50 mL/min is a level that affects $1,25(OH)_2D$ production.[18] Because many people older than 80 have a GFR less than 50 mL/min, decreased production of $1,25(OH)_2D$ in this age group is common. To examine the effect of age and GFR on the 25OHD-$1,25(OH)_2D$ axis, we infused PTH for 24 hours in women of different ages. The increase in serum $1,25(OH)_2D$ was about 50% lower in the older subjects, indicating decreased renal responsiveness to PTH with age (**Fig. 3**).[19]

Measurement of serum $1,25(OH)_2D$ in elderly people shows the impact clinically of declining renal production. In a study of women aged 80 to 95 years who were residents of nursing homes and had normal 25OHD levels, the serum $1,25(OH)_2D$ levels were much lower than in women aged 65 to 75 years (**Fig. 4**).

In summary,

- There is an age-related decrease in calcium absorption that is partly dependent and partly independent of $1,25(OH)_2D$.
- Serum $1,25(OH)_2D$ levels decrease as a result of an age-related decline in renal function.

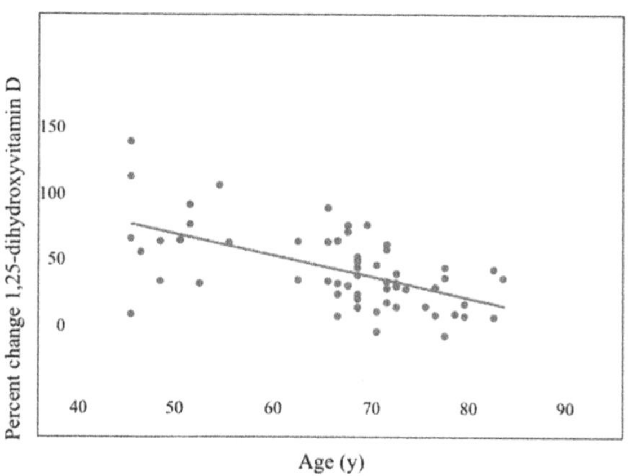

Fig. 3. Decreased renal production of serum $1,25(OH)_2D$ with age after PTH stimulation.

- Reduced levels of serum $1,25(OH)_2D$ likely further reduce calcium absorption, causing secondary hyperparathyroidism and increased bone resorption.
- Secondary hyperparathyroidism persistently stimulates renal $1,25(OH)_2D$ production until the kidney can no longer respond effectively.

Decreased Skin Production

Aging reduces vitamin D production in skin. There is a decrease in the concentration of 7-dehydrocholesterol in the epidermis in old compared with young individuals and a reduced response to UV light, resulting in a 50% decrease in the formation of previtamin D3.[20]

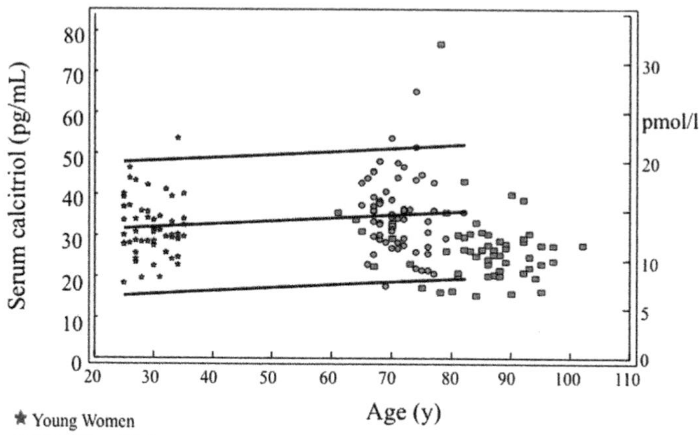

Fig. 4. Serum $1,25(OH)_2D$ levels in women of different ages. (*Data from* Kinyamu HK, Gallagher JC, Balhorn KE, et al. Serum vitamin D metabolites and calcium absorption in normal and elderly free-living women and in women in nursing homes. Am J Clin Nutr 1997;65:790–7.)

Substrate Deficiency of Vitamin D

All age-related changes in vitamin D metabolism are magnified if there is concomitant vitamin D deficiency, because it limits the substrate supply for 25OHD and ultimately $1,25(OH)_2D$. Substrate deficiency is a common problem in the elderly and is important to recognize because it is preventable and treatable. There may be deficiency of vitamin D either from diet or from lack of sunlight, and the decrease in serum 25OHD further limits $1,25(OH)_2D$ production, especially when there is also renal dysfunction. Serum $1,25(OH)_2D$ levels decrease when serum the 25OHD level falls below 10 ng/mL in both younger[21] and older[22] people.

VITAMIN D NUTRITION IN THE ELDERLY

Vitamin D is a unique nutrient because its requirement is met from diet and skin. The dietary intake of vitamin D can be estimated from dietary food tables and is usually between 100 and 400 IU daily. Dietary surveys in North America in the National Health and Nutrition Examination Survey (NHANES) show that dietary intake of vitamin D is low, averaging 200 IU daily (**Table 1**), and, unless one eats a lot of fish with high vitamin D content, daily intake is unlikely to exceed 400 IU daily. Vitamin D intake increases with age because elderly people consume more multivitamins that contain vitamin D.[23,24]

The production of vitamin D in skin cannot be measured directly; however, the change in serum 25OHD gives an estimate of the effect of sun if diet remains constant. In the Midwest at latitude 40°, serum 25OHD increases by 50% from 20 to 30 ng/mL in summer[25]; this change is equivalent to a daily oral vitamin D dose of 2000 IU daily. The UV spectrum is effective only when the sun is more than 30° above the horizon. Below that level, ground pollution filters out the UV rays. In the Midwestern section of North America, effective UV light occurs only between late April and early September.

Table 1
Vitamin D intake and serum 25 hydroxyvitamin D (25OHD) for the United States, 2005–2006

	Vitamin D Intake (IU/d) (mean ± SE)		
Age Group (y)	Diet Alone[a]	Total Intake[b]	Serum 25OHD ng/mL (mean ± SE)
Males			
14–18	244 ± 16	276 ± 20	24 ± 0.6
19–30	204 ± 12	264 ± 16	23 ± 0.5
31–50	216 ± 12	316 ± 12	24 ± 0.4
51–70	204 ± 12	352 ± 16	24 ± 0.5
>70	224 ± 16	428 ± 28	24 ± 0.4
Females			
14–18	152 ± 8	200 ± 20	24 ± 0.7
19–30	144 ± 12	232 ± 12	25 ± 0.8
31–50	176 ± 12	308 ± 20	23 ± 0.5
51–70	156 ± 16	404 ± 40	23 ± 0.4
>70	180 ± 8	400 ± 20	23 ± 0.4

[a] Data for foods.
[b] Data for food + supplements.

Adapted from Bailey RL, Dodd KW, Goldman JA, et al. Estimation of total usual calcium and vitamin D intakes in the United States. J Nutr 2010;140(4):817–22; and Institute of Medicine. Dietary reference intakes for calcium and vitamin D. Washington, DC: The National Academies Press; 2011. Available at: http://www.ncbi.nlm.nih.gov/books/NBK56072.

Effective UV exposure time is 2 months less in Canada and 2 months more in Florida. Vitamin D supplementation should be increased in winter.

VITAMIN D NUTRITIONAL STATUS: VITAMIN D DEFICIENCY/INSUFFICIENCY

It is now recognized that serum 25OHD is the best measure of vitamin D nutritional status because it represents input from diet and skin. In the past, vitamin D *deficiency* was defined as a serum 25OHD level lower than 10 ng/mL because both $1,25(OH)_2D$ and calcium absorption decline at this threshold.[21,22] In 2003, the World Health Organization defined vitamin D *insufficiency* as serum 25OHD lower than 20 ng/mL and normal as 20 to 30 ng/mL.[26] The Institute of Medicine (IOM) reiterated that recommendation in 2011.[24] The Endocrine Society suggested an alternative, defining insufficiency as lower than 30 ng/mL and normal as higher than 30 ng/mL.[27] Why does it matter if the recommended cutoff for insufficiency is 20 ng/mL or 30 ng/mL? The reason is that meeting this target serum 25OHD changes the Recommended Dietary Allowance (RDA).

If a serum 25OHD lower than 20 ng/mL is used as a cutoff for vitamin D *insufficiency*, then surveys worldwide show that vitamin D insufficiency occurs in many people and more in the elderly. In the North American survey NHANES, 24% had serum 25OHD lower than 20 ng/mL and 8% had serum 25OHD lower than 10 ng/mL.[28] However, if one takes into account the within-person variability of the accuracy of the test, the variance of the population data reduces the prevalence of insufficiency to 19%.[29] In another North American study of 490 free-living and nursing home elderly women, approximately 28% of women screened in winter had serum 25OHD levels lower than 20 ng/mL and 4% had serum 25OHD lower than 10 ng/mL.[13] In a multicenter study from Europe and Australia, 80% of 80-year-old institutionalized women had serum 25OHD levels lower than 20 ng/mL,[30] and in a national survey from Ireland of 1500 people, 40% had serum 25OHD levels lower than 20 ng/mL in winter and 36% in summer.[31]

If a serum 25OHD lower than 10 to 12 ng/mL is used as a cutoff for vitamin D *deficiency*, then the prevalence in free-living people varies from 4% to 33% depending on location, whereas in institutionalized elderly, the proportion is much higher at 45% to 36%.[32] The higher prevalence in institutionalized elderly suggests that lack of sun exposure is the most important factor, as diets are intrinsically low in vitamin D. In Denmark, average serum 25OHD levels were only 3 ng/mL in women covering their body and face with a Burka. Compared with 8 ng/mL in women without, even though dietary vitamin D was 600 IU daily.[33]

WHY WAS A SERUM 25OHD LEVEL LOWER THAN 20 NG/ML AND NOT LOWER THAN 30 NG/ML SELECTED TO DEFINE INSUFFICIENCY?

The IOM determined in their 2011 report that much of the data that related serum 25OHD levels higher than 30 ng/mL to diseases other than bone was based on association studies and was not supported by clinical trials.[24] The IOM selected a serum 25OHD level of 20 ng/mL to define vitamin D insufficiency, whereas a serum 25OHD level of 30 ng/mL was suggested to define insufficiency in an Endocrine Society guideline.[27]

The data presented in the Endocrine Society guideline to support a sufficiency level of 30 ng/mL were based on 2 laboratory test–based premises. First, serum PTH was used as a biomarker to define vitamin D insufficiency, with a threshold serum 25OHD of 30 ng/mL used because high levels of PTH decreased and reached a plateau at that level; however, this was based on a selected dataset of 3 studies.[27] An additional 70 studies that were not analyzed did not confirm the 30 ng/mL plateau.[34] A recent study of 350,000 PTH/serum 25OHD samples from a laboratory database showed no evidence of a plateau in serum PTH even at a serum 25OHD of 100 ng/mL.[35] In addition, up to 50% of people with a very low serum 25OHD of 5 to 15 ng/mL have low serum PTH.[36] Thus, the value of serum PTH as an absolute indicator of vitamin D insufficiency is questionable. Second, it was suggested that calcium absorption reaches a maximum at 32 ng/mL, although this was based on modeled, not actual data. Two other studies of calcium absorption show that absorption reaches a maximal threshold at serum 25OHD levels between 5 and 10 ng/mL.[22,37] Thus, neither the PTH plateau nor calcium absorption tests support a 30 ng/mL threshold.

The data that IOM cites as support for a serum 25OHD level of 20 ng/mL are based on a number of studies with bone outcomes. Several prospective cohort studies relate serum 25OHD lower than 20 ng/mL to an increase in hip fracture rates,[24] with no significant increase in hip fractures when serum 25OHD exceeds 20 ng/mL. An analysis of bone markers and serum 25OHD showed that bone resorption markers decrease and plateau at a serum 25OHD level of 18 ng/mL.[34] Subsequently, a large study of rates of bone loss in men (the Mr Os study) showed increased bone loss in the hip only in the groups with serum 25OHD lower than 20 ng/mL.[38]

To estimate what dosage of vitamin D was needed to exceed a serum 25OHD level of 20 ng/mL, the IOM performed an analysis of various individual dose studies of vitamin D and showed that a dosage of 600 to 800 IU daily would exceed a serum 25OHD level of 20 ng/mL.[24] This result has been determined experimentally in a recent dose-ranging study and the findings are identical (**Fig. 5**).[39] This study is the first to show that serum 25OHD is regulated and is most likely attributable to formation of 24,25$(OH)_2$D, the inactive metabolite. Formation of 24,25$(OH)_2$D is the essential step preventing vitamin D intoxication from a high intake, another regulatory step in skin

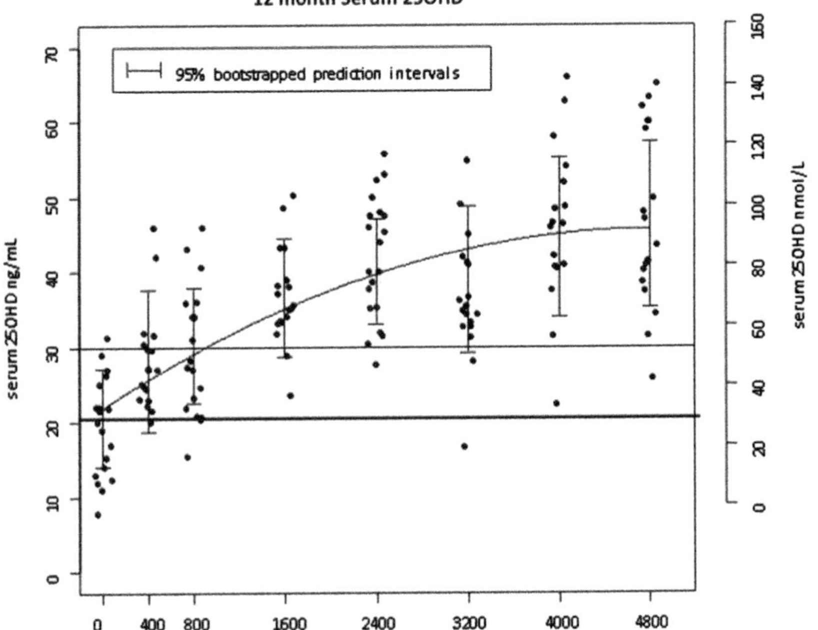

Fig. 5. Dose response of vitamin D on serum 25OHD.

prevents vitamin D intoxication from sunlight. Because serum 25OHD levels plateau at a mean serum 25OHD level of 45 ng/mL, it would appear that the homeostatic vitamin D system does not need higher levels in healthy people. If reaching a serum 25OHD level higher than 20 ng/mL is the objective, then 600 to 880 IU will achieve this point in 97.5% of people, satisfying the criteria for the RDA, and 400 IU will meet the needs of 50% of the population (Estimated Average Requirement [EAR]).

Other supporting data were derived from fracture studies. A vitamin D dosage of 800 IU with calcium was shown to be effective in reducing fractures in the most recent meta-analysis performed for the IOM.[40] Thus, the evidence suggests that an 800 IU vitamin D dosage with calcium increases serum 25OHD to higher than 20 ng/mL and reduces fractures, and that it is not necessary to exceed a serum level of 30 ng/mL for bone efficacy. The preceding discussion applies only to the calcium and bone and may not apply to other diseases of interest, such as cancer and diabetes. Only clinical trials using different vitamin D dosages together with measurement of serum 25OHD can provide an answer in the future.

In Europe, the issue of severe vitamin D deficiency is more of a problem because average serum 25OHD levels are much lower, at approximately 10 to 15 ng/mL. In a recent study of bone biopsies performed at autopsy, 97.5% of cases of osteomalacia occurred at a serum 25OHD level lower than 20 ng/mL.[41] Interestingly, most bone biopsies did not show osteomalacia at serum 25OHD levels lower than 5 ng/mL for unclear reasons, although it is possible that in many of these cases, a high dietary intake of calcium and phosphorus prevented osteomalacia. The evidence-based recommendations by the IOM for the new dietary reference intakes (DRIs) are provided in **Table 2**.

TOXICITY OF VITAMIN D

Vitamin D intoxication can occur at dosages of more than 20,000 IU daily over the long term or a serum 25OHD level of 200 ng/mL, overwhelming the 24,24$(OH)_2$D inactivation step. The resultant hypercalcemia suppresses PTH, acting as a second regulatory step against developing vitamin D intoxication by decreasing 1,25$(OH)_2$D production. However, if the high vitamin D dosage is continued, it appears that at very high levels, serum 25OHD can bind to the VDR and simulate the effect of 1,25$(OH)_2$D.

Table 2
Calcium and vitamin D intake recommendations for those older than 50 years

Vitamin D	EAR IU/d	RDA IU/d
Men, 51–70 y	400	600
Women, 51–70 y	400	600
Men + women >70 y	400	800
Calcium	**EAR mg/d**	**RDA mg/d**
Men, 51–70 y	800	1000
Women, 51–70 y	1000	1200
>70 y	1000	1200

Abbreviations: EAR, Estimated Average Requirement; RDA, Recommended Dietary Allowance.
Data from Institute of Medicine. Dietary reference intakes for calcium and vitamin D. Washington, DC: The National Academies Press; 2011. Available at: http://www.ncbi.nlm.nih.gov/books/NBK56072.

Most data on vitamin D intoxication are derived from case studies of accidental vitamin D overdosing. In deriving a Tolerable Upper Limit (TUL) for vitamin D, the IOM agreed that 20,000 IU daily or more would increase the chance of vitamin D intoxication, and that because of safety concerns and reports that serum 25OHD levels higher than 50 ng/mL were associated with increased mortality rates,[42,43] 4000 IU should represent the TUL. The TUL should not be confused with the recommended dose. It is possible that the TUL is less in older people, those with impaired renal function, or those who take calcium supplements.

EFFECT OF VITAMIN D AND CALCIUM ON OSTEOPOROSIS AND FRACTURES

Osteoporosis is a one of the common diseases of aging. Management of osteoporosis using vitamin D and calcium has been in practice for almost 30 years. However, the role of vitamin D and calcium in fracture prevention is an area of controversy, with varying results of meta-analyses depending on their criteria for inclusion. The most recent meta-analysis was based on an analysis performed for the IOM report,[40] although it was essentially the same as a previously reported analysis, because only 2 more studies were included.[44]

There have been 12 studies of vitamin D plus calcium and 5 of vitamin D alone compared with a placebo or calcium control group. In the vitamin D plus calcium trials, there was a difference between community free-living adults and institutionalized individuals in the findings. In the community trials, the effect of vitamin D plus calcium reduction on fractures was nonsignificant, with a relative risk of 0.89 (95% confidence interval 0.76–1.04). In the institutional studies, there was a significant reduction in hip fractures of almost 30%, with a relative risk of 0.71 (95% confidence interval 0.57–0.89). The vitamin D dose varied from 300 to 800 IU across studies, but the 800 IU dose was most commonly used and the calcium dose was usually 1000 mg; therefore, vitamin D 800 IU and calcium 1000 mg are the standard daily recommended doses.

ARE THE EFFECTS OF VITAMIN D AND CALCIUM ON FRACTURES RELATED TO SERUM 25OHD?

Most evidence suggests that a serum 25OHD higher than 20 ng/mL is sufficient for skeletal health. This conclusion is based on 5 large studies totaling 6562 subjects that show a higher rate of hip fracture in women and men with serum 25OHD lower than 20 ng/mL.[45] The evidence linking clinical nonvertebral fractures to low serum 25OHD differs between men and women and by ethnicity. In men, nonhip fractures are more frequent only in those with serum 25OHD lower than 20 ng/mL.[46] In white women, nonhip fractures are significantly lower in groups with serum 25OHD of higher than 20 ng/mL compared with lower than 20 ng/mL.[47] However, the opposite is found in African American and Asian women, namely fracture events are more common in the groups when serum 25OHD is higher than 20 ng/mL compared with lower than 20 ng/mL. These results are based on cohort studies and the accuracy of reporting fractures is approximately 80%. Larger prospective studies are needed to confirm these results.

Evidence to link a specific serum 25OHD threshold to treatment with vitamin D is not clear. In half the studies, the baseline serum 25OHD level was higher than 20 ng/mL, and efficacy does not appear to differ whether the baseline starts above or below 20 ng/mL. Another issue is that almost all studies used a single dose, so that a threshold dose cannot be defined. Furthermore, meta-analyses that try to define a threshold response based on serum 25OHD measurements are challenging because serum 25OHD values have been performed with different assays over 30 years and no external independent standards were common to these assays.

FALLS

Although there has been a claim that vitamin D reduces falls, these studies have been affected by the same problems as fracture studies, including small numbers, variable duration from 6 weeks to 1 year, differing doses of vitamin D, and variation in amounts of calcium supplements. The analytic design of a meta-analysis that showed a positive effect of vitamin D on falls has been questioned, and the IOM analysis of the same data did not a significant effect of vitamin D on falls.[24] An adequately powered trial is required to answer this question definitively. There is some evidence that calcitriol reduces falls, especially in older people with a GFR less than 60 mL/min,[48–50] and it may be that in those older than 80 years, reduced conversion of vitamin D to calcitriol reduces the effect of vitamin D on falls.

SUMMARY

Age-related changes affect vitamin D metabolism and reduce the nutritional status of the elderly. A vitamin D supplement is recommended in the elderly. The optimal total calcium intake is unclear. In the absence of adequate safety data, it is suggested that total calcium intake be limited to 1000 to 1200 mg daily, because of a 35% incidence of hypercalciuria or hypercalcemia in women taking low doses of vitamin D who have a total calcium intake of 1200 mg daily.[39] Increasing calcium from dietary sources may be safer than supplements, and requires increasing the intake of dairy products or other vitamin D and calcium-fortified foods. The RDA value is listed on every food and vitamin either as the actual amount or as a percentage of the RDA. For example, if the RDA for vitamin D is 800 IU and a multivitamin contains 1000 IU, the multivitamin provides 125% of the RDA. It has been common practice to supplement dairy products in the United States, Canada, and Scandinavian countries. In North America, milk is fortified with 400 IU per quart. An 8-oz glass of milk provides 80 IU of vitamin D and 250 mg calcium. Evidence suggests that vitamin D and calcium nutrition can be improved in the elderly by increasing the vitamin D intake to 800 IU daily together with calcium 1000 mg daily. This combination is a simple inexpensive strategy that can reduce fractures in institutionalized individuals by 30%.

REFERENCES

1. DeLuca HF. Overview of general physiologic features and functions of vitamin D. Am J Clin Nutr 2004;80:1689S–96S.
2. Bullamore JR, Gallagher JC, Wilkinson R, et al. Effect of age on calcium absorption. Lancet 1970;II:535–7.
3. Ireland P, Fordtran JS. Effect of dietary calcium and age on jejunal calcium absorption in human studies by intestinal perfusion. J Clin Invest 1973;52:2672–81.
4. Gallagher JC, Riggs BL, Eisman J, et al. Intestinal calcium absorption and serum vitamin D metabolites in normal subjects and osteoporotic patients. J Clin Invest 1979;64:729–36.
5. Pike JW. Vitamin D3 receptors: structure and function in transcription. Annu Rev Nutr 1991;11:189–216.
6. Li YC, Pirro AE, Amling M, et al. Targeted ablation of the vitamin D receptor: an animal model of vitamin D-dependent rickets type II with alopecia. Proc Natl Acad Sci U S A 1997;94:9831–5.

7. Sheikh MS, Ramirez A, Emmett M, et al. Role of vitamin D dependent and vitamin D independent mechanisms in absorption of food calcium. J Clin Invest 1988;81: 126–32.
8. Akhter S, Kutuzova GD, Christakos S, et al. Calbindin D9k is not required for 1,25-dihydroxyvitamin D3-mediated Ca2+ absorption in small intestine. Arch Biochem Biophys 2007;460(2):227–32.
9. Kutuzova GD, Sundersingh F, Vaughan J, et al. TRPV6 is not required for 1alpha,25-dihydroxyvitamin D3-induced intestinal calcium absorption in vivo. Proc Natl Acad Sci U S A 2008;105(50):19655–9.
10. Benn BS, Ajibade D, Porta A, et al. Active intestinal calcium transport in the absence of transient receptor potential vanilloid type 6 and calbindin-D9k. Endocrinology 2008;149(6):3196–205.
11. Fujita H, Sugimoto K, Inatomi S, et al. Tight junction proteins claudin-2 and -12 are critical for vitamin D-dependent Ca2+ absorption between enterocytes. Mol Biol Cell 2008;19(5):1912–21.
12. Francis RM, Peacock M, Taylor GA, et al. Calcium malabsorption in elderly women with vertebral fractures: evidence for resistance to the action of vitamin D metabolites on the bowel. Clin Sci (Lond) 1984;66:103–7.
13. Kinyamu HK, Gallagher JC, Balhorn KE, et al. Serum vitamin D metabolites and calcium absorption in normal and elderly free-living women and in women in nursing homes. Am J Clin Nutr 1997;65:790–7.
14. Gallagher JC, Jerpbak CM, Jee WS, et al. 1,25-Dihydroxyvitamin D3: short- and long-term effects on bone and calcium metabolism in patients with postmenopausal osteoporosis. Proc Natl Acad Sci U S A 1982;79(10):3325.
15. Horst RL, Goff JP, Reinhardt TA. Advancing age results in reduction of intestinal and bone 1,25-dihydroxyvitamin D receptor. Endocrinology 1990;126:1053–7.
16. Ebeling PR, Sandgren ME, DiMagno EP, et al. Evidence of an age-related decrease in intestinal responsiveness to vitamin D: relationship between serum 1,25-dihydroxyvitamin D3 and intestinal vitamin D receptor concentrations in normal women. J Clin Endocrinol Metab 1992;75:176–82.
17. Kinyamu HK, Gallagher JC, Prahl JM, et al. Association between intestinal vitamin D receptor, calcium absorption, and serum 1,25 dihydroxyvitamin D in normal young and elderly women. J Bone Miner Res 1996;11:1400–5.
18. Tsai KS, Heath H III, Kumar R, et al. Impaired vitamin D metabolism with aging in women. Possible role in pathogenesis of senile osteoporosis. J Clin Invest 1984; 73:1668–72.
19. Kinyamu HK, Gallagher JC, Petranick KM, et al. Effect of parathyroid hormone (hPTH[1-34]) infusion on serum 1,25-dihydroxyvitamin D and parathyroid hormone in normal women. J Bone Miner Res 1996;11(10):1400–5.
20. MacLaughlin J, Holick MF. Aging decreases the capacity of human skin to produce vitamin D3. J Clin Invest 1985;76:1536–8.
21. Bouillon RA, Auwerx JH, Lissens WD, et al. Vitamin D status in the elderly: seasonal substrate deficiency causes 1,25-dihydroxycholecalciferol deficiency. Am J Clin Nutr 1987;45:755–63.
22. Need AG, O'Loughlin PD, Morris HA, et al. Vitamin D metabolites and calcium absorption in severe vitamin D deficiency. J Bone Miner Res 2008;23:1859–63.
23. Bailey RL, Dodd KW, Goldman JA, et al. Estimation of total usual calcium and vitamin D intakes in the United States. J Nutr 2010;140(4):817–22.
24. Institute of Medicine. Dietary reference intakes for calcium and vitamin D. Washington, DC: The National Academies Press; 2011. Available at: http://www.ncbi.nlm.nih.gov/books/NBK56072.

25. Rapuri PB, Kinyamu HK, Gallagher JC, et al. Seasonal changes in calciotropic hormones, bone markers, and bone mineral density in elderly women. J Clin Endocrinol Metab 2002;87:2024–32.
26. WHO Scientific Group on the Prevention and Management of Osteoporosis. Prevention and management of osteoporosis: report of a WHO scientific group. Geneva (Switzerland): World Health Organization; 2003.
27. Holick MF, Binkley NC, Bischoff-Ferrari HA, et al. Evaluation, treatment, and prevention of vitamin D deficiency: an Endocrine Society clinical practice guideline. J Clin Endocrinol Metab 2011;96:1911–30.
28. Looker AC, Johnson CL, Lacher DA, et al. Vitamin D status: United States (2001–2006). NCHS data brief, no 59. Hyattsville (MD): National Center for Health Statistics; 2011.
29. Taylor CL, Carriquiry AL, Bailey RL, et al. Appropriateness of the probability approach with a nutrient status biomarker to assess population inadequacy: a study using vitamin D. Am J Clin Nutr 2012;97(1):72–8.
30. Bruyere O, Decock C, Delhez M, et al. Highest prevalence of vitamin D inadequacy in institutionalized women compared with non-institutionalized women: a case–control study. Womens Health (Lond Engl) 2009;5(1):49–54.
31. Cashman KD, Muldowney S, McNulty B, et al. Vitamin D status of Irish adults: findings from the National Adult Nutrition Survey. Br J Nutr 2012;10:1–9.
32. Gaugris S, Heaney RP, Boonen S, et al. Vitamin D inadequacy among postmenopausal women: a systematic review. QJM 2005;98(9):667–76.
33. Glerup H, Mikkelsen K, Poulsen L, et al. Commonly recommended daily intake of vitamin D is not sufficient if sunlight exposure is limited. J Intern Med 2000;247:260–8.
34. Sai AJ, Walters RW, Fang X, et al. Relationship between vitamin D, parathyroid hormone and bone health. J Clin Endocrinol Metab 2011;18:1101–12.
35. Valcour A, Blocki F, Hawkins DM, et al. Effects of age and serum 25-OH-Vitamin D on serum parathyroid hormone levels. J Clin Endocrinol Metab 2012;97:3989–99.
36. Sahota O, Mundey MK, San P, et al. The relationship between vitamin D and parathyroid hormone: calcium homeostasis, bone turnover, and bone mineral density in postmenopausal women with established osteoporosis. Bone 2004;35:312–9.
37. Gallagher JC, Yalamanchili V, Smith LM. The effect of vitamin D on calcium absorption in older women. J Clin Endocrinol Metab 2012;97(10):3550–6.
38. Ensrud KE, Taylor BC, Paudel ML, et al. Osteoporotic Fractures in Men Study Group. Serum 25-hydroxyvitamin D levels and rate of hip bone loss in older men. J Clin Endocrinol Metab 2009;94:2773–80.
39. Gallagher JC, Sai AJ, Templin TJ, et al. Dose response to vitamin D supplementation in postmenopausal women 2011 A randomized clinical trial. Ann Intern Med 2012;156:425–37.
40. Chung M, Lee J, Terasawa T, et al. Vitamin D with or without calcium supplementation for prevention of cancer and fractures: an updated meta-analysis for the U.S. Preventive Services Task Force. Ann Intern Med 2011;155(12):827–38.
41. Priemel M, von Domarus C, Klatte TO, et al. Bone mineralization defects and vitamin D deficiency: histomorphometric analysis of iliac crest bone biopsies and circulating 25-hydroxyvitamin D in 675 patients. J Bone Miner Res 2010;25:305–11.
42. Melamed ML, Michos ED, Post W, et al. Serum 25-Hydroxyvitamin D levels and the risk of mortality in the general population. Arch Intern Med 2008;168:1629–37.

43. Durup D, Jørgensen HL, Christensen J, et al. A reverse J-shaped association of all-cause mortality with serum 25-hydroxyvitamin D in general practice: the CopD study. J Clin Endocrinol Metab 2012;97(8):2644–52.
44. Ward CA, Moher D, Hanley DA, et al. Effectiveness and safety of Vitamin D in relation to bone health. Evidence report/technology assessment No. 158. (Prepared by the University of Ottawa. Evidence-based Practice Center (UO-EPC) under Contract No. 290-02-0021). AHRQ Publication No. 07-E013. Rockville (MD): Agency for Healthcare Research and Quality; 2007.
45. Gallagher JC, Sai AJ. Vitamin D insufficiency, deficiency, and bone health. J Clin Endocrinol Metab 2010;95:2630–3.
46. Cauley JA, Parimi N, Ensrud KE, et al. Osteoporotic fractures in men research G. Serum 25-hydroxyvitamin D and the risk of hip and nonspine fractures in older men. J Bone Miner Res 2012;25:545–53.
47. Cauley JA, Danielson ME, Boudreau R, et al. Serum 25-hydroxyvitamin D and clinical fracture risk in a multiethnic cohort of women: the Women's Health Initiative (WHI). J Bone Miner Res 2011;26:2378–88.
48. Francis RM, Peacock M, Barkworth SA. Renal impairment and its effects on calcium metabolism in elderly women. Age Ageing 1984;13:14–22.
49. Gallagher JC, Rapuri P, Smith L. Falls are associated with decreased renal function and insufficient calcitriol production by the kidney. J Steroid Biochem Mol Biol 2007;103:610–3.
50. Dukas L, Schacht E, Runge M. Independent from muscle power and balance performance, a creatinine clearance below 65 ml/min is a significant and independent risk factor for falls and fall-related fractures in elderly men and women diagnosed with osteoporosis. Osteoporos Int 2012;21:1237–45.

Diabetes and Altered Glucose Metabolism with Aging

Rita Rastogi Kalyani, MD, MHS[a,*], Josephine M. Egan, MD[b]

KEYWORDS

• Diabetes • Aging • Insulin resistance • Beta-cell dysfunction

KEY POINTS

- Adults aged 60 and over have more than twice the prevalence of diabetes compared with younger age groups. The number of older persons with diabetes will continue to grow as the population ages.
- Abnormal glucose metabolism is associated with aging but is not a necessary component.
- Older persons with diabetes and/or abnormal glucose metabolism may be at higher risk of developing adverse geriatric syndromes, such as accelerated muscle loss, functional disability, and frailty.
- Goals of care for older persons with diabetes need to be individualized and consider treatment of symptomatic hyperglycemia, prevention of long-term complications, avoidance of hypoglycemia, and preservation of quality of life.
- Lifestyle modifications, in particular, regular exercise as tolerated, and pharmacologic therapies that account for the presence of comorbid renal and hepatic impairments or physical and cognitive limitations are important components of diabetes management in older adults.

EPIDEMIOLOGY OF DIABETES AND IMPAIRED GLUCOSE STATES WITH AGING

Diabetes in older adults is a growing public health concern, with almost one-third of US adults over the age of 60 years having diabetes, of whom approximately half are undiagnosed; an additional one-third of older adults have prediabetes.[1] Diabetes prevalence in older adults is more than twice that of middle-aged adults.[1] It is projected that the numbers of elderly persons will approximately double by the year

Funding Sources: This work is supported in part by the National Institute of Diabetes and Digestive and Kidney Diseases (R.R. Kalyani; K23DK093583) and the Intramural Research Program/National Institutes of Health, and the National Institute on Aging (J.M. Egan).
Conflict of Interest: None.
[a] Division of Endocrinology and Metabolism, Department of Medicine, Johns Hopkins University School of Medicine, The Johns Hopkins University, 1830 East Monument Street, Suite 333, Baltimore, MD 21287, USA; [b] National Institute on Aging/National Institutes of Health, Suite 100, Room 8C222, 251 Bayview Boulevard, Baltimore, MD 21224, USA
* Corresponding author.
E-mail address: rrastogi@jhmi.edu

Endocrinol Metab Clin N Am 42 (2013) 333–347
http://dx.doi.org/10.1016/j.ecl.2013.02.010 **endo.theclinics.com**
0889-8529/13/$ – see front matter

2030.[2,3] In addition, the number of people in nursing homes with diabetes continues to increase.[4] Consequently, the burden of diabetes in the elderly is significant and growing.

Glucose intolerance is associated with aging.[1,5–7] Aging has been associated with elevated levels of both glucose and insulin after oral glucose challenge testing.[8] The 2-hour plasma glucose during an oral glucose tolerance test (OGTT) rises much more steeply than fasting glucose levels with aging.[8–10] As a result, elderly individuals are more likely to be classified as having abnormal glucose status compared with younger adults using similar diagnostic criteria for diabetes.[11] Some investigators have suggested that the diagnosis of diabetes can be made many years earlier using OGTT versus fasting glucose levels alone in older persons.[12] Data from the Baltimore Longitudinal Study of Aging demonstrate an age-related increase in progression rate from normal glucose status to impaired glucose tolerance that is almost twice the progression rate from normal to impaired fasting glucose after 20 years of follow-up.[12] These findings suggest that OGTT, in particular, is important to consider when characterizing abnormal glucose status in the elderly.

ALTERED GLUCOSE METABOLISM WITH AGING

Using hyperinsulinemic-euglycemic clamp methodology as a method for quantification of insulin effectiveness in regulating glucose transport into tissues, whole-body insulin sensitivity is demonstrably reduced in older versus younger adults.[13,14] Impaired intracellular whole-body rates of glucose oxidation in elderly versus young adults have also been reported.[15] Potential explanations for reduced insulin effectiveness with aging include (1) increased abdominal fat mass, (2) decreased physical activity, (3) sarcopenia, (4) mitochondrial dysfunction, (5) hormonal changes (ie, lower insulinlike growth factor 1 and dehydroepiandrosterone), and (6) increased oxidative stress and inflammation.[16] Nonetheless, insulin sensitivity decreases with age even after adjustment for differences in adiposity, fat distribution, and physical activity.[17]

Beta-cell dysfunction with aging is also a significant contributing factor to abnormal glucose metabolism. Insulin secretion is most commonly tested using an OGTT; it is standardized, simple to administer, and widely used in longitudinal studies. An oral load of 75 g of glucose is delivered as a rapid bolus to the gut and can trigger neural and incretin responses, over and beyond stimulus by the glucose per se, to the insulin-secreting β-cells. Responses to physiologic stimuli, such as a meal containing complex carbohydrates, fat, and protein, may be different from that of a glucose load. With those limitations in mind, there is a gradual decline with aging in insulin secretion during the first hour in response to an oral glucose load, despite older adults having higher glucose levels after the glucose challenge.[18,19] Once plasma glucose levels reach the diabetic range, however, insulin secretion is severely compromised.[20]

β-Cell function has also been evaluated using the hyperglycemic clamp, in which plasma glucose levels are increased in a square wave fashion and maintained at this level for a fixed duration of time in a controlled manner. The final attained stable (or clamped) plasma glucose level can be varied and insulin secretion studied with clamped plasma glucose levels as high as 450 mg/dL.[13] The β-cell response to a hyperglycemic clamp is stereotypical in that there is a first-phase insulin secretion that occurs within 2 to 3 minutes of the initiation of the square wave of infused glucose, followed by a slower plateau phase that reaches stability in approximately 100 to 120 minutes. In general, among older adults with normal glucose tolerance based on the OGTT, deficits in insulin secretion are seen only when high plasma glucose levels are achieved when compared with the young. But, as with all patients with type 2 diabetes mellitus, once an elderly patient has developed diabetes, the first-phase insulin secretion in response to the square wave of a hyperglycemic clamp is defective to absent,[13] and the plateau-phase insulin secretion is less than in nondiabetic subjects.

Insulin secretion falls under 2 types: constitutive (sometimes called basal) and stimulated (such as occurs after a meal, an OGTT, or hyperglycemic clamp), with constitutive insulin accounting for approximately 50% of the total 24-hour insulin output. Insulin secretion is pulsatile in nature. Using 1-minute blood sampling and highly sensitive insulin assays, rapid, low-amplitude insulin pulses occurring approximately every 8 to 14 minutes and larger-amplitude ultradian pulses occurring every 60 to 140 minutes can be elucidated.[21] The rapid pulses persist even in isolated islets and are independent of circulating glucose levels whereas the ultradian pulses are tightly coupled to glucose, by which they are entrained. In the fasting state, elderly subjects without diabetes have disorderly pulsatile insulin secretion, with reduced amplitude and mass of the rapid pulses and decreased frequency of the ultradian pulses. Scheen and colleagues[22] and Meneilly and colleagues[23] studied pulsatile insulin secretion in young and elderly subjects under conditions of sustained experimentally induced hyperglycemia. Overall, the findings were similar to the fasting state; specifically, older subjects displayed reduced amplitude and mass of the rapid insulin pulses, and the ultradian pulses were more irregular with lower amplitude compared to younger subjects. The investigators also found that glucose infusion for up to 53 hours[22] was not capable of normalizing pulsatile insulin secretion in older individuals. Pulsatile insulin secretion is important for regulating glucose output from the liver and may be involved in maintaining skeletal muscle in a state of metabolic readiness, such as maintaining insulin receptors and glucose transporters in a primed state. The disordered pulsatile insulin secretion seen in the elderly may play a role in the previously described decrease in insulin sensitivity observed with aging. In type 2 diabetes mellitus, severe disorderliness is found because the oscillatory pattern of insulin secretion is almost totally disrupted. The rapid pulses are replaced by irregular pulses of short duration, and the ultradian pulses are disrupted, chaotic, and uncoupled from glucose, because glucose fails to control the periodicity of the ultradian pulses.[24]

Rising plasma glucose accounts for approximately 50% of the secreted insulin after a meal or OGTT; the remaining 50% is due to incretin hormones released from the enteroendocrine cells lining the gut.[25] Incretins are peptide hormones, of which there are 2 main types: gastric inhibitory polypeptide (GIP) and glucagon-like peptide 1 (GLP-1). Their effect on β-cells is to increase glucose-dependent insulin secretion. There is no evidence that secretion of incretins, as measured by plasma levels after OGTT, is defective in aging per se, although the β-cell may be less responsive to their stimulatory effects. In an elegant study, Elahi and colleagues[26] combined the hyperglycemic clamp with oral glucose (to stimulate endogenous GIP secretion) and found that, in older individuals, GIP secretion in response to the oral glucose was increased compared with that in younger participants but led to slightly lower insulin secretion in response to the endogenous GIP. Hyperglycemic clamps at 100 mg/dL and 230 mg/dL above basal have been performed in young and elderly subjects[27] with combined GIP infusions. At the lower clamped plasma glucose level, the potentiation of glucose-induced insulin secretion by GIP was reduced by half in the elderly compared with the young, whereas at the higher clamped plasma glucose level, insulin response to GIP was similar in both age groups. Becuase the lower clamped plasma glucose level is more physiologic, however, this probably reflects a true decline in GIP effectiveness with aging. In type 2 diabetes mellitus, GIP no longer potentiates glucose-induced insulin secretion and also increases glucagon secretion, which exacerbates hyperglycemia[28]; however, GIP secretion is not lower in type 2 diabetes mellitus compared with nondiabetic subjects.[25] The data on GLP-1 secretion with increasing age and onset of type 2 diabetes mellitus are similar to those of GIP in that secretion of GLP-1 is not necessarily decreased with older age or the presence of diabetes but, unlike GIP, GLP-1 is still a powerful stimulus to insulin secretion—hence, the robust development of several agents for treating type 2 diabetes mellitus that activate the GLP-1 receptor on β-cells (ie, exenatide and liragulatide). Also, unlike GIP, use of GLP-1 receptor agonists leads to a decrease in glucagon secretion.[25]

The enzyme, dipeptidyl-peptidase 4 (DPP 4), inactivates both GIP and GLP-1 and has decreasing activity with older age,[29] which may explain the higher GIP levels observed in the elderly.[26] The recent development of DPP 4 inhibitors (ie, sitagliptin, saxagliptin, and linagliptin) as therapeutic agents may also have a role for treatment of diabetes in the elderly.

COMPLICATIONS OF DIABETES IN THE ELDERLY

Microvascular and macrovascular complications of diabetes occur in older patients, similar to younger persons, although the absolute risk of cardiovascular disease is much higher in older adults.[30] Diabetes in the older adult population, however, is heterogeneous and includes individuals with both middle age–onset and elderly-onset diabetes,[31] with the latter group accounting for up to one-third of older adults with diabetes. Middle age–onset adults may have worse glycemic control and are more likely to be taking glucose-lowering medications. Whereas the prevalence of macrovascular diseases (stroke, coronary heart disease, and peripheral arterial disease) may be similar between the middle age–onset and elderly-onset diabetes groups, the burden of microvascular disease (particularly retinopathy) may be greater in the former.[31,32] Thus, the age of diabetes onset may have an impact on the burden of disease and diabetic complications present in elderly patients with diabetes, but more studies need to be done.

GERIATRIC SYNDROMES ASSOCIATED WITH DIABETES

Descriptions of otherwise healthy centenarians without impaired glucose uptake suggest that insulin resistance is not a necessary component of the aging process.[33,34] Instead, older adults with abnormal glucose status and diabetes likely represent a vulnerable subset at high risk for adverse outcomes. Geriatric syndromes that have been described to occur more frequently in persons with diabetes include loss of muscle function, functional limitations and disability, and frailty—all of which can have a significant impact on quality of life in older patients—in addition to early mortality (**Fig. 1**). Diabetes also increases the risk of other common geriatric syndromes, such as depression, cognitive dysfunction, chronic pain, injurious falls, urinary incontinence, and polypharmacy,[30] but is not specifically discussed in this article.

Loss of Muscle Function

Previous studies of older adults with diabetes have demonstrated decreased muscle strength and mass, especially in the lower extremities.[35] Older adults with type 2 diabetes mellitus have approximately 50% more rapid decline in knee extensor strength than those without diabetes over a 3-year period,[36] suggesting that decreased muscle strength is a consequence of type 2 diabetes mellitus, with similar findings for muscle mass.[37] Disease duration and severity may have a role in the decreased muscle strength observed among persons with diabetes. Park and colleagues[35] reported that leg muscle quality was lowest in older adults with diabetes (mean age 74 years)

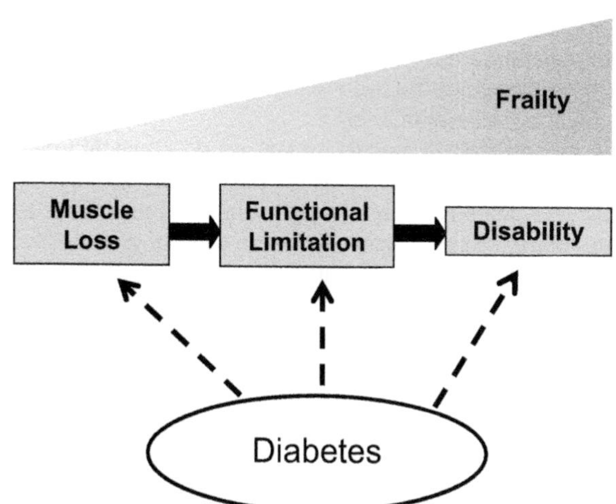

Fig. 1. Diabetes and the pathway to disability. Proposed associations of diabetes with each step in the pathway to disability are depicted. Accelerated loss of muscle mass and strength, particularly in the lower extremities, may lead to functional limitations in routine tasks of daily living, which may ultimately result in physical disability among older persons with diabetes. Frailty is a geriatric syndrome that encompasses the full spectrum of the disability process and is also more common with impaired glucose states and diabetes.

who had the longest diabetes duration (≥6 years) or most severe hyperglycemia (hemoglobin A_{1c} [HbA_{1c}] >8%). Even among persons without diabetes, associations between hyperglycemia and insulin resistance with decreased muscle mass and strength, have been described.[38–40]

In older adults, skeletal muscle protein synthesis may be resistant to the anabolic action of insulin.[41,42] Insulin resistance is also associated with activation of muscle proteolysis pathways,[43] which may further lead to muscle loss. In turn, muscle is the primary site for insulin-dependent glucose uptake, and reduced muscle surface area for insulin-mediated glucose uptake may aggravate peripheral insulin resistance, leading to a vicious cycle. Oral insulin sensitizers have been reported to preserve muscle mass[44] although similar associations for muscle strength have yet to be investigated. Skeletal muscle mitochondrial function is reduced in type 2 diabetes mellitus and may be improved with peripheral insulin sensitization.[45,46]

Potential pathways underlying the association of diabetes with reduced muscle function include the presence of comorbidities, such as peripheral neuropathy, which may mediate these associations[47,48]; however, decreased leg muscle strength is present even after accounting for lower extremity nerve dysfunction in diabetes.[49] Diabetes is associated with inflammatory markers, which in turn may also lead to impaired muscle function.[50,51]

Functional Limitations and Physical Disability

In the general population, muscle strength is a predictor of functional limitations and disability.[52] Persons with diabetes perform worse on objective measures of lower extremity physical performance, such as walking, chair stands, and tandem stand.[53] Slower walking speed in persons with type 2 diabetes mellitus has been demonstrated.[53,54] The greatest differences have been observed, however, at maximal walking speeds.[55] There is some evidence that impaired muscle function mediates the association of diabetes with lower gait speed in older adults.[54] Severe hyperglycemia and insulin resistance have also been associated, however, with walking difficulties and poorer performance-based measures of lower extremity function both in persons with and without diabetes.[53,56,57]

Similarly, diabetes can have a significant impact on physical functioning, such as lower extremity mobility, potentially mediated through effects on muscle function.[58] Functional disability or difficulty in performing routine physical tasks is more common in older adults with diabetes compared with those without diabetes.[57–64] Older adults with diabetes have significantly greater difficulty in a range of routine physical activities, including walking a quarter mile, climbing stairs, reaching overhead, doing housework, bathing, eating, and participating in leisure activities compared with their counterparts. Up to 70% of adults with diabetes have difficulties performing these tasks of everyday living.[64]

The higher prevalence of functional disability in older adults with diabetes may be related to the presence of comorbidities, such as cardiovascular disease, vision loss, obesity, and arthritis.[59,63,64] These comorbidities may be associated with decreased cardiopulmonary reserve or restricted physical movement, which contributes to physical disability. These factors, however, do not consistently explain the association of diabetes with disability; the degree of glycemic control is also related to disability among older adults with diabetes.[57,64,65] Support for an association between hyperglycemia and disability comes from previous studies reporting a significant correlation between higher HbA_{1c} levels and disability.[57,65] Alternatively, physical and cognitive impairment may affect ability to self-manage diabetes and lead to poorer glycemic control; thus, the relationship between hyperglycemia and disability is likely bidirectional and requires further investigation.

Frailty Syndrome

Diabetes has been associated with the presence of frailty, a geriatric condition of physiologic vulnerability to stressors associated with adverse outcomes, such as disability and mortality.[66–69] Frailty increases with age and is distinguished by a characteristic phenotype. A common definition includes the presence of 3 or more of the following criteria: unintentional weight loss, self-reported exhaustion, muscle weakness (poor grip strength), slow walking speed, or low physical activity.[67]

Recent literature has suggested an association between insulin resistance and frailty[16,70] in cross-sectional studies of persons with and without diabetes. Altered glucose-insulin dynamics has also been reported in frail women compared with their counterparts with 120-minute post-OGTT levels of both glucose and insulin discriminating frailty status better compared with fasting values.[71,72] Similar alterations in glucose dynamics have also been described in frail older adults who underwent a mixed meal test and had a more exaggerated and prolonged glucose response after 2 hours compared with nonfrail older adults.[73] These studies suggest relative insulin resistance in frail older adults compared with nonfrail older adults.

The presence of hyperglycemia and insulin resistance is also temporally related to the subsequent development of frailty in longitudinal cohort studies.[53,74] In the Cardiovascular Health Study, homeostasis model–insulin resistance was calculated based on fasting glucose and insulin levels. For every standard deviation increment in homeostasis model–insulin resistance, the adjusted hazard ratio for frailty was 1.15 (95% CI, 1.02–1.31).[74] Individuals who eventually developed frailty were also more likely, in parallel, to develop diabetes compared with older adults who never developed frailty (8.6% vs 4.2%). Thus, the association between frailty and abnormal glucose status is likely bidirectional. In the Women's Health and Aging Study, older vomen in the highest HbA_{1c} category (≥8%) compared with lowest HbA_{1c} category <5.5%) had a significant 3-fold increased risk for the development of frailty, with nost events occurring in the highest HbA_{1c} category.[53] These findings suggest that ıyperglycemia, particularly in the diabetic range, can predict the onset of incident railty less than a decade later.[53]

The underlying physiologic mechanisms relating insulin resistance to the develop-nent of frailty remain unclear. Frail older adults have a higher burden of inflammatory narkers that may also affect glucose metabolism.[71,75,76] Hyperglycemia may further ıctivate inflammatory pathways that subsequently cause muscle catabolism and lisability as part of the frailty process.[77] Frail women on average are also more likely o be obese, which may be associated with chronic inflammation.[72,78] One study ɔund that only frail obese adults, but not frail lean adults, had reduced insulin sensi-ivity versus nonfrail counterparts.[16] Another study found, however, that associations of insulin resistance and frailty are independent of obesity.[72] In addition, chronic ıyperglycemia may be a risk factor for cardiovascular disease, which, in turn, has een associated with frailty[79]; however, the presence of cardiovascular disease loes not fully explain these associations. Thus, underlying mechanisms linking hyper-glycemia with frailty remain unclear but are likely multifactorial.[80]

'arly Mortality

)iabetes in older adults is associated with increased disability, frailty, and accelerated nuscle loss. These adverse geriatric syndromes can be associated with both ncreased health care expenditures[81,82] and early mortality.[66,69,83] On average, ersons with diabetes have an almost 2-fold increased risk of death from any cause, vith 40% of this difference in survival due to nonvascular deaths.[84] Results from the 3altimore Longitudinal Study of Aging demonstrate higher total and cardiovascular nortality even in older adults with impaired glucose tolerance compared with those vith normal glucose metabolism.[85,86] A J-shaped association of HbA_{1c} with mortality ıas also been described, with increased mortality rates seen at higher levels of HbA_{1c} ut also, to a lesser degree, at lower HbA_{1c} levels.[87,88] Reduced length and activity of he telomerase enzyme, which maintains stability of chromosomes with aging, has een linked to impaired glucose-stimulated insulin islet secretion and may also nderlie these epidemiologic associations but is currently still an area of active nvestigation.[89]

'REATMENT OF DIABETES IN THE ELDERLY

iuidelines

'he goals of diabetes care in older patients with diabetes include (1) control of hyper-glycemia, (2) prevention and treatment of macrovascular and microvascular complica-ions of diabetes, (3) avoidance of hypoglycemia, and (4) preservation of quality of life. ılthough the goals are similar to those in younger adults, older adults with diabetes are ıeterogeneous in their physical and cognitive functioning capacity, multiple comor-idities, and life expectancy. Otherwise robust older adults with expected life expec-ancy over 10 years might benefit from similar glycemic goals as younger adults (ie, HbA_{1c} <7%) to prevent diabetic complications. For frail older adults with multiple comorbidities and limited life expectancy, however, avoidance of hypoglycemia and ymptomatic hyperglycemia and preservation of quality of life are arguably just as nportant, and less stringent targets (ie, HbA_{1c} <8%) may be more appropriate. 'urthermore, patient preferences must also be recognized in decisions related to diabetes management. Thus, treatment often requires an individualized approach for older patients with diabetes.

Current glycemic targets of HbA_{1c} less than 7% are based on older studies (eg, United Kingdom Prospective Diabetes Study) that showed a significantly reduced risk of developing diabetic microvascular complications with intensive versus standard glucose control.[90] Long-term follow-up of the United Kingdom Prospective Diabetes Study demonstrated further benefits of early and intensive glucose control in reducing long-term risk of developing macrovascular disease.[90] Elderly individuals were excluded from the United Kingdom Prospective Diabetes Study, however, and there have been few other clinical trials examining the benefits of intensive glycemic control in older individuals; thus, extrapolation of previous results of clinical trials to elderly patients is challenging.[91] Recent clinical trials studying the effect of intensive glucose control that included older patients with diabetes failed to show a clear benefit of intensive glucose control on mortality and demonstrated potential harm with too aggressive glucose lowering (ie, HbA_{1c} <6%).[92–94] As a result, recent recommendations from the American Diabetes Association and the American Geriatrics Society recognize that a patient-centered approach may be more appropriate for older adults with diabetes.[11,95,96] Cardiovascular risk factor control (ie, lowering blood pressure, treating dyslipidemia, smoking cessation, and aspirin therapy) is also recommended for the majority of adults with diabetes based on health status.

Management of older patients with diabetes is complex and often individualized. Avoiding hypoglycemia and preserving functional independence are additional considerations for older patients with diabetes. Alternatively, an evolving area of research is exploring the degree to which hyperglycemia may be associated with the presence of adverse geriatric syndromes, such as physical disability, accelerated muscle loss, and frailty, and may ultimately have an impact on glycemic goals in the elderly. Current guidelines recognize the need to account for the presence of limited life expectancy and/or multiple comorbidities in treatment decisions for this vulnerable and growing population of individuals with diabetes.

Treatment

Lifestyle recommendations for older adults with prediabetes or diabetes can be tailored to physical function ability and are more appropriate for obese elderly individuals than those who are underweight. Encouragingly, the oldest age group in the Diabetes Prevention Program (>60 years at of age at baseline) had the most dramatic improvement in glycemic control over time with lifestyle modification programs and was associated with better adherence to lifestyle programs compared with younger age groups.[97,98] In prescribing dietary modification, additional factors to consider in elderly patients with diabetes include social factors, such as whether patients are eating alone (easier to eat precooked meals) and the presence of depression. Impaired perception of sweet and salty occurs with age, so using potassium chloride for saltiness and using sucralose or stevia for sweetness may be preferred because they are perceived as saltier and sweeter than sodium chloride or sucrose.[99] A sedentary lifestyle in older patients might signify the need for a reduced intake of total calories. Alcohol consumption is also associated with a significant number of calories and should be ascertained when formulating a lifestyle modification program.

Daily exercise, as part of activities of daily living, is necessary for older patients with diabetes. Weight-bearing exercises can improve insulin sensitivity. In older patients with diabetes, usual recommendations for aerobic and resistance exercise can be prescribed as tolerated in the context of other medical conditions (ie, arthritis and heart disease) that may otherwise limit exercise tolerance or participation in physical activities.[100]

The choice of pharmacologic therapy for older patients with diabetes may be affected by changes in renal and hepatic functions with aging and the physical and cognitive abilities of each patient, in addition to other coexisting comorbidities. **Fig. 2** outlines the sites of action for common glucose-lowering therapies used in diabetes management. Special considerations in the elderly include the need to monitor renal function using both creatinine and glomerular filtration rate when prescribing metformin due to risk of lactic acidosis; hypoglycemia with sulfonylureas, which work by increasing endogenous insulin secretion, and often require dose reductions when used with insulin and in patients with renal insufficiency (short-acting glimepiride and glipizide may be preferred); and the use of weight-neutral agents, such as DPP 4 inhibitors, which increase endogenous levels of incretins, and may be appropriate in cachetic older adults. Thiazolidenediones, which are *peroxisome proliferator-activated receptor* γ-activators, may exacerbate underlying heart failure and are associated with increased risk of bone fractures, so they should be avoided in persons with underlying bone disease, but they are less likely to result in hypoglycemia. GLP-1 receptor agonists are injectable agents that can slow gastric motility and lead to weight loss. Thus, these agents may be useful for obese older patients with diabetes but not in those with complications, such as gastroparesis. Endogenous insulin clearance may also be decreased with aging[101,102] and, perhaps, exogenous insulin clearance as well, although this has not been consistently described.[103] Insulin clearance is particularly affected by changes in renal function, which may affect dosing.

Monitoring of blood glucose in older patients with diabetes is similar to that in younger adults. HbA_{1c} may rise by approximately 0.1% with each decade of age independent of changes in blood glucose and potentially affect the interpretability of HbA_{1c}

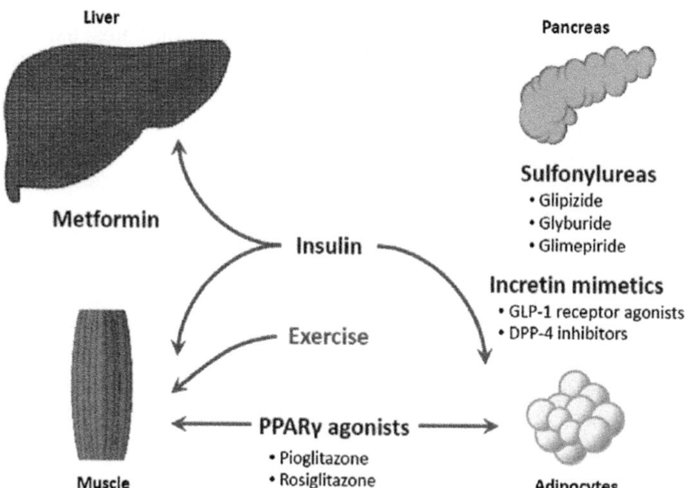

Fig. 2. Sites of action for common glucose-lowering therapies. The sites of action for common glucose-lowering therapies used in persons with type 2 diabetes mellitus are illustrated. The different mechanisms by which these drugs improve blood glucose, along with potential benefits and side effects, are important considerations in the management of older patients with diabetes. Exercise, in particular, muscle-strengthening or resistance activities, can have additional benefits on glucose uptake by skeletal muscle. PPARγ, *peroxisome proliferator-activated receptor* γ.

in older patients.[104] Self-monitoring of blood glucose can be considered based on a patient's cognitive ability, functional status, and risk of hypoglycemia.

SUMMARY

Diabetes and altered glucose metabolism commonly occur with aging. OGTT may help characterize abnormal glucose status in the elderly population. Diabetes in this population is heterogeneous, with middle age–onset versus elderly-onset individuals possibly representing groups at different risks for the development of microvascular complications. Geriatric syndromes, such as muscle loss, disability, and frailty, are more prevalent in older patients with diabetes and may be related to the presence of hyperglycemia or insulin resistance but more research is needed. Treatment of diabetes in the elderly includes lifestyle recommendations, when appropriate, and the use of pharmacologic therapies that account for the presence of comorbidities, especially renal and hepatic impairment, as well as the physical and cognitive abilities of patients, while seeking to minimize hypoglycemia. Ultimately, goals of care need to be individualized for elderly patients with diabetes.

ACKNOWLEDGMENTS

We thank David Liu (National Institute on Aging) for help with **Fig. 2** illustration.

REFERENCES

1. Cowie CC, Rust KF, Ford ES, et al. Full accounting of diabetes and pre-diabetes in the U.S. population in 1988-1994 and 2005-2006. Diabetes Care 2009;32: 287–94.
2. Centers for Disease Control and Prevention (CDC). Public health and aging: trends in aging—United States and worldwide. JAMA 2003;289:1371–3.
3. Wild S, Roglic G, Green A, et al. Global prevalence of diabetes: estimates for the year 2000 and projections for 2030. Diabetes Care 2004;27:1047–53.
4. Zhang X, Decker FH, Luo H, et al. Trends in the prevalence and comorbidities of diabetes mellitus in nursing home residents in the United States: 1995-2004. J Am Geriatr Soc 2010;58:724–30.
5. Shimokata H, Muller DC, Fleg JL, et al. Age as an independent determinant of glucose tolerance. Diabetes 1991;40:44–51.
6. DeFronzo RA. Glucose intolerance and aging. Diabetes Care 1981;4:493–501.
7. Ferrannini E, Vichi S, Beck-Nielsen H, et al. Insulin action and age. European Group for the Study of Insulin Resistance (EGIR). Diabetes 1996;45:947–53.
8. Davidson MB. The effect of aging on carbohydrate metabolism. Metabolism 1979;28:688–705.
9. Elahi D, Muller DC, Egan JM, et al. Glucose tolerance, glucose utilization and insulin secretion in ageing. Novartis Found Symp 2002;242:222–42.
10. Elahi D, Muller DC. Carbohydrate metabolism in the elderly. Eur J Clin Nutr 2000;54(Suppl 3):S112–20.
11. American Diabetes Association. Standards of medical care in diabetes—2012. Diabetes Care 2012;35(Suppl 1):S11–63.
12. Meigs JB, Muller DC, Nathan DM, et al. The natural history of progression from normal glucose tolerance to type 2 diabetes in the Baltimore Longitudinal Study of Aging. Diabetes 2003;52:1475–84.
13. DeFronzo RA, Tobin JD, Andres R. Glucose clamp technique: a method for quantifying insulin secretion and resistance. Am J Physiol 1979;237:E214–23.

14. Defronzo RA. Glucose intolerance and aging: evidence for tissue insensitivity to insulin. Diabetes 1979;28:1095–101.
15. Gumbiner B, Thorburn AW, Ditzler TM, et al. Role of impaired intracellular glucose metabolism in the insulin resistance of aging. Metabolism 1992;41: 1115–21.
16. Goulet ED, Hassaine A, Dionne IJ, et al. Frailty in the elderly is associated with insulin resistance of glucose metabolism in the postabsorptive state only in the presence of increased abdominal fat. Exp Gerontol 2009;44:740–4.
17. Elahi D, Muller DC, McAloon-Dyke M, et al. The effect of age on insulin response and glucose utilization during four hyperglycemic plateaus. Exp Gerontol 1993; 28:393–409.
18. Chen M, Halter JB, Porte D Jr. The role of dietary carbohydrate in the decreased glucose tolerance of the elderly. J Am Geriatr Soc 1987;35:417–24.
19. Muller DC, Elahi D, Tobin JD, et al. The effect of age on insulin resistance and secretion: a review. Semin Nephrol 1996;16:289–98.
20. Tabák AG, Jokela M, Akbaraly TN, et al. Trajectories of glycaemia, insulin sensitivity, and insulin secretion before diagnosis of type 2 diabetes: an analysis from the Whitehall II study. Lancet 2009;373:2215–21.
21. Polonsky KS, Given BD, Van Cauter E. Twenty-four-hour profiles and pulsatile patterns of insulin secretion in normal and obese subjects. J Clin Invest 1988; 81:442–8.
22. Scheen AJ, Sturis J, Polonsky KS, et al. Alterations in the ultradian oscillations of insulin secretion and plasma glucose in aging. Diabetologia 1996;39:564–72.
23. Meneilly GS, Veldhuis JD, Elahi D. Disruption of the pulsatile and entropic modes of insulin release during an unvarying glucose stimulus in elderly individuals. J Clin Endocrinol Metab 1999;84:1938–43.
24. O'Meara NM, Sturis J, Van Cauter E, et al. Lack of control by glucose of ultradian insulin secretory oscillations in impaired glucose tolerance and in non-insulin-dependent diabetes mellitus. J Clin Invest 1993;92:262–71.
25. Kim W, Egan JM. The role of incretins in glucose homeostasis and diabetes treatment. Pharmacol Rev 2008;60:470–512.
26. Elahi D, Andersen DK, Muller DC, et al. The enteric enhancement of glucose-stimulated insulin release. The role of GIP in aging, obesity, and non-insulin-dependent diabetes mellitus. Diabetes 1984;33:950–7.
27. Meneilly GS, Ryan AS, Minaker KL, et al. The effect of age and glycemic level on the response of the beta-cell to glucose-dependent insulinotropic polypeptide and peripheral tissue sensitivity to endogenously released insulin. J Clin Endocrinol Metab 1998;83:2925–32.
28. Chia CW, Carlson OD, Kim W, et al. Exogenous glucose-dependent insulinotropic polypeptide worsens post prandial hyperglycemia in type 2 diabetes. Diabetes 2009;58:1342–9.
29. Meneilly GS, Demuth HU, McIntosh CH, et al. Effect of ageing and diabetes on glucose-dependent insulinotropic polypeptide and dipeptidyl peptidase IV responses to oral glucose. Diabet Med 2000;17:346–50.
30. Chiniwala N, Jabbour S. Management of diabetes mellitus in the elderly. Curr Opin Endocrinol Diabetes Obes 2011;18:148–52.
31. Selvin E, Coresh J, Brancati FL. The burden and treatment of diabetes in elderly individuals in the U.S. Diabetes Care 2006;29:2415–9.
32. Wang Y, Qin MZ, Liu Q, et al. Clinical analysis of elderly patients with elderly-onset type 2 diabetes mellitus in China: assessment of appropriate therapy. J Int Med Res 2010;38:1134–41.

33. Barbieri M, Rizzo MR, Manzella D, et al. Age-related insulin resistance: is it an obligatory finding? The lesson from healthy centenarians. Diabetes Metab Res Rev 2001;17:19–26.
34. Paolisso G, Gambardella A, Ammendola S, et al. Glucose tolerance and insulin action in healty centenarians. Am J Physiol 1996;270:E890–4.
35. Park SW, Goodpaster BH, Strotmeyer ES, et al. Decreased muscle strength and quality in older adults with type 2 diabetes: the health, aging, and body composition study. Diabetes 2006;55:1813–8.
36. Park SW, Goodpaster BH, Strotmeyer ES, et al. Health, aging, and body composition study. Accelerated loss of skeletal muscle strength in older adults with type 2 diabetes: the health, aging, and body composition study. Diabetes Care 2007;30:1507–12.
37. Park SW, Goodpaster BH, Lee JS, et al. Health, aging, and body composition study. Excessive loss of skeletal muscle mass in older adults with type 2 diabetes. Diabetes Care 2009;32:1993–7.
38. Barzilay JI, Cotsonis GA, Walston J, et al, Health ABC Study. Insulin resistance is associated with decreased quadriceps muscle strength in nondiabetic adults aged ≥70 years. Diabetes Care 2009;32:736–8.
39. Lazarus R, Sparrow D, Weiss ST. Handgrip strength and insulin levels: cross-sectional and prospective associations in the Normative Aging Study. Metabolism 1997;46:1266–9.
40. Kalyani RR, Metter EJ, Ramachandran R, et al. Glucose and insulin measurements from the oral glucose tolerance test and relationship to muscle mass. J Gerontol A Biol Sci Med Sci 2012;67:74–81.
41. Rasmussen BB, Fujita S, Wolfe RR, et al. Insulin resistance of muscle protein metabolism in aging. FASEB J 2006;20:768–9.
42. Volpi E, Mittendorfer B, Rasmussen BB, et al. The response of muscle protein anabolism to combined hyperaminoacidemia and glucose-induced hyperinsulinemia is impaired in the elderly. J Clin Endocrinol Metab 2000;85:4481–90.
43. Wang X, Hu Z, Hu J, et al. Insulin resistance accelerates muscle protein degradation: activation of the ubiquitin-proteasome pathway by defects in muscle cell signaling. Endocrinology 2006;147:4160–8.
44. Lee CG, Boyko EJ, Barrett-Connor E, et al, Osteoporotic Fractures in Men (MrOS) Study Research Group. Insulin sensitizers may attenuate lean mass loss in older men with diabetes. Diabetes Care 2011;34:2381–6.
45. Phielix E, Schrauwen-Hinderling VB, Mensink M, et al. Lower intrinsic ADP-stimulated mitochondrial respiration underlies in vivo mitochondrial dysfunction in muscle of male type 2 diabetic patients. Diabetes 2008;57:2943–9.
46. Rabøl R, Boushel R, Almdal T, et al. Opposite effects of pioglitazone and rosiglitazone on mitochondrial respiration in skeletal muscle of patients with type 2 diabetes. Diabetes Obes Metab 2010;12:806–14.
47. Strotmeyer ES, de Rekeneire N, Schwartz AV, et al, Health ABC Study. Sensory and motor peripheral nerve function and lower-extremity quadriceps strength: the health, aging and body composition study. J Am Geriatr Soc 2009;57:2004–10.
48. Andersen H, Nielsen S, Mogensen CE, et al. Muscle strength in type 2 diabetes. Diabetes 2004;53:1543–8.
49. Volpato S, Bianchi L, Lauretani F, et al. Role of muscle mass and muscle quality in the association between diabetes and gait speed. Diabetes Care 2012;35:1672–9.
50. Van Hall G, Steensberg A, Fischer C, et al. Interleukin-6 markedly decreases skeletal muscle protein turnover and increases nonmuscle amino acid utilization in healthy individuals. J Clin Endocrinol Metab 2008;7:2851–8.

51. Duncan BB, Schmidt MI, Pankow JS, et al. Low-grade systemic inflammation and the development of type 2 diabetes: the atherosclerosis risk in communities study. Diabetes 2003;52:1799–805.
52. Visser M, Kritchevsky SB, Goodpaster BH, et al. Leg muscle mass and composition in relation to lower extremity performance in men and women aged 70 to 79: the health, aging and body composition study. J Am Geriatr Soc 2002;50: 897–904.
53. Kalyani RR, Tian J, Xue QL, et al. Hyperglycemia and incidence of frailty and lower extremity mobility limitations in older women. J Am Geriatr Soc 2012;60: 1701–7.
54. Volpato S, Blaum C, Resnick H, et al, Women's Health and Aging Study. Comorbidities and impairments explaining the association between diabetes and lower extremity disability: the Women's Health and Aging Study. Diabetes Care 2002;25:678–83.
55. Ko SU, Stenholm S, Chia CW, et al. Gait pattern alterations in older adults associated with type 2 diabetes in the absence of peripheral neuropathy—results from the Baltimore Longitudinal Study of Aging. Gait Posture 2011;34:548–52.
56. Kuo HK, Leveille SG, Yen CJ, et al. Exploring how peak leg power and usual gait speed are linked to late-life disability: data from the National Health and Nutrition Examination Survey (NHANES), 1999-2002. Am J Phys Med Rehabil 2006;85: 650–8.
57. De Rekeneire N, Resnick HE, Schwartz AV, et al, Health, Aging, and Body Composition Study. Diabetes is associated with subclinical functional limitation in nondisabled older individuals: the Health, Aging, and Body Composition study. Diabetes Care 2003;26:3257–63.
58. Sinclair AJ, Conroy SP, Bayer AJ. Impact of diabetes on physical function in older people. Diabetes Care 2008;31:233–5.
59. Gregg EW, Beckles GL, Williamson DF, et al. Diabetes and physical disability among older U.S. adults. Diabetes Care 2000;23:1272–7.
60. Volpato S, Ferrucci L, Blaum C, et al. Progression of lower-extremity disability in older women with diabetes: the Women's Health and Aging Study. Diabetes Care 2003;26:70–5.
61. Ryerson B, Tierney EF, Thompson TJ, et al. Excess physical limitations among adults with diabetes in the U.S. population, 1997-1999. Diabetes Care 2003; 26:206–10.
62. Egede LE. Diabetes, major depression, and functional disability among U.S. adults. Diabetes Care 2004;27:421–8.
63. Maty SC, Fried LP, Volpato S, et al. Patterns of disability related to diabetes mellitus in older women. J Gerontol A Biol Sci Med Sci 2004;59:148–53.
64. Kalyani RR, Saudek CD, Brancati FL, et al. The Association of Diabetes, Comorbidities, and Hemoglobin A1c with Functional Disability in Older Adults: results from the National Health and Nutrition Examination Survey (NHANES), 1999-2006. Diabetes Care 2010;33:1055–60.
65. Bossoni S, Mazziotti G, Gazzaruso C, et al. Relationship between instrumental activities of daily living and blood glucose control in elderly subjects with type 2 diabetes. Age Ageing 2008;37:222–5.
66. Boyd CM, Xue QL, Simpson CF, et al. Frailty, hospitalization, and progression of disability in a cohort of disabled older women. Am J Med 2005;118:1225–31.
67. Fried LP, Tangen CM, Walston J, et al, Cardiovascular Health Study. Frailty in older adults: evidence for a phenotype. J Gerontol A Biol Sci Med Sci 2001; 56:M146–56.

68. Bandeen-Roche K, Xue QL, Ferrucci L, et al. Phenotype of frailty: characterization in the women's health and aging studies. J Gerontol A Biol Sci Med Sci 2006;61:262–6.
69. Wolinsky FD, Callahan CM, Fitzgerald JF, et al. Changes in functional status and the risks of subsequent nursing home placement and death. J Gerontol 1993; 48:S94–101.
70. Blaum CS, Xue QL, Tian J, et al. Is hyperglycemia associated with frailty status in older women? J Am Geriatr Soc 2009;57:840–7.
71. Walston J, McBurnie MA, Newman A, et al, Cardiovascular Health Study. Frailty and activation of the inflammation and coagulation systems with and without clinical comorbidities: results from the Cardiovascular Health Study. Arch Intern Med 2002;162:2333–41.
72. Kalyani RR, Varadhan R, Weiss CO, et al. Frailty status and altered glucose-insulin dynamics. J Gerontol A Biol Sci Med Sci 2012;67:1300–6.
73. Serra-Prat M, Palomera E, Clave P, et al. Effect of age and frailty on ghrelin and cholecystokinin responses to a meal test. Am J Clin Nutr 2009;89:1410–7.
74. Barzilay JI, Blaum C, Moore T, et al. Insulin resistance and inflammation as precursors of frailty: the Cardiovascular Health Study. Arch Intern Med 2007; 167:635–41.
75. Senn JJ, Klover PJ, Nowak IA, et al. IL-6 induces cellular insulin resistance in hepatocytes. Diabetes 2002;51:3391–9.
76. Lee CC, Adler AI, Sandhu MS, et al. Association of C-reactive protein with type 2 diabetes: prospective analysis and meta-analysis. Diabetologia 2009;52:1040–7.
77. Barbieri M, Ferrucci L, Ragno E, et al. Chronic inflammation and the effect of IGF-I on muscle strength and power in older persons. Am J Physiol Endocrinol Metab 2003;284:E481–7.
78. Hubbard RE, Lang IA, Llewellyn DJ, et al. Frailty, body mass index, and abdominal obesity in older people. J Gerontol A Biol Sci Med Sci 2010;65:377–81.
79. Newman AB, Gottdiener JS, Mcburnie MA, et al, Cardiovascular Health Study Research Group. Associations of subclinical cardiovascular disease with frailty. J Gerontol A Biol Sci Med Sci 2001;56:M158–66.
80. Fried LP, Xue QL, Cappola AR, et al. Nonlinear multisystem physiological dysregulation associated with frailty in older women: implications for etiology and treatment. J Gerontol A Biol Sci Med Sci 2009;64:1049–57.
81. Fried TR, Bradley EH, Williams CS, et al. Functional disability and health care expenditures for older persons. Arch Intern Med 2001;161:2602–7.
82. Janssen I, Shepard DS, Katzmarzyk PT, et al. The healthcare costs of sarcopenia in the United States. J Am Geriatr Soc 2004;52:80–5.
83. Newman AB, Kupelian V, Visser M, et al. Strength, but not muscle mass, is associated with mortality in the health, aging and body composition study cohort. J Gerontol A Biol Sci Med Sci 2006;61:72–7.
84. Emerging Risk Factors Collaboration, Seshasai SR, Kaptoge S, Thompson A, et al. Diabetes mellitus, fasting glucose, and risk of cause-specific death. N Engl J Med 2011;364:829–41.
85. Metter EJ, Windham BG, Maggio M, et al. Glucose and insulin measurements from the oral glucose tolerance test and mortality prediction. Diabetes Care 2008;31:1026–30.
86. Sorkin JD, Muller DC, Fleg JL, et al. The relation of fasting and 2-h postchallenge plasma glucose concentrations to mortality: data from the Baltimore Longitudinal Study of Aging with a critical review of the literature. Diabetes Care 2005;28:2626–32.

87. Selvin E, Steffes MW, Zhu H, et al. Glycated hemoglobin, diabetes, and cardiovascular risk in nondiabetic adults. N Engl J Med 2010;362:800–11.
88. Huang ES, Liu JY, Moffet HH, et al. Glycemic control, complications, and death in older diabetic patients: the diabetes and aging study. Diabetes Care 2011;34: 1329–36.
89. Kuhlow D, Florian S, von Figura G, et al. Telomerase deficiency impairs glucose metabolism and insulin secretion. Aging (Albany NY) 2010;2:650–8.
90. UK Prospective Diabetes Study (UKPDS) Group. Intensive blood-glucose control with sulphonylureas or insulin compared with conventional treatment and risk of complications in patients with type 2 diabetes (UKPDS 33). Lancet 1998;352:837–53.
91. Finucane TE. "Tight control" in geriatrics: the emperor wears a thong. J Am Geriatr Soc 2012;60:1571–5.
92. Action to Control Cardiovascular Risk in Diabetes Study Group, Gerstein HC, Miller ME, et al. Effects of intensive glucose lowering in type 2 diabetes. N Engl J Med 2008;358:2545–59.
93. Patel A, MacMahon S, Chalmers J, et al, ADVANCE Collaborative Group. Intensive blood glucose control and vascular outcomes in patients with type 2 diabetes. N Engl J Med 2008;358:2560–72.
94. Duckworth W, Abraira C, Moritz T, et al. Glucose control and vascular complications in veterans with type 2 diabetes. N Engl J Med 2009;360:129–39.
95. Durso SC. Using clinical guidelines designed for older adults with diabetes mellitus and complex health status. JAMA 2006;295:1935–40.
96. Brown AF, Mangione CM, Saliba D, et al. Guidelines for improving the care of the older person with diabetes mellitus. J Am Geriatr Soc 2003;51:S265–80.
97. Knowler WC, Barrett-Connor E, Fowler SE, et al, Diabetes Prevention Program Research Group. Reduction in the incidence of type 2 diabetes with lifestyle intervention or metformin. N Engl J Med 2002;346:393–403.
98. Wing RR, Hamman RF, Bray GA, et al, Diabetes Prevention Program Research Group. Achieving weight and activity goals among diabetes prevention program lifestyle participants. Obes Res 2004;12:1426–34.
99. Shin YK, Cong WN, Cai H, et al. Age-related changes in mouse taste bud morphology, hormone expression, and taste responsivity. J Gerontol A Biol Sci Med Sci 2012;67:336–44.
100. Colberg SR, Sigal RJ, Fernhall B, et al, American College of Sports Medicine, American Diabetes Association. Exercise and type 2 diabetes: the American College of Sports Medicine and the American Diabetes Association: joint position statement executive summary. Diabetes Care 2010;33:2692–6.
101. McGuire EA, Tobin JD, Berman M, et al. Kinetics of native insulin in diabetic, obese, and aged men. Diabetes 1979;28:110–20.
102. Fink RI, Revers RR, Kolterman OG, et al. The metabolic clearance of insulin and the feedback inhibition of insulin secretion are altered with aging. Diabetes 1985;34:275–80.
103. Mooradian AD. Special considerations with insulin therapy in older adults with diabetes mellitus. Drugs Aging 2011;28:429–38.
104. Pani LN, Korenda L, Meigs JB, et al. Effect of aging on A1C levels in individuals without diabetes: evidence from the Framingham Offspring Study and the National Health and Nutrition Examination Survey 2001-2004. Diabetes Care 2008;31:1991–6.

Age-Associated Abnormalities of Water Homeostasis

Laura E. Cowen, MD[a], Steven P. Hodak, MD[b],
Joseph G. Verbalis, MD[a,*]

KEYWORDS

- Aging • Arginine vasopressin • Homeostasis • Elderly • Hypernatremia
- Hyperosmolality • Hyponatremia • Hypoosmolality

KEY POINTS

- Alterations in the regulation of water homeostasis in the elderly result from multiple consequences of aging including changes in body composition, diminished renal function, and alterations in hypothalamic-pituitary regulation of thirst and secretion of arginine vasopressin.
- As a result of these multiple changes, the elderly have an increased frequency and severity of hypoosmolality and hyperosmolality, manifested by hyponatremia and hypernatremia as well as hypovolemia and hypervolemia.
- The syndrome of inappropriate antidiuretic hormone secretion is the most common cause of hyponatremia in elderly populations; unlike in younger populations, this is often idiopathic with no identifiable etiology.
- Hyponatremia in the elderly population is associated with many clinically significant adverse outcomes including neurocognitive deficits, gait instability, falls, osteoporosis, as well as increased incidence of bone fractures, hospital readmission, and need for long-term care.
- It is incumbent on all who care for the elderly to realize the more limited nature of the compensatory and regulatory mechanisms that maintain normal fluid homeostasis in elderly patients, and to incorporate this understanding into the diagnosis and clinical interventions that must be made to provide optimal care for this uniquely susceptible group of patients.

INTRODUCTION

Findley[1] first proposed the presence of age-related dysfunction of the hypothalamic-neurohypophyseal-renal axis more than 60 years ago. His hypothesis was based on clinical observations that predated the first assays for arginine vasopressin (AVP).

[a] Division of Endocrinology and Metabolism, Georgetown University Medical Center, 4000 Reservoir Road Northwest, Washington, DC 20007, USA; [b] Center for Diabetes and Endocrinology, University of Pittsburgh Medical Center, 3601 Fifth Avenue, Suite 3B, Pittsburgh, PA 15213, USA
* Corresponding author.
E-mail address: verbalis@georgetown.edu

Endocrinol Metab Clin N Am 42 (2013) 349–370
http://dx.doi.org/10.1016/j.ecl.2013.02.005
endo.theclinics.com

More sophisticated scientific methodologies have largely corroborated Findley's hypothesis of age-related dysfunction of the hypothalamic-neurohypophyseal-renal axis, and have further revealed the underlying physiologies that are part of the aging process. As a result, it is now clear that multiple abnormalities in water homeostasis occur commonly with aging, and that the elderly are uniquely susceptible to disorders of body volume and osmolality. This article summarizes the distinct points along the hypothalamic-neurohypophyseal-renal axis where these changes have been characterized, as well as the clinical significance of these changes, with special attention to effects on cognition, gait instability, osteoporosis, fractures, and morbidity and mortality. This article represents a comprehensive update of the authors' previously published review on this topic.[2]

PHYSIOLOGIC OVERVIEW OF DISTURBANCES OF WATER METABOLISM

The ratio of solute content to body water determines the osmolality of body fluids, including plasma. As the most abundant extracellular electrolyte, the serum sodium concentration ([Na^+]) is the single most important determinant of plasma osmolality under normal circumstances. Although the regulation of water and sodium balance is closely interrelated, it is predominantly the homeostatic control of water, rather than of sodium, that determines serum [Na^+], and therefore plasma osmolality. On the other hand, homeostatic controls of sodium metabolism and sodium-driven shifts in extracellular fluids more directly regulate the volume status of body-fluid compartments rather than their osmolality. Isolated shifts in body water unaccompanied by shifts in body solute do not typically result in clinically significant changes in volume status. These isolated shifts in total body water, however, can result in dramatic changes in serum [Na^+] and plasma osmolality.[3] For example, in a 70-kg adult, a 10% increase in total body water would cause a significant decrease in serum [Na^+] of approximately 14 mmol/L. Such a change could easily result in clinically significant hyponatremia and hypoosmolality. However, this same 10% gain of total body water would only cause an increase in intravascular volume of approximately 400 mL. Such a mild increase in circulating volume would not be expected to cause observable clinical findings. Similarly, the reverse situation of a 10% water loss would result in an increase in serum [Na^+] and clinically significant hyperosmolality, but without clinically significant hypovolemia[3]; such is the case with uncompensated diabetes insipidus.

Physiologic processes that occur with aging are associated with changes in water metabolism and sodium balance, leading to alterations in plasma osmolality and body-fluid compartment volumes. As a result of these changes, the elderly have increased frequency and severity of hypoosmolality and hyperosmolality, manifested by hyponatremia and hypernatremia, as well as hypovolemia and hypervolemia. Although the processes of water and sodium metabolism cannot be completely separated from each other, this article focuses mainly on the effects of aging on water balance and plasma osmolality.

CLINICAL OVERVIEW OF HYPONATREMIA

Hyponatremia is the most common electrolyte disorder encountered in clinical practice.[4] Such hyponatremia becomes clinically significant when accompanied by plasma hypoosmolality. When hyponatremia is defined as a serum [Na^+] level of less than 135 mmol/L, the inpatient incidence is reported to be between 15% and 22%. Studies that define hyponatremia as serum [Na^+] of less than 130 mmol/L demonstrate a lower, but still significant, incidence of 1% to 4%.[5] Determination of a true incidence and prevalence of hyponatremia in the elderly is problematic. Several excellent observational studies examining this issue have been published, but the literature has lacked a uniform threshold for defining hyponatremia. The definition of the term "elderly" and criteria for age, stratification by serum [Na+], medication use, and clinical setting vary widely between studies, making direct comparisons among such clinical series difficult. A recent review illustrates the disparate nature of the existing literature by pointing out that the incidence of hyponatremia in elderly populations has been reported to vary between 0.2% and 29.8%, depending on the criteria used to define both hyponatremia and elderly.[6]

Miller and colleagues[7] have published numerous observational studies on the elderly and hyponatremia. In a retrospective study of 405 ambulatory elderly patients with a mean age of 78 years, the incidence of serum [Na+] of less than 135 mmol/L was 11% over a 24-month observational period. These results are analogous to an earlier study by Caird and colleagues,[8] which reported that among healthy patients aged 65 years or older living at home, the incidence of serum [Na+] less than 137 mmol/L was 10.5%. Miller[9] has also observed that the incidence of hyponatremia doubled to approximately 22% among elderly who reside in long-term institutional settings. He further noted that during a 1-year observational period, 53% of such institutional populations experienced 1 or more hyponatremic episodes. Another study by Anpalahan[10] found similar results: 25% of patients aged 65 years and older who resided in an acute geriatric rehabilitation hospital had hyponatremia, defined as serum [Na+] less than 135 mmol/L. Although the true incidence of hyponatremia in the elderly is difficult to define given differing diagnostic criteria across studies, it is nonetheless clear that this problem cannot be considered to be an uncommon occurrence.

The syndrome of inappropriate antidiuretic hormone secretion (SIADH) is the most common cause of hyponatremia in elderly populations. Cases of SIADH were first described by Bartter and colleagues[11] in 1957, and the defining characteristics of the syndrome were summarized by the same investigators 10 years later.[12] The defining criteria presented in this landmark publication remain valid and clinically relevant today. SIADH can be caused by many types of diseases and injuries common in the elderly, including central nervous system injury, pulmonary disease, malignancies, nausea, and pain. An idiopathic form of SIADH associated with aging has also been described. Several studies have demonstrated that SIADH accounts for approximately half (50%–58.7%) of the hyponatremia observed in some elderly populations,[7,10,13] and one-quarter to one-half (26%–60%) of elderly patients with SIADH appear to have the idiopathic form of this disorder.[7,10,13]

CLINICAL IMPLICATIONS OF HYPONATREMIA

Hyponatremia is a strong independent predictor of mortality, reported to be as high as 60% in some series.[14,15] Recent data have confirmed that hyponatremia in the elderly population is associated with multiple clinically significant outcomes with regard to neurocognitive effects and falls,[16] osteoporosis,[17] incidence of bone fractures,[18] and hospital readmission and need for long-term care.[19]

Terzian and colleagues[15] studied the occurrence of admission hyponatremia and its association with in-hospital mortality in a geriatric patient cohort older than 65 years who were admitted to a community teaching hospital. Serum [Na+] of less than 130 mmol/L within 24 hours of admission was the cutoff for inclusion. Of the 4123 patients studied, 3.5% were hyponatremic. Higher prevalence rates were noted in women (4.6% vs 2.6%), patients who had not undergone operation (4.0% vs 2.4%), and those who had more than 3 diagnoses on admission (4.3% vs 1.9%). It was noted that 16% of patients with admission hyponatremia died in the hospital, compared with

8% without hyponatremia. The relative risk of in-hospital mortality associated with admission hyponatremia was significantly increased at 2.0. This relative risk of mortality was higher for men than women, patients younger than 75 years, and patients with malignancy or digestive disease. There was evidence of a linear association between in-hospital mortality and sodium level, with mortality increasing as sodium levels decreased. Although this study could not establish the chronicity of hyponatremia at admission nor the underlying metabolic derangement, it suggested that the degree of hyponatremia may be an important indicator of poor prognosis for elderly hospitalized patients.[15]

More recently, Wald and colleagues[19] examined the entire spectrum of in-hospital hyponatremia in a group of adults presenting to a community academic hospital. This retrospective cohort study divided the patients into 3 categories: community-acquired hyponatremia (CAH; [Na^+] <138 mEq/L at the time of admission), hospital-aggravated hyponatremia (HAH; further decline in [Na^+] of at least 2 mEq/L in the first 48 hours of a CAH admission), and hospital-acquired hyponatremia (nadir serum [Na^+] <138 mEq/L developing after hospital admission). The relationship between serum [Na^+] and predicted inpatient mortality is represented by a U-shaped curve (**Fig. 1**), with [Na^+] of 140 mEq/L associated with the lowest risk of mortality. Increased mortality was significantly associated with [Na^+] less than 138 mEq/L and greater than 142 mEq/L. CAH occurred in 37.9% of hospitalizations and was associated with an adjusted odds ratio of 1.52 for in-hospital mortality, 1.12 for discharge to a short-term or long-term care facility, and a 14% increase in length of stay. HAH occurred in 38.2% of admissions and was associated with adjusted odds ratios of 1.66 for in-hospital mortality, 1.64 for discharge to a facility, and a 64% increase in length of stay. The strength of the associations increased along with severity of hyponatremia.

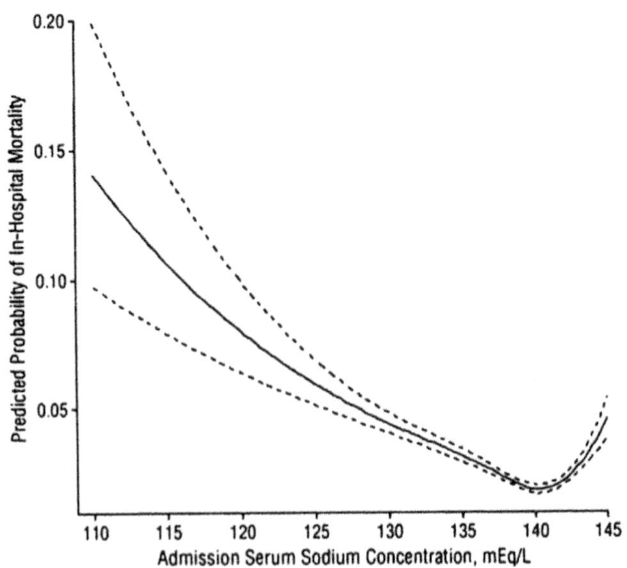

Fig. 1. Restrictive cubic spline depicting the unadjusted relationship between hospital admission serum sodium concentrations and predicted probability of in-hospital mortality. Dashed lines represent the 95% confidence interval. (*From* Wald R, Jaber BL, Price LL, et al. Impact of hospital-associated hyponatremia on selected outcomes. Arch Intern Med 2010;170(3):295; with permission.)

Overall, this study highlighted the burden of hyponatremia on both patient outcomes and use of health care resources.

In addition to increases in inpatient mortality, recent studies have also demonstrated an increase in outpatient mortality associated with hyponatremia. Hoorn and colleagues[20] examined the effect of hyponatremia on all-cause mortality within the framework of the Rotterdam Study, an ongoing prospective longitudinal cohort study among outpatients older than 55 years living in the Netherlands. A subset of 5208 patients with baseline data on sodium concentration was included in their analysis. All-cause mortality was higher in subjects with hyponatremia than in those without (51.6% vs 32.6%, $P<.001$). This increased risk remained after adjustment for age, sex, and body mass index (BMI). After further adjustment for baseline comorbidities, the hazard ratio (HR) of all-cause mortality was 1.21 (95% confidence interval [CI] 1.03–1.43, $P = .022$).[20] This study suggests that hyponatremia should no longer be considered a benign condition in the outpatient elderly population.

Renneboog and colleagues[16] conducted a case-control study to determine the functional significance of so-called asymptomatic mild chronic hyponatremia on cognitive impairment and falls. In this study, 122 Belgian patients with $[Na^+]$ between 115 and 132 mEq/L, all judged to be asymptomatic at the time of presentation to the emergency department (ED), were compared with 244 age-, sex-, and disease-matched controls presenting during the same time period. All patients were assessed as to the primary reason for the ED visit. Twenty-one percent of the hyponatremic patients presented because of a recent fall, compared with only 5% of controls, resulting in an adjusted odds ratio of 67 for hyponatremic patients presenting to an ED because of a fall. These data clearly demonstrated an increased incidence of falls in hyponatremic patients.

Renneboog and colleagues[16] also evaluated the clinical implications of asymptomatic hyponatremia on attention deficits and gait instability. Sixteen patients with hyponatremia secondary to SIADH had comprehensive neurocognitive testing both before and after correction of their hyponatremia to normal ranges. When performing a series of attention tests, hyponatremic patients (mean $[Na^+] = 128 \pm 3$ mEq/L) had prolonged median response latencies by 74 milliseconds, compared with the same patients after correction of their hyponatremia (mean $[Na^+] = 138 \pm 2$ mEq/L); this effect proved to be greater than the 25-millisecond decrease in response latency induced in normal volunteers by acute alcohol ingestion (blood alcohol concentration $= 0.6 \pm 0.2$ g/L). These impairments suggested a global decrease of attentional capabilities in hyponatremic patients that is greater than or equivalent to alcohol ingestion.[16] A subset of 12 patients with $[Na^+]$ in the range of 124 to 130 mEq/L was also tested for gait stability. The patients were asked to walk a tandem gait on a computerized platform that measured the center of gravity on the ball of their foot. Deviation from the straight line was measured as total traveled way. The hyponatremic patients wandered markedly off the tandem gait line in terms of their center of balance, but straightened their walk significantly once their hyponatremia was corrected (**Fig. 2**). As with the neurocognitive testing, this effect was greater than the gait instability induced in normal volunteers by acute alcohol ingestion. These results suggest that even mild degrees of hyponatremia can cause a significant gait instability that normalizes following correction of the hyponatremia, which may contribute to the increased incidence of falls in the elderly.

Four independent international studies have now demonstrated increased fracture rates in hyponatremic patients.[21] Gankam Kengne and colleagues[18] investigated the association between bone fracture, falls, and clinically asymptomatic hyponatremia in an ambulatory elderly population. A total of 513 patients older than 65 years who presented to the hospital with a bone fracture following an incidental fall was compared

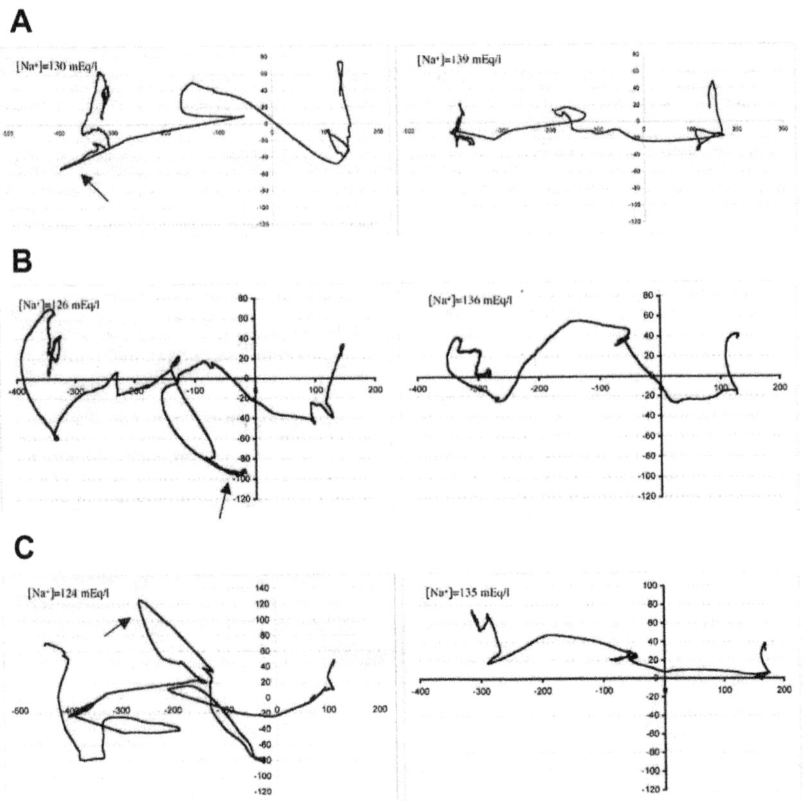

Fig. 2. Total traveled way measured by the center of pressure during a dynamic walking test consisting of 3 stereotyped steps "in tandem," eyes open, in 3 patients (*A–C*) with mild asymptomatic hyponatremia before (*left*) and after (*right*) correction. Patients are walking from right to left. Markedly irregular paths of the center of pressure were observed in the hyponatremia condition (*arrows*). (*From* Renneboog B, Musch W, Vandemergel X, et al. Mild chronic hyponatremia is associated with falls, unsteadiness, and attention deficits. Am J Med 2006;119(1):71; with permission.)

with 513 control subjects admitted during the same period but without a bone fracture. The prevalence of hyponatremia ([Na^+] <135 mEq/L) was 13.1% in patients with bone fractures, compared with only 3.9% in the control patients, resulting in an adjusted odds ratio for bone fracture associated with hyponatremia of 4.16.

A retrospective study by Sandhu and colleagues[22] showed similar findings. Investigators compared patients aged 65 years and older presenting to the ED with fracture with those presenting for other reasons. Of 364 patients identified with fracture, 9.1% were hyponatremic, accounting for a 2-fold increase in fracture risk compared with the control group. Of note, 24.2% of the hyponatremic patients were using selective serotonin reuptake inhibitors (SSRIs), compared with 0% of controls. SSRIs may cause hyponatremia, and can cause both sensorium and mobility deficits, contributing further to increased fracture risk.[22]

Kinsella and colleagues[23] also explored the association between hyponatremia and fracture, and confirmed the findings of the 2 prior studies. Their study used a database that had been used previously to examine the association between self-reported fracture occurrence and chronic kidney disease. Of the 1400 individuals included in the database, 4.2% were hyponatremic with mean serum [Na^+] 132.2 mmol/L. Compared with normonatremic patients, the hyponatremic patients were older and had a higher prevalence of osteoporosis. Hyponatremia was more common than normonatremia in the subset of patients experiencing fracture (8.7% vs 3.2%, $P<.001$). Further regression models were tested, indicating that the association between hyponatremia and fracture was independent of osteoporotic risk factors and osteoporosis treatment.[23]

Finally, Hoorn and colleagues[20] examined the relationship between mild hyponatremia and incidence of fracture within the framework of the prospective Rotterdam longitudinal aging study. Of the 5208 patients mentioned previously, 399 patients (7.7%) were noted to be hyponatremic with mean serum [Na^+] of 133.4 mmol/L. Subjects with hyponatremia were older, had more recent falls, had increased prevalence of type 2 diabetes mellitus, and used more diuretics than the normonatremic controls. Hyponatremia was associated with increased risk of incident nonvertebral fractures (HR 1.39, 95% CI 1.11–1.73; $P = .004$) after adjustment for age, sex, and BMI. Further adjustments for comorbidities and falls did not modify these results. Hyponatremic patients also demonstrated an increased risk of vertebral fractures at baseline, but no association with bone mineral density (BMD). This increased risk of fracture was independent of falls, pointing toward a possible effect of hyponatremia on bone quality.[20]

Verbalis and colleagues[17] explored the effect of hyponatremia and bone quality, and demonstrated a link between chronic hyponatremia and metabolic bone loss. This study used a rat model of SIADH to study the effects of hyponatremia on bone at the level of resorption and mineralization. Dual-energy x-ray absorptiometry (DXA) analysis of excised femurs established that hyponatremia for 3 months significantly reduced BMD by approximately 30% in comparison with normonatremic control rats. Moreover, micro–computed tomography and histomorphometric analyses indicated that hyponatremia markedly reduced both trabecular and cortical bone via increased bone resorption and bone formation. The most striking histologic finding was an increase in the number of osteoclast numbers per bone area and osteoclast surface per bone surface in the hyponatremic rats. This study demonstrated that chronic hyponatremia causes a significant reduction of bone mass at the cellular level. Follow-up studies confirmed that this process occurred in aging animals as well, though to somewhat lesser degrees than in the younger animals (**Fig. 3**). The suggested reason for this phenomenon is that one-third of total body sodium is stored in bone, and release of this sodium from bone during prolonged deprivation requires resorption of bone matrix.

To address the potential clinical relevance of this animal study, Verbalis and colleagues[17] analyzed human data from the National Health and Nutrition Examination Survey NHANES III, a cross-sectional survey that provided information on sodium concentrations and BMD of the hip in a nationally representative sample of United States adults. The mean serum [Na^+] of the hyponatremic cohort of NHANES III was 133.0 mmol/L, compared with 141.4 mmol/L in the normonatremic group. A statistically significant positive linear association between serum [Na^+] and femoral neck BMD was observed in hyponatremic subjects. Among hyponatremic subjects, serum [Na^+] explained 14.7% of the variation in total hip BMD, and total hip BMD decreased by 0.037 g/cm^2 for every 1 mmol/L decrease in serum [Na^+]. The adjusted odds of osteoporosis at the femoral neck and total hip were significantly higher among participants with hyponatremia than in normonatremic subjects. The NHANES III data in humans support the experimental data in rodents, and suggest direct clinical implications for these findings. Hyponatremia-induced bone resorption and osteoporosis are unique in that they represent attempts of the body to preserve sodium homeostasis at the expense of structural integrity of bone. Finally, subsequent animal studies have implicated hyponatremia in the pathology of other organ systems,[24] including the

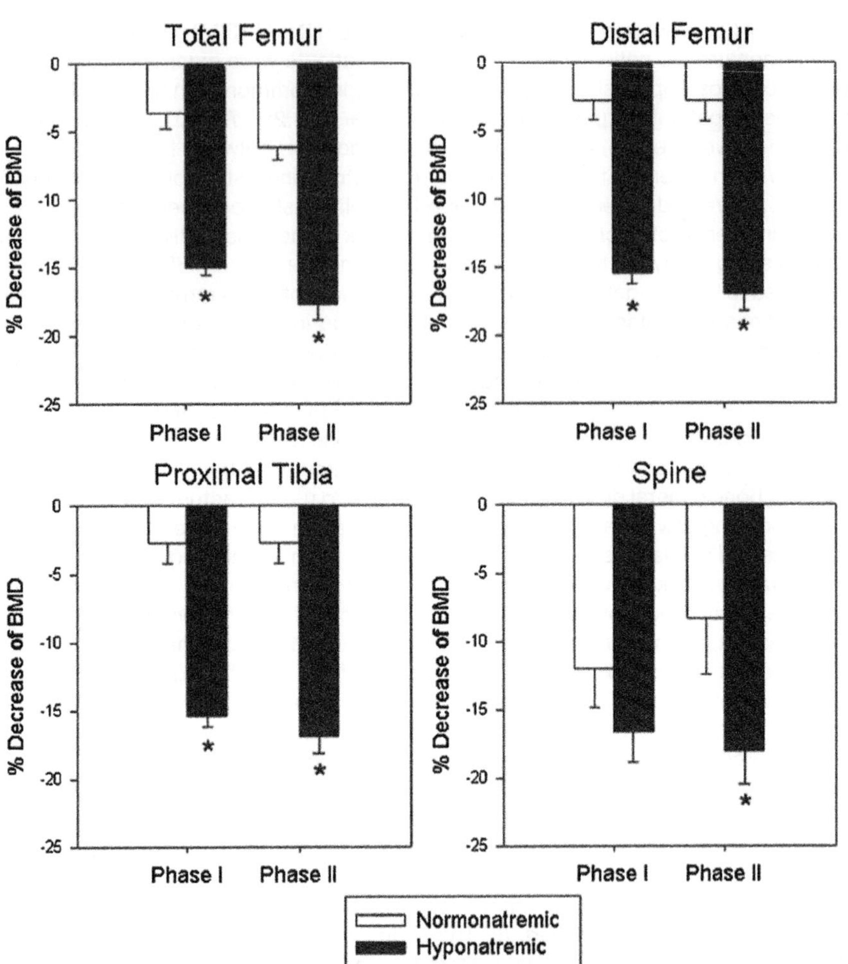

Fig. 3. Changes of bone mineral density (BMD) at multiple sites at the end of phase I (10 weeks) and phase II (18 weeks) in normonatremic (*open bars*) and hyponatremic (*closed bars*) aged F344BN rats (22 months old at the start of the study). The BMD decreases from baseline were significantly greater in the hyponatremic rats than in the normonatremic rats ($P<.001$). During phase II, hyponatremic rats received high-dose vitamin D supplement that mitigated further declines of BMD. Asterisks indicate statistically significant differences from the normonatremic controls.

heart (**Fig. 4**), skeletal muscle, and gonads. This finding has led to the provocative hypothesis that hyponatremia may exacerbate multiple aspects of senescence, including osteoporosis, cardiomyopathy, sarcopenia, hypogonadism, and changes in body composition.[24]

CLINICAL OVERVIEW OF HYPERNATREMIA

Hypernatremia necessarily reflects an increase in plasma osmolality. Cross-sectional studies of both hospitalized elderly patients and elderly residents of long-term care facilities show incidences of hypernatremia that vary between 0.3% and 8.9%.[6,14]

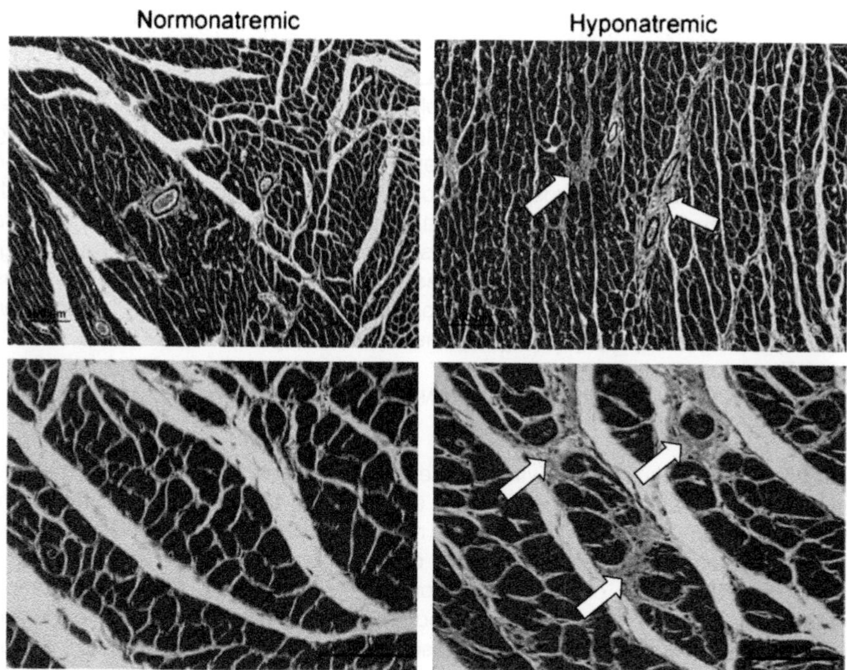

Fig. 4. Histology of hearts from normonatremic and chronically hyponatremic aged F344BN rats. Representative low-power (*upper panels*; original magnification ×20) and high power (*lower panels*; original magnification ×40) microscopic images of 5-μm sections from the hearts stained with Masson trichrome protocol that marks collagen fibers. Note increased interstitial and perivascular collagen deposits (*arrows*) in micrographs of the left ventricle from hyponatremic rats (*right panels*) compared with micrographs from normonatremic rats (*left panels*).

Though a common presenting diagnosis in the elderly, 60% to 80% of hypernatremia in elderly populations occurs after hospital admission.[14] By the same token, up to 30% of elderly nursing home patients experience hypernatremia following hospital admission.[25]

The clinical implications of hypernatremia in hospitalized elderly are significant. In a retrospective study, Snyder and colleagues[26] reviewed outcomes in 162 hypernatremic elderly patients, representing 1.1% of all elderly patients admitted for acute hospital care to a community teaching hospital. All patients were at least 60 years of age with a serum [Na^+] greater than 148 mmol/L. Forty-three percent of these patients presented with hypernatremia at admission and the remaining 57% developed hypernatremia after admission. Hypernatremia discovered at the time of admission was associated with greater age (mean age 81 years) and female sex, and was more common in patients admitted from a nursing home. All-cause mortality in the hypernatremic elderly patients was 42%, which was 7 times greater than age-matched normonatremic patients. Furthermore, 38% of the hypernatremic patients who survived to discharge had a significantly decreased ability to provide self-care. Mortality among patients who presented with hypernatremia on admission was lower (29%) than mortality among patients who developed hypernatremia after admission (52%), despite higher peak serum [Na^+] in the former in comparison with the latter group.[26]

Wald and colleagues[19] confirmed this association (see **Fig. 1**), noting a similar association between hypernatremia and increased predicted mortality risk in hospitalized patients with [Na^+] greater than 142 mEq/L.

As hypernatremia develops, the normal physiologic response integrates renal water conservation through osmotically stimulated secretion of AVP and accompanying potent stimulation of thirst.[27] Although renal water conservation can forestall the development of severe hyperosmolality, only appropriate stimulation of thirst with subsequent increase in water ingestion can replace body fluid deficits and reverse existing hyperosmolality.[3] This entire physiologic response is impaired with aging. Thus, the elderly have a greatly increased susceptibility to a variety of situations that can induce hypernatremia and hyperosmolality, with the attendant increases in morbidity and mortality that accompany the disorder.[26,28]

MECHANISMS INVOLVED WITH DISTURBANCES OF WATER METABOLISM IN THE ELDERLY

Alterations in the regulation of water homeostasis in the elderly result from multiple consequences of aging: changes in body composition, alterations in renal function, and changes in hypothalamic-pituitary regulation of thirst and AVP secretion (**Box 1**). The cumulative effect of these changes is a diminution of homeostatic reserve, as well as loss of appropriate corrective responses to environmental and metabolic stressors.[29,30] Each of these potential mechanisms is considered separately, then combined into an integrated discussion of the etiology of disorders of water metabolism in the elderly.

Changes in Body Composition with Aging

Aging typically leads to a 5% to 10% increase in total body fat, and a decrease in total body water of equal magnitude. In an elderly 70-kg man, this can account for a reduction of total body water of as much as 7 to 8 L compared with a young man of the same weight.[29] With aging, plasma volume has also been shown to decrease by as much as 21% relative to body weight and surface area in older men when compared with younger controls.[31] The consequence of these changes is that an equivalent acute loss, or gain, of body water will cause a greater degree of flux in osmolality in elderly compared with younger individuals. Thus, states of relatively mild dehydration or volume overload in the elderly are more likely to cause clinically significant shifts in concentration of body solutes, such as sodium. This process was unequivocally

Box 1
Multiple factors that impair maintenance of normal body fluid homeostasis with aging

Altered Body Composition:

Reduced plasma volume

Increased osmolal flux

Kidney Effects:

Impaired free water excretion

Decreased urine concentrating ability

Brain Effects:

Decreased thirst perception

Increased AVP secretion

demonstrated by Rolls and Phillips[30] in a study that compared plasma osmolality in elderly and young subjects before and after equivalent degrees of fluid deprivation. Despite identical weight loss and similar changes in indices of plasma volume, the elderly clearly sustained a significantly greater increase in plasma osmolality than did the younger controls (**Fig. 5**). A similar process likely accounts for the much higher prevalence of hyponatremia in the elderly as a result of retention of relatively smaller volumes of water.

Changes in Renal Function with Aging

Many aspects of renal function related to water homeostasis are under neurohormonal control via secretion of AVP from the posterior pituitary. However, intrinsic renal mechanisms that play a key role in the derangement of water balance in aging also exist. Typical age-associated changes in the kidney include loss of parenchymal mass, progressive glomerulosclerosis, tubulopathy, interstitial fibrosis, and the development of afferent-efferent arteriolar shunts.[32] By age 80 years, the normal kidney loses up to 25% of its mass and develops a histopathologic appearance similar to that seen in chronic tubulointerstitial disease.[28] Beck[28,29] has described the resulting functional changes as an "inelasticity" in fluid homeostasis. Such defects may not be of immediate consequence during states of health, but in the elderly, especially under conditions of stress, disease, dehydration, or volume overload, such moderate impairments in normal renal physiology may cause significant imbalances in water and solute homeostasis.[28] The clinical result is the development of depletional or dilutional states such as hyperosmolality and hypoosmolality.

Age-associated changes in glomerular filtration rate

The Baltimore Longitudinal Study of Aging showed that up to 30% of healthy aged adults maintain a normal glomerular filtration rate (GFR). However, with few exceptions, in the remaining 70% of subjects, GFR was noted to decrease by approximately 1 mL/min/1.73 m^2 per year after age 40 years. A further acceleration in the rate of decline after age 65 years was also noted.[28,32,33] Whether these changes are an inevitable consequence of aging or are the result of subtle pathologic states remains uncertain. The consequences of such changes, however, are well established. Reductions in GFR increase proximal renal tubular fluid absorption, which leads to a decrease in tubular delivery of free water to the distal diluting segments of the

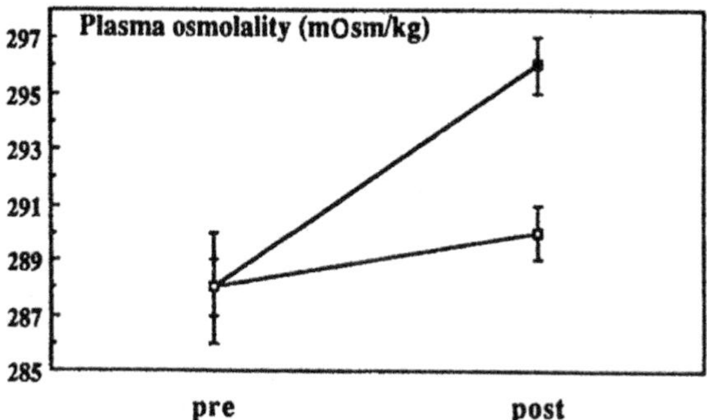

Fig. 5. Mean changes, prefluid and postfluid deprivation in young (*open boxes*) and elderly (*closed boxes*) subjects after equivalent degrees of induced weight loss. (*From* Rolls BJ, Phillips PA. Aging and disturbances of thirst and fluid balance. Nutrition Reviews 1990;48:137; with permission.)

nephron.[14] The result is a loss of the dilutional capacity of the kidney, manifested by an impaired ability to excrete a free water load.[25,30] Faull and colleagues[34] studied free water excretion among elderly subjects (mean age 68 years) in a comparison with young controls. This study showed that although the older group was able to achieve normal excretion following a standard water load of 20 mL/kg body weight, a significant decrement in maximal free water clearance in the older group was present. Work by Clark and colleagues[35] has suggested that this may, in part, be caused by decreased distal renal tubular delivery of water attributable to reduced prostaglandin production in the elderly. Such impairment in the ability to excrete excess body water has direct implications for the susceptibility of the elderly to dilutional states that predispose to hypoosmolality and hyponatremia.

Loss of urinary concentrating ability

Concomitant with the loss of diluting capacity, the aging kidney also loses the ability to maximally conserve body water during states of dehydration.[36] In such a volume-depleted state, in the absence of fluid ingestion, maximal urinary concentration is the only means by which further losses of body water can be reduced. By age 80 years, maximal urinary concentration typically declines from a youthful peak of 1100 to 1200 mOsm/kg H_2O to the range of 400 to 500 mOsm/kg H_2O.[25] Phillips and colleagues[37] established that following 24 hours of water deprivation, older subjects demonstrated significantly less urinary concentrating ability compared with younger controls, despite higher levels of plasma osmolality. This effect was also noted to occur despite higher plasma AVP levels in the elderly, suggesting that the concentrating defect is predominantly due to intrinsic renal factors. The clinical implications of this age-acquired defect in the maintenance of normal plasma osmolality are clear. Loss of urinary concentrating ability contributes to the exacerbation of numerous conditions common in the elderly such as diarrhea, vomiting, decreased thirst, and poor oral intake, thus worsening the resulting dehydration, hyperosmolality, and hypovolemia.

Changes in Centrally Mediated Control of Water Homeostasis with Aging

Central neuroendocrine control of AVP secretion and thirst are the major regulators of normal water balance in subjects with relatively normal renal function. Despite large variations in fluid intake, plasma osmolality is maintained within narrow limits via the secretion of AVP, the renal response to AVP secretion, and the appropriate control of thirst. Each of these processes is significantly affected by aging.

Regulation of AVP secretion in aging

AVP has a central role in the regulation of renal water excretion through its control of membrane insertion and abundance of the water channel aquaporin-2 (AQP2) in the distal nephron.[38] These effects are mediated through AVP interaction with the type 2 vasopressin receptor (V2R) expressed in the renal collecting ducts. Increased membrane-bound AQP2 increases water permeability of the collecting duct, and thereby induces a decrease in renal free water excretion, or antidiuresis. AVP is a nonapeptide synthesized by the cell bodies of the supraoptic and paraventricular nuclei of the hypothalamus. AVP is packaged in granules with its carrier protein neurophysin, and transported down axons terminating in the posterior pituitary where it is stored and ultimately secreted in response to specific stimuli.[27] The secretion of AVP is under exquisite, moment-to-moment control of osmoreceptors located in and around the organum vasculosum of the lamina terminalis and the anterior wall of the third ventricle. For any given individual an osmotic threshold, or set point, for AVP release typically exists within a relatively narrow normal range. An increase in plasma smolality as small as 1% to 2% is sufficient to cause an increase in plasma AVP con-entration of 1 pg/mL. Such an increase is able to rapidly and significantly decrease ee water excretion and reduce urine flow.[27] Any increase in plasma osmolality above he set point induces a linear increase in the secretion of AVP,[14] with maximum anti-liuresis occurring with plasma AVP concentrations higher than 5 pg/mL.[27] This xtraordinarily sensitive mechanism is able to maintain plasma osmolality within the ange 275 to 295 mOsm/kg H_2O. A secondary hemodynamic and volume-lependent regulatory mechanism for AVP secretion also exists. This mechanism is ontrolled by baroreceptors located in the cardiac atria and large arteries. In contrast o the exquisitely sensitive osmotic regulation of AVP secretion, the AVP response to a olume or hemodynamic stimulus does not occur until effective arterial volume is ecreased by approximately 8% to 10%.[14,27] The interaction of osmoreceptor and aroreceptor regulation of AVP secretion produces an integrated AVP secretory pro-le that is linear, but with a variable slope that is modulated by changes in volume and emodynamic status.[14]

Secretion and end-organ effects of AVP are also affected by aging. A majority of tudies has found that basal AVP levels in healthy elderly subjects are at least equal o, or more typically greater than those of young controls. However, a small number f studies have reported no differences in basal AVP levels in the elderly,[39] and at least ne study has suggested that basal AVP levels may be lower in older subjects.[40] Regardless of basal AVP levels, most of the literature regarding water homeostasis as demonstrated that the elderly have a greater augmentation of AVP secretion er unit change in plasma osmolality than do younger subjects. This finding is consis-ent with an increase in osmoreceptor sensitivity in the elderly.[40] Helderman and col-eagues[36] first made this observation more than 35 years ago in studies of dehydrated lderly patients subjected to hypertonic saline infusions (**Fig. 6**). Subsequent studies ave repeatedly confirmed this observation.[37,40,41] However, despite general

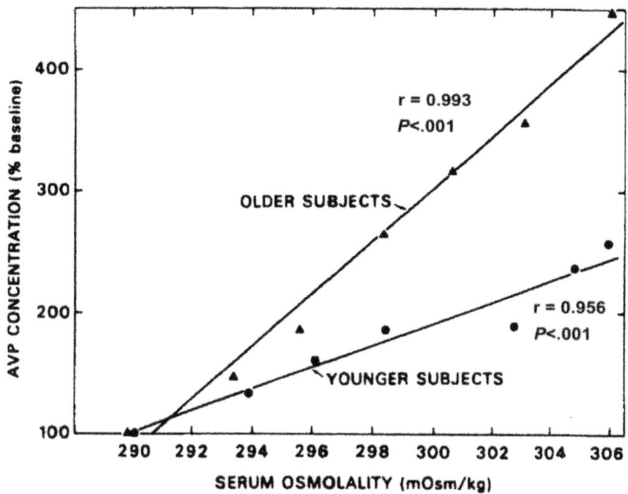

ig. 6. Correlation between serum osmolality and arginine vasopressin (AVP) concentration 8 young and 8 older subjects during a 2-hour 3% saline infusion following mild dehydra-on. The older subjects had significantly higher plasma levels of AVP per unit increase in lasma osmolality, strongly suggesting an enhanced osmotically stimulated secretion. *rom* Helderman JH. The response of arginine vasopressin to intravenous ethanol and hy-ertonic saline in man: the impact of aging. J Gerontol 1978;33(1):39–47; with permission.)

agreement, a few notable exceptions exist. The early work of Phillips and colleagues[37] showed a threefold increase in secretion of AVP per unit change in osmolality in the elderly, but later work by the same group indicated that AVP secretion in response to osmolar stimulus is maintained rather than augmented.[42,43] One isolated study demonstrating the absence of a correlation between AVP secretion and osmolality in the elderly has also been published.[44] Nonetheless, preservation or, more commonly, augmentation of osmoreceptor sensitivity has been repeatedly confirmed in the elderly.

Several mechanistic explanations for observed age-associated changes in AVP secretion have been proposed. Rowe and colleagues[45] studied AVP secretory responses to orthostatic maneuvers in young and elderly subjects, and found that 11 of 12 young subjects augmented AVP secretion in response to a position change from supine to erect. However, only 8 of 15, or just over half, of the elderly patients had a similar response.[45] The study also demonstrated an appropriate increase in sympathetic nervous system discharge of norepinephrine in response to positional changes regardless of AVP secretory status. This finding suggests that aging may not affect AVP secretion through impairment of the baroreceptor afferent-efferent loop. Rather, the study concludes that aging may result in a loss of appropriate transmission of postural stimuli from the vasomotor centers of the brainstem where these stimuli are received, to the hypothalamus where secretion of AVP is controlled. Such a defect would thereby impair normal secretion of AVP in response to position changes. Based on these results, Rowe and colleagues[45] have speculated that the increased AVP secretion in response to osmolar stimuli, which has been verified in the majority of studies performed in the elderly, may represent a compensatory response to the loss of normal baroreceptor-mediated control of AVP secretion in response to hemodynamic changes.

Whereas Rowe and colleagues[45] suggest that the loss of baroreceptor influence on AVP secretion occurs because of the loss of a neurologic pathway between the vasomotor center and the hypothalamus, Stachenfeld and colleagues[41] make an argument for a role of atrial natriuretic peptide (ANP) as an important mediator of AVP secretion. These investigators used studies of isosmotic central blood volume expansion during head-out water immersion (HOI) and measured AVP responses in healthy elderly and young cohorts. In addition to the loss of normal baroreceptor response to increases in central pressure, the elderly also demonstrated more exuberant secretion of ANP. Stachenfeld and colleagues[41] postulate that increased secretion of ANP may directly suppress AVP secretion during HOI. This hypothesis is consistent with earlier reports that exogenous ANP infusion suppresses osmotically stimulated AVP release in both young and elderly subjects.[46] However, other work has cast doubt on the relationship between ANP infusion and AVP secretion.[47] Thus, the question of whether ANP exerts significant physiologic control over AVP secretion in the elderly remains unclear.

Regulation of AVP function in aging

AVP V2 receptors, the site of AVP action in the kidney, are members of the 7-transmembrane domain G-protein–coupled receptor family. Activation of the receptor by AVP induces production of the intracellular second-messenger cyclic adenosine monophosphate (cAMP) via activation of adenylyl cyclase. Through activation of the cAMP pathway, new aquaporin-2 (AQP2) water channels are synthesized, and existing AQP2s are shuttled from intracellular storage vesicles and inserted into the apical plasma membrane of the renal collecting duct cells.[48] Once inserted into the apical membrane, AQP2s form channels through which water molecules can be absorbed from the lumen of the collecting duct into the renal medullary interstitium driven by the medullary osmotic gradient. The resulting antidiuresis is capable of concentrating urine to an osmolality equivalent to that at the tip of the inner renal medulla.[27]

Because AVP levels are generally found to be elevated in the elderly, a pituitary secretory defect is unlikely to explain the decreased renal response to AVP noted in aging. A more likely explanation is a decrease in normal renal responsivity to AVP. Decreased V2R receptor expression and/or decreased second-messenger response to AVP-V2R signaling would both result in loss of maximal urinary concentration. Both types of defects have been suggested in rat models of aging. A study in F344BN rats demonstrated an age-related impairment of renal concentrating ability after a moderate water restriction despite a normal AVP secretory response.[38] This study found lower basal levels of AQP2 water-channel expression in aging rats, and an inability of aging rats to normally upregulate AQP2 synthesis and mobilization despite appropriate AVP secretion. Other animal studies have suggested that decreased AVP-V2R signaling in the thick ascending limb and collecting ducts may also have deleterious effects on generation of the medullary concentrating gradient required for maximal urine concentration.[49,50] Human studies have not been possible to date, therefore the presence of such age-related changes in human kidneys remains speculative.

In addition to age-related changes in V2R expression and function, it has recently become clear that sex-related changes are clinically important. Studies in experimental animals have documented a 2.6-fold greater mRNA and 1.7-fold greater protein expression of the AVP V2R in female mice and rats in comparison with males.[51] This finding is postulated to be a result of the location of the V2R on the X chromosome, in a position that is predictive of incomplete inactivation of the V2R gene, based on X-inactivation tests in heterozygous human fibroblasts.[52] Clinical use of the AVP V2R agonist desmopressin for the treatment of enuresis in children and nocturia in adults has resulted in a small but significant incidence of hyponatremia,[53,54] which has occurred predominantly in elderly women. Recent clinical studies have demonstrated a greater sensitivity of women to smaller doses of desmopressin,[55] consistent with the studies in experimental animals. The combined clinical and experimental studies therefore suggest that increased V2R expression in women may cause greater sensitivity to the renal effects of exogenously administered AVP or desmopressin, and raises the possibility of similarly increased sensitivity to endogenously stimulated AVP, thereby leading more frequently to hyponatremia from SIADH, particularly in elderly women who manifest other factors that limit water excretion.

Regulation of thirst in aging

Stimulation of thirst osmoreceptors produces signals that are conveyed to the higher cerebral cortex, resulting in the perception of thirst and water-seeking behavior.[3] The osmotic threshold for thirst is 5 to 10 mOsm/kg H_2O above that for AVP release. This small difference in the set points regulating AVP secretion and manifestation of the thirst response has important physiologic consequences. Small osmolar excursions relative to an individual's osmotic set point induce changes only in AVP secretion and AVP-mediated changes in renal water excretion to maintain normal plasma osmolality. Only larger osmolar excursions are able to trigger the robust thirst response that either increases or decreases thirst to restore normal plasma osmolality. The important behavioral consequence of this mechanism is that the primary and earliest response to increased plasma osmolality involves an unconscious increase in AVP-mediated augmentation of renal concentration that occurs below the level of awareness. Only more pronounced increases in plasma osmolality are able to induce the potent and potentially disruptive behavioral response of water seeking.

Intrinsic defects in thirst clearly develop with aging. Phillips and colleagues[56] showed that older men deprived of hydration for 24 hours showed no subjective increase in thirst or mouth dryness and drank less water than young controls, despite significant increases in serum [Na^+] and plasma osmolality.[37] Furthermore, in contrast to the young controls, when allowed free access to water elderly subjects drank less and were unable to restore serum [Na^+] to predeprivation levels (**Fig. 7**). These data suggest a blunted thirst response to osmotic changes in the elderly. One explanation for these findings has been offered by Mack and colleagues.[57] This study showed that although a blunted thirst response was present in the elderly, the rate of fluid intake in healthy elderly and young controls was equivalent for equivalent degrees of thirst. Thus, elderly subjects appeared to have a higher osmolar set point for thirst that results in a decrease in the degree of perceived thirst for any given level of plasma osmolality, leading to a net decrease in the amount of fluid ingested owing to a decrease in the thirst response.[57] By contrast, other studies of thirst in the elderly that used hypertonic saline infusions and HOI have suggested that the response of thirst to an osmotic stimulus unaccompanied by a change in plasma volume is not appreciably affected by normal aging.[40,41] Instead, these studies demonstrated a diminution of baroreceptor-mediated regulation of thirst in response to changes in plasma volume.[58] Studies using HOI have supported the concept that control of thirst by volume shifts may actually take priority and override contradictory osmotic stimuli, at least in young subjects.[59] Using this same method, Stachenfeld and colleagues[41] demonstrated that in carefully selected healthy dehydrated participants, HOI caused a greater suppression of thirst and drinking response in the young than in elderly subjects. This study found that although net thirst was not different between the elderly and the young, this was due to relatively greater baroreceptor-mediated suppression of more exuberant thirst in the young compared with the elderly subjects. These combined data, therefore, provide further evidence of an intrinsic defect in thirst with normal aging.

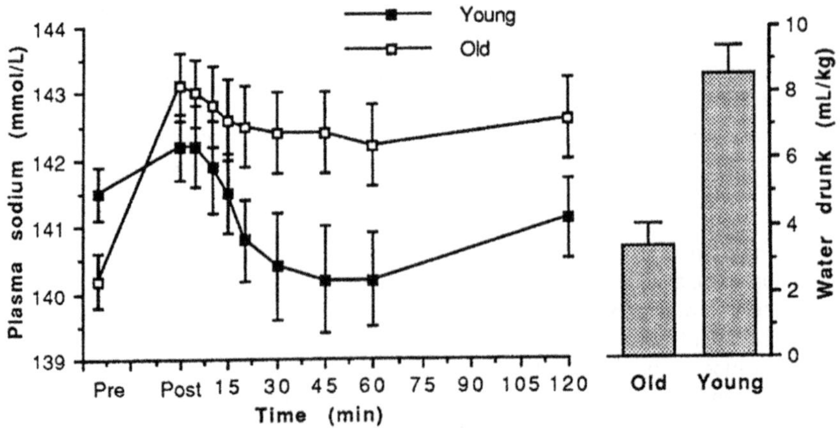

Fig. 7. Plasma sodium concentration and total water intake in healthy elderly and young subjects following 24 hours of dehydration. Baseline sodium concentrations before dehydration (Pre) and after dehydration (Post) are shown. Free access to water was allowed for 60 minutes following dehydration starting at time = 0 minutes. Cumulative water intake during the free drinking period by young and old subjects is depicted in the bar graph. Despite a greater initial increase in serum [Na^+], elderly subjects drank significantly less water, resulting in lesser correction of the elevated serum [Na^+]. (*From* Phillips PA, Johnston CI, Gray L. Disturbed fluid and electrolyte homeostasis following dehydration in elderly people. Age and Aging 1993;22(suppl 1):S26–S33; with permission.)

The subjective sensation of thirst requires unimpaired transmission of efferent signals from hypothalamic osmoreceptors to the cerebral cortex where thirst is perceived. Although the neural pathways that conduct these signals are not well characterized, it is likely that one of the major factors responsible for age-related changes in thirst is impairment of these poorly defined efferent pathways.[42] Subtle and cumulative brain injury caused by age-associated illness rather than aging, per se, may play an active role in such a process. It has been suggested that elderly patients who had many types of mild chronic illness may not have been adequately excluded from study populations previously described as "healthy." How the possible inclusion of such patients may have colored early studies of aging is difficult to assess.[39,40] Nonetheless, well-controlled studies on highly selected groups of healthy elderly subjects appear to corroborate the early findings of the presence of intrinsic defects in thirst with normal aging. Most studies confirm that aging is accompanied by decreased thirst. However, the relationships among osmolar changes, volume status, and other stimuli, and how these interact to mediate thirst with aging, remains incompletely understood. Thirst is a complex response to multiple and frequently interrelated physiologic stimuli. The literature provides observations of numerous stimulus response mechanisms involved in the generation and perception of thirst, and changes associated with aging. The exact mechanisms by which these changes occur, and whether they are an unavoidable consequence of normal aging, remain to be ascertained.

INTEGRATION OF CHANGES IN AVP SECRETION, THIRST, AND KIDNEY FUNCTION WITH AGING

Beck's conceptualization of "homeostatic inelasticity" aptly describes the consequences of the spectrum of physiologic changes that occur with aging.[28] Aging causes distinct changes that affect normal water homeostasis at several discrete locations along the neurorenal axis responsible for maintaining normal water balance. As a result of these changes, the elderly experience a loss of homeostatic reserve to compensate for both decreases and increases in body fluids and osmolality. The net effect is increased susceptibility to pathologic and iatrogenic causes of disturbed water homeostasis, and a decreased ability both to conserve and obtain fluids, leading to dehydration and hyperosmolality, and to excrete fluids, leading to overhydration and hypoosmolality.

The primary threat to dehydration and hyperosmolality seems to be a reduced sensation of thirst, leading to a compromised drinking response to thirst in the elderly. It is likely, as Phillips and colleagues[43] have suggested, that part of this defect is through loss of normal neural pathways that convey sensory input to the higher cortical centers where thirst is perceived, and from which the thirst response emanates. A clear age-related deficit in the thirst response appears to arise from decreased sensitivity to osmolar stimulation. The early work of Phillips and colleagues[56] demonstrated the presence of such a defect, and subsequent studies by Mack and colleagues[57] suggest that this defect is due to a higher osmotic set point leading to a blunted thirst response in the elderly. Most importantly, the loss of an appropriate thirst response compromises the critical compensatory mechanisms responsible for the drive to replace lost body fluid, and the only true physiologic means of correcting a hyperosmolar state.

Impaired GFR and resultant loss of maximal urinary concentrating ability also contribute to the threat of dehydration and hyperosmolality with aging. Decreased renal function is a common, if not certain, consequence of aging.[33,60] Although it seems that the development of such a deficit is not inevitable, how to discern which elderly are most likely to suffer such a loss is not easily determined. Because most otherwise "normal" elderly patients manifest such a decrement in renal function, the argument regarding whether such a change is inevitable may be overly academic. It may, on the other hand, be appropriate to assume that such a defect is probable, although some elderly who age more "successfully" than others may maintain reasonably normal renal function. Whatever the onset and progression of this process, its consequence is clear: decreased GFR causes an inability to maximally conserve free water and favors development of inappropriate body-water deficits. In addition to decrements in GFR, animal studies have unequivocally indicated an accompanying age-acquired end-organ insensitivity to the effects of AVP,[61] which would have the effect of magnifying renal water losses with aging. These combined effects likely initiate the pathophysiologic pathway leading to mild hyperosmolality in the elderly, which is then exacerbated by impaired thirst and drinking in response to the hyperosmolality, leading to more clinically pathologic degrees of hypernatremia and hyperosmolality.

The primary threat to overhydration and hypoosmolality seems to be a decrement in maximal water excretion that paradoxically also occurs in the elderly.[34,35] Such a defect would have significant clinical consequences in situations of inadvertent or forced overhydration. The elderly are at a higher risk of developing diseases such as congestive heart failure, which are associated with volume overload. So, too, are the elderly at risk for inadvertent iatrogenic overhydration from intravenous and enteral hydration therapy. Any inability to appropriately excrete an excessive fluid load would predispose elderly individuals to the development of overhydration and hypoosmolality. The secretion and end-organ effects of AVP account for 2 of the most interesting, and perhaps least well understood aspects of water regulation in the elderly. Although a few exceptions exist, most agree that basal AVP secretion is at least maintained, and more likely increased, with normal aging.[27] Furthermore, the AVP secretory response (ie, the osmoreceptor sensitivity to osmolar stimuli) is also increased in normal aging.[40] Thus, AVP secretion represents one of the few endocrine responses that increase rather than decrease with age. Although renal responsiveness to AVP may be reduced with aging, it is certainly not entirely eliminated. This fact may underlie the increased incidence of idiopathic SIADH occurring in the elderly that often cannot be explained by identifiable pathology.[7] The authors hypothesize that enhanced secretion of AVP in the elderly and inability to appropriately suppress AVP secretion during fluid intake,[43] combined with an intrinsic inability to maximally excrete free water,[34,35] increases the likelihood that SIADH will occur in this group of patients. The authors believe that these factors may explain the unusually high incidence of idiopathic SIADH noted in elderly populations. Direct experimental proof of this hypothesis is still required. Nonetheless, the preponderance of existing experimental data suggests that this assumption is well founded.

Although excessive fluid intake is likely not the major cause of hypoosmolality in most elderly patients, it may nonetheless also contribute to the threat of overhydration and hypoosmolality with aging. Stachenfeld and colleagues[41] have clearly demonstrated that plasma-volume expansion in elderly subjects does not generate the normal suppression of thirst found in the young. Thus, absent suppression of thirst would be likely to aggravate the effects of excessive renal water retention in elderly patients, leading to more pathologic degrees of hyponatremia and hypoosmolality in the elderly.

In conclusion, much has been learned in the 6 decades since Findley's original reflections about the effects of aging on water homeostasis. Since then, clearly demonstrated deficits in renal function, thirst, and responses to osmotic and volume stimulation have been repeatedly demonstrated in the elderly population. Although much is already known about the renal actions of AVP at the V2 receptor, this area remains an active field of study with regard to age-induced changes in renal concentrating ability, including how these effects interact with sex-related differences in V2R expression and function. The lessons learned over the past 6 decades of research serve to emphasize the fragile nature of water balance that is characteristic of aging. The elderly are at increased risk for disturbances of water homeostasis resulting from both intrinsic disease and iatrogenic causes. Recent studies have now shown that these disturbances have real-life clinical implications in terms of neurocognitive effects, falls, osteoporosis, bone fractures, hospital readmission, the need for long-term care, and morbidity and mortality. It is therefore incumbent on all those who care for the elderly to realize the more limited nature of the compensatory and regulatory mechanisms that maintain normal fluid homeostasis in elderly patients, and to incorporate this understanding into the diagnosis and clinical interventions that must be made to provide optimal care for this uniquely susceptible group of patients.

REFERENCES

1. Findley T. Role of the neurohypophysis in the pathogenesis of hypertension and some allied disorders associated with aging. Am J Med 1949;7(1):70–84.
2. Hodak SP, Verbalis JG. Abnormalities of water homeostasis in aging. Endocrinol Metab Clin North Am 2005;34(4):1031–46, xi.
3. Palevsky PM. Hypernatremia. Semin Nephrol 1998;18(1):20–30.
4. Janicic N, Verbalis JG. Evaluation and management of hypo-osmolality in hospitalized patients. Endocrinol Metab Clin North Am 2003;32(2):459–81, vii.
5. Verbalis JG. Hyponatremia and hypo-osmolar disorders. In: Greenberg A, Cheung AK, Coffman TM, et al, editors. Primer on kidney diseases. 5th edition. Philadelphia: Saunders Elsevier; 2009. p. 52–9.
6. Hawkins RC. Age and gender as risk factors for hyponatremia and hypernatremia. Clin Chim Acta 2003;337(1–2):169–72.
7. Miller M, Hecker MS, Friedlander DA, et al. Apparent idiopathic hyponatremia in an ambulatory geriatric population. J Am Geriatr Soc 1996;44(4):404–8.
8. Caird FI, Andrews GR, Kennedy RD. Effect of posture on blood pressure in the elderly. Br Heart J 1973;35(5):527–30.
9. Miller M. Hyponatremia: age-related risk factors and therapy decisions. Geriatrics 1998;53(7):32–3, 37–8, 41–2:assim.
10. Anpalahan M. Chronic idiopathic hyponatremia in older people due to syndrome of inappropriate antidiuretic hormone secretion (SIADH) possibly related to aging. J Am Geriatr Soc 2001;49(6):788–92.
11. Schwartz WB, Bennett W, Curelop S, et al. A syndrome of renal sodium loss and hyponatremia probably resulting from inappropriate secretion of antidiuretic hormone. 1957. J Am Soc Nephrol 2001;12(12):2860–70.
12. Bartter FC, Schwartz WB. The syndrome of inappropriate secretion of antidiuretic hormone. Am J Med 1967;42:790–806.
13. Hirshberg B, Ben-Yehuda A. The syndrome of inappropriate antidiuretic hormone secretion in the elderly. Am J Med 1997;103(4):270–3.
14. Fried LF, Palevsky PM. Hyponatremia and hypernatremia. Med Clin North Am 1997;81(3):585–609.
15. Terzian C, Frye EB, Piotrowski ZH. Admission hyponatremia in the elderly: factors influencing prognosis. J Gen Intern Med 1994;9:89–91.

16. Renneboog B, Musch W, Vandemergel X, et al. Mild chronic hyponatremia is associated with falls, unsteadiness, and attention deficits. Am J Med 2006; 119(1):71.
17. Verbalis JG, Barsony J, Sugimura Y, et al. Hyponatremia-induced osteoporosis. J Bone Miner Res 2010;25(3):554–63.
18. Gankam Kengne F, Andres C, Sattar L, et al. Mild hyponatremia and risk of fracture in the ambulatory elderly. QJM 2008;101(7):583–8.
19. Wald R, Jaber BL, Price LL, et al. Impact of hospital-associated hyponatremia on selected outcomes. Arch Intern Med 2010;170(3):294–302.
20. Hoorn EJ, Rivadeneira F, van Meurs JB, et al. Mild hyponatremia as a risk factor for fractures: the Rotterdam Study. J Bone Miner Res 2011;26(8):1822–8.
21. Hoorn EJ, Liamis G, Zietse R, et al. Hyponatremia and bone: an emerging relationship. Nat Rev Endocrinol 2011;8(1):33–9.
22. Sandhu HS, Gilles E, DeVita MV, et al. Hyponatremia associated with large-bone fracture in elderly patients. Int Urol Nephrol 2009;41(3):733–7.
23. Kinsella S, Moran S, Sullivan MO, et al. Hyponatremia independent of osteoporosis is associated with fracture occurrence. Clin J Am Soc Nephrol 2010;5(2):275–80.
24. Barsony J, Manigrasso MB, Xu Q, et al. Chronic hyponatremia exacerbates multiple manifestations of senescence in male rats. Age (Dordr) 2012. [Epub ahead of print].
25. Beck LH. Changes in renal function with aging. Clin Geriatr Med 1998;14(2): 199–209.
26. Snyder NA, Feigal DW, Arieff AI. Hypernatremia in elderly patients. A heterogeneous, morbid, and iatrogenic entity. Ann Intern Med 1987;107(3):309–19.
27. Wong LL, Verbalis JG. Systemic diseases associated with disorders of water homeostasis. Endocrinol Metab Clin North Am 2002;31(1):121–40.
28. Beck LH. The aging kidney. Defending a delicate balance of fluid and electrolytes. Geriatrics 2000;55(4):26–8.
29. Beck LH, Lavizzo-Mourey R. Geriatric hypernatremia [corrected]. Ann Intern Med 1987;107(5):768–9.
30. Rolls BJ, Phillips PA. Aging and disturbances of thirst and fluid balance. Nutr Rev 1990;48(3):137–44.
31. Davy KP, Seals DR. Total blood volume in healthy young and older men. J Appl Physiol 1994;76(5):2059–62.
32. Lamb EJ, O'Riordan SE, Delaney MP. Kidney function in older people: pathology, assessment and management. Clin Chim Acta 2003;334(1–2):25–40.
33. Lindeman RD. Assessment of renal function in the old. Special considerations. Clin Lab Med 1993;13(1):269–77.
34. Faull CM, Holmes C, Baylis PH. Water balance in elderly people: is there a deficiency of vasopressin? Age Ageing 1993;22(2):114–20.
35. Clark BA, Shannon RP, Rosa RM, et al. Increased susceptibility to thiazide-induced hyponatremia in the elderly. J Am Soc Nephrol 1994;5(4):1106–11.
36. Helderman JH, Vestal RE, Rowe JW, et al. The response of arginine vasopressin to intravenous ethanol and hypertonic saline in man: the impact of aging. J Gerontol 1978;33:39–47.
37. Phillips PA, Rolls BJ, Ledingham JG, et al. Reduced thirst after water deprivation in healthy elderly men. N Engl J Med 1984;311(12):753–9.
38. Abramow M, Beauwens R, Cogan E. Cellular events in vasopressin action. Kidney Int Suppl 1987;21:S56–66.
39. Duggan J, Kilfeather S, Lightman SL, et al. The association of age with plasma arginine vasopressin and plasma osmolality. Age Ageing 1993;22(5):332–6.

40. Davies I, O'Neill PA, McLean KA, et al. Age-associated alterations in thirst and arginine vasopressin in response to a water or sodium load. Age Ageing 1995; 24(2):151–9.
41. Stachenfeld NS, DiPietro L, Nadel ER, et al. Mechanism of attenuated thirst in aging: role of central volume receptors. Am J Physiol 1997;272(1 Pt 2): R148–57.
42. Phillips PA, Bretherton M, Risvanis J, et al. Effects of drinking on thirst and vasopressin in dehydrated elderly men. Am J Physiol 1993;264(5 Pt 2): R877–81.
43. Phillips PA, Johnston CI, Gray L. Disturbed fluid and electrolyte homoeostasis following dehydration in elderly people. Age Ageing 1993;22(1):S26–33.
44. Johnson AG, Crawford GA, Kelly D, et al. Arginine vasopressin and osmolality in the elderly. J Am Geriatr Soc 1994;42(4):399–404.
45. Rowe JW, Minaker KL, Sparrow D, et al. Age-related failure of volume-pressure-mediated vasopressin release. J Clin Endocrinol Metab 1982;54:661–4.
46. Clark BA, Elahi D, Fish L, et al. Atrial natriuretic peptide suppresses osmostimulated vasopressin release in young and elderly humans. Am J Physiol 1991; 261(2 Pt 1):E252–6.
47. Wazna-Wesly JM, Meranda DL, Carey P, et al. Effect of atrial natriuretic hormone on vasopressin and thirst response to osmotic stimulation in human subjects. J Lab Clin Med 1995;125(6):734–42.
48. Nielsen S, Fror J, Knepper MA. Renal aquaporins: key roles in water balance and water balance disorders. Curr Opin Nephrol Hypertens 1998;7(5):509–16.
49. Catudioc-Vallero J, Sands JM, Klein JD, et al. Effect of age and testosterone on the vasopressin and aquaporin responses to dehydration in Fischer 344/ Brown-Norway F1 rats. J Gerontol A Biol Sci Med Sci 2000;55(1):B26–34.
50. Combet S, Geffroy N, Berthonaud V, et al. Correction of age-related polyuria by dDAVP: molecular analysis of aquaporins and urea transporters. Am J Physiol Renal Physiol 2003;284(1):F199–208.
51. Liu J, Sharma N, Zheng W, et al. Sex differences in vasopressin V(2) receptor expression and vasopressin-induced antidiuresis. Am J Physiol Renal Physiol 2011;300(2):F433–40.
52. Carrel L, Willard HF. X-inactivation profile reveals extensive variability in X-linked gene expression in females. Nature 2005;434(7031):400–4.
53. Glazener CM, Evans JH. Desmopressin for nocturnal enuresis in children. Cochrane Database Syst Rev 2000;(2):CD002112.
54. Zong H, Yang C, Peng X, et al. Efficacy and safety of desmopressin for treatment of nocturia: a systematic review and meta-analysis of double-blinded trials. Int Urol Nephrol 2012;44(2):377–84.
55. Juul KV, Klein BM, Sandstrom R, et al. Gender difference in antidiuretic response to desmopressin. Am J Physiol Renal Physiol 2011;300(5):F1116–22.
56. Phillips PA, Bretherton M, Johnston CI, et al. Reduced osmotic thirst in healthy elderly men. Am J Physiol 1991;261(1 Pt 2):R166–71.
57. Mack GW, Weseman CA, Langhans GW, et al. Body fluid balance in dehydrated healthy older men: thirst and renal osmoregulation. J Appl Physiol 1994;76(4): 1615–23.
58. Stachenfeld NS, Mack GW, Takamata A, et al. Thirst and fluid regulatory responses to hypertonicity in older adults. Am J Physiol 1996;271(3 Pt 2): R757–65.
59. Wada F, Sagawa S, Miki K, et al. Mechanism of thirst attenuation during head-out water immersion in men. Am J Physiol 1995;268(3 Pt 2):R583–9.

60. Lindeman RD, Tobin J, Shock NW. Longitudinal studies on the rate of decline in renal function with age. J Am Geriatr Soc 1985;33(4):278–85.
61. Tian Y, Serino R, Verbalis JG. Downregulation of renal vasopressin V2 receptor and aquaporin-2 expression parallels age-associated defects in urine concentration. Am J Physiol Renal Physiol 2004;287(4):F797–805.

Sleep and Hormonal Changes in Aging

Georges Copinschi, MD, PhD[a,*], Anne Caufriez, MD, PhD[b]

KEYWORDS

• Sleep • Aging • Growth hormone • Cortisol • Gonadotropins • Testosterone
• Glucose tolerance

KEY POINTS

- Most frequently, endocrinometabolic function is partly dependent on sleep-wake homeostasis. Because major modifications of the sleep-wake homeostasis occur during normal aging, it can be expected that age-related hormonal alterations follow a similar pattern.
- Age-related dramatic decrease in GH secretion is closely associated with simultaneous decrease in the amount of SW sleep.
- Alterations of sleep architecture in the elderly could amplify the age-related decrease in the resiliency of the hypothalamic-pituitary-adrenal axis, resulting in a deleterious elevation of evening cortisol concentrations. Conversely, increased hypothalamic-pituitary-adrenal activity could inhibit SW sleep and promote nocturnal awakenings. This feed-forward cascade of negative events, generated by sleep and hypothalamic-pituitary-adrenal alterations, is likely to accelerate the development and enhance the severity of several age-related central and peripheral disorders.
- Hormonal alterations might contribute, directly or indirectly, to sleep disruptions observed in postmenopausal women, but these sleep disruptions play no role in the development of hormonal alterations.
- A feed-forward cascade of negative events generated by testicular and sleep disruptions could accelerate the senescence process in otherwise healthy normal men.
- Sleep curtailment is likely to accelerate the age-related deterioration of glucose tolerance.

INTRODUCTION

A prominent feature of hormonal regulation in humans is its high degree of temporal organization. Indeed, circulating hormonal levels undergo temporal oscillations ranging in period from a few minutes to 1 year. This organization provides the endocrine system with a high degree of flexibility. Hormonal variations in the circadian range (ie,

The authors have nothing to disclose.
[a] Laboratory of Physiology and Physiopathology, Université Libre de Bruxelles, CP 604, 808 route de Lennik, Brussels B-1070, Belgium; [b] Laboratory of Physiology, Physiopathology, and CHU Saint-Pierre, Université Libre de Bruxelles, CP 604, 808 route de Lennik, Brussels B-1070, Belgium
* Corresponding author.
E-mail address: gcop@ulb.ac.be

Endocrinol Metab Clin N Am 42 (2013) 371–389
http://dx.doi.org/10.1016/j.ecl.2013.02.009 endo.theclinics.com
0889-8529/13/$ – see front matter

approximately once per 24 hours) and in the ultradian range (ie, once per 60–120 minutes) are ubiquitous in hormonal systems. The menstrual cycle (approximately once per 28 days) belongs to the infradian range (periods longer than 24 hours).[1]

The organization of hormonal secretions during the 24-hour cycle results from the interaction in the central nervous system of two time-keeping mechanisms: the endogenous "circadian pacemaker"; and the sleep-wake homeostasis, a mechanism relating the timing and the intensity of sleep to the duration of prior wakefulness. The "master circadian clock" is located in the hypothalamic paired suprachiasmatic nucleus.[2] The suprachiasmatic nucleus controls the timing of most circadian rhythms (including hormonal rhythms), and partly regulates the sleep-wake cycle. In turn, the sleep-wake cycle regulates the timing of many hormonal rhythms. Thus, for most hormones, the 24-hour profiles result from the interaction of the circadian clock with sleep-wake homeostasis[3] and reflect the superposition of 24-hour periodicities on an ultradian, or pulsatile, pattern of release.

However, the 24-hour sleep-wake cycle is driven partially by the circadian pacemaker and partially by the homeostatic regulation of sleep pressure. Sleep itself involves two states of distinct brain activity, generated in specific brain regions: the rapid eye movement (REM) and the non-REM stages. REM sleep and non-REM sleep are characterized by different patterns of cerebral and peripheral activity. Non-REM sleep and REM sleep occur in alternating cycles, each lasting approximately 90 minutes. Each cycle is normally initiated by light non-REM stages (stages I and II), followed by deeper non-REM stages (stages III and IV), then by REM sleep. During REM sleep, eye movements are present, muscle tone is inhibited, and the electroencephalogram (EEG) is similar to that of active waking. Therefore, REM sleep is also referred to as paradoxical sleep. During deep non-REM sleep, the EEG is synchronized with high-amplitude, low-frequency waveforms, referred to as slow waves (SW). Therefore, deep non-REM sleep is currently referred to as SW sleep. The intensity of SW sleep, or SW activity, may be quantified by spectral analysis of the EEG. SW sleep is considered to be the most restorative sleep stage.[1] Dreams mainly occur during REM sleep.[4]

In young healthy subjects, normal sleep involves four to six successive cycles: the first cycle successively includes 10 to 20 minutes of light non-REM sleep, nearly 60 minutes of deep non-REM sleep, and a few minutes of REM sleep. As the night progresses, non-REM sleep becomes shallower, the duration of REM episodes progressively becomes longer, and the number and duration of transient awakenings increase. Approximately 50% of a normal night is spent in stages I and II, 20% in SW sleep, 25% in REM sleep, and 5% in wake. Typical individual sleep pattern in a healthy 20-year-old man is shown in **Fig. 1**.

Major modifications of the sleep-wake pattern occur during normal aging. Elderly healthy subjects frequently complain of shallow sleep with frequent transient awakenings during the night, early morning awakening, and unwanted daytime naps.[5–7] These alterations in subjective sleep quality reflect important alterations in sleep architecture.[8–16] The total sleep period (ie, the time interval between initial sleep onset and final morning awakening) remains relatively stable across adulthood. However, the total sleep time (ie, the total sleep period minus the total duration of transient nocturnal awakenings) decreases after 50 years of age, reflecting sleep fragmentation.[14–17] From early adulthood (16–25 years) to midlife (35–50 years), a spectacular decrease in SW sleep occurs. This decrease is compensated by an increase in lighter non-REM sleep (stages I and II), whereas there is no significant modification in REM sleep, nor in time spent awake.[17] From midlife to old age (70–80 years), no additional decline in SW sleep occurs, but light non-REM sleep and REM sleep progressively decrease, resulting in a mirror increase in wake time.[17] The decrease in the duration of REM

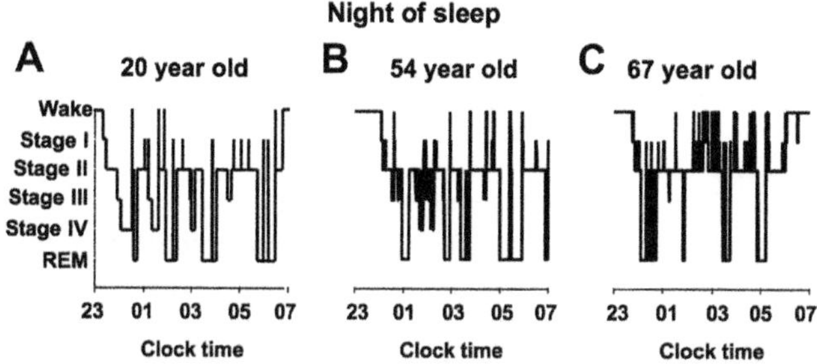

Fig. 1. Hypnograms recorded in healthy men aged 20, 54, and 67 years during nocturnal sleep from 23 to 07 hours. (*A, Young man*) Note the progressive decrease in deep slow-wave sleep (stages III and IV), the progressive increase in the duration of REM episodes, and in the number and duration of awakenings as the night progresses. (*B, Middle-aged man*) Note the replacement of slow-wave sleep by lighter non-REM sleep (stages I and II) compared with the young man. (*C, Old man*) Note the decrease in REM sleep and the increase in the number and duration of awakenings, compared with the middle-aged man. (Rachel Leproult, PhD, personal communication, 2012.)

sleep is associated with a redistribution of REM stages across the sleep period, with a shift of REM stages toward the early part of the night. Typical individual sleep patterns in healthy 20-, 54-, and 67-year-old men are shown in **Fig. 1**. The time course of age-related modifications of sleep architecture in a large group of healthy men, aged 16 to 83 years, is illustrated in **Fig. 2**.

Older women have more frequent and important subjective sleep complaints than men,[18–20] and the quality of non-REM sleep seems to be better preserved with aging in men than in women.[21]

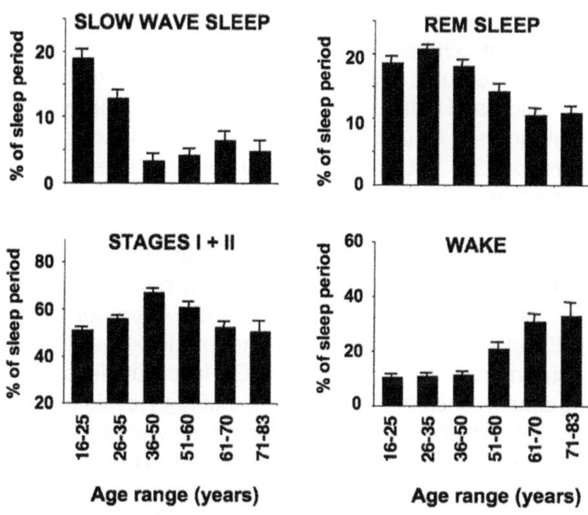

Fig. 2. Slow-wave sleep (stages III and IV), light non-REM sleep (stages I and II), REM sleep, and wake during sleep as a function of age in 149 healthy men, aged 16 to 83 years. For each age group, values shown are mean (+SEM). (*Data from* Van Cauter E, Leproult R, Plat L. Age-related changes in slow wave sleep and REM sleep and relationship with growth hormone and cortisol levels in healthy men. JAMA 2000;284:861.)

The mechanisms of sleep-hormonal interactions, and therefore the endocrinometabolic consequences of age-related sleep alterations, which markedly differ from one hormone to another, are reviewed in the following sections.

GROWTH HORMONE

In normal young adults, the 24-hour profile of circulating growth hormone (GH) levels is characterized by stable low levels abruptly interrupted by secretory episodes. The most reproducible pulse occurs shortly after sleep onset and is temporally associated with the first phase of SW sleep.[22] In men, the sleep-onset GH peak is generally the largest pulse observed over the 24-hour span. This pulse is also present in healthy cycling young women but daytime pulses are larger and more frequent, resulting in higher 24-hour GH levels than in men.[23] Daytime GH secretion was found to be higher during the luteal than during the follicular phase, and this increase correlated positively with progesterone (but not with estradiol) levels.[24]

The temporal organization of GH secretion is primarily dependent on the sleep-wake homeostasis.[25] A close temporal and quantitative association between SW sleep or SW activity and GH secretion is consistently found, even when sleep is advanced, delayed, or fragmented.[26–28] GH secretion is inhibited by transient awakenings.[29] The mechanisms underlying the relationship between SW sleep and GH secretion seem to involve synchronous activity of at least two populations of GH-releasing hormone (GHRH) neurons in the hypothalamus.[30] Indeed, inhibition of endogenous GHRH secretion, either by immunoneutralization or by administration of a specific GHRH antagonist, inhibits GH secretion and SW activity.[31] In rodents, GHRH injections stimulate REM and non-REM sleep in intact animals, but only non-REM sleep in hypophysectomized animals.[32,33] Those findings suggest that the effects of GHRH on REM sleep (but not the effects on non-REM sleep) are mediated by GH. In healthy humans, GHRH injections during sleep, at a dose eliciting GH responses within the physiologic range, may stimulate SW sleep and, although to a lesser extent, REM sleep.[34,35] Conversely, the somatostatin analog octreotide inhibits GH secretion and stage IV sleep.[36] On the other hand, enhancement of SW sleep by a low dose of γ-hydroybutyrate (a natural metabolite of γ-aminobutyric acid used in the treatment of narcolepsy) or by ritanserin (a selective serotonin antagonist) results in simultaneous and correlated increases in nocturnal GH secretion.[26,37] Thus, a robust and complex interaction exists between sleep and GH secretion.

Aging is associated with major decreases in GH[17,23,38] and in insulin-like growth factor-I[39,40] levels. Mean GH profiles in young and old healthy men are illustrated in **Fig. 3**. The reduction in GH secretion results from a decrease in amplitude, rather than in frequency, of GH pulses.[38,41,42] Maximal GH secretion is observed during the pubertal spurt. Between young adulthood and middle age, GH secretion rapidly decreases in an exponential fashion. At midlife, GH levels are less than half the values obtained in young adults, despite the persistence of high levels of sex steroids. From midlife to old age, GH secretion declines at a much slower rate. Not surprisingly, the age-related decrease of GH secretion during sleep follows the same chronology as the decrease observed for SW sleep (**Fig. 4**).[17] A cross-sectional study, conducted in 114 healthy men to examine the variance of GH secretion in relation to age and to SW sleep, found that SW sleep and the interaction between SW sleep and age accounted for most of the variance, whereas the effects of age per se were not significant.[17] The progressive decline in circulating insulin-like growth factor-I levels is linear from young adulthood to old age.[40]

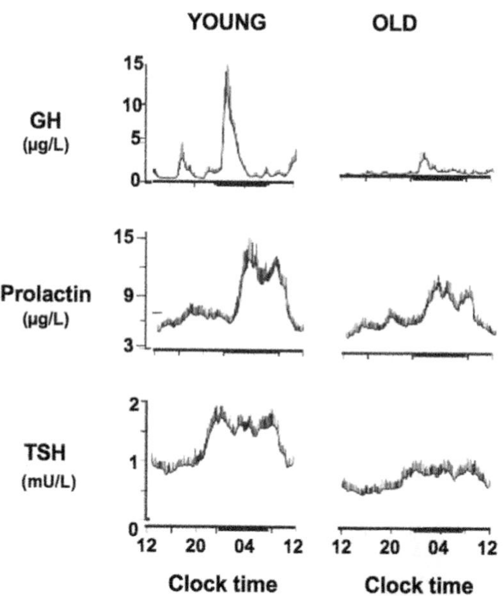

ig. 3. Mean (+SEM) 24-hour profiles of plasma growth hormone (GH), prolactin, and thyro- ropin (TSH) in eight young (20–27 years) and eight old (67–84 years) healthy men. The *black ars* denote the mean sleep periods. (*Data from* Van Coevorden A, Mockel J, Laurent E, et al. Jeuroendocrine rhythms and sleep in aging men. Am J Physiol 1991;260:E651.)

ROLACTIN

he sleep-wake homeostasis also seems to play a major role in the temporal organi- ation of prolactin secretion.[25] Under normal conditions, the 24-hour profile of circu- ating prolactin levels exhibits relatively low daytime concentrations, followed by major nocturnal elevation starting shortly after sleep onset and culminating around nid-sleep at levels corresponding to an average elevation of 200% above minimum ay levels.[43,44] Sleep onset is consistently associated with a rise in prolactin secretion, respective of the time of the day, and shifts in the sleep-wake cycle are immediately ollowed by parallel shifts in the diurnal prolactin rhythm.[22] A close temporal relation- hip has been evidenced between increased prolactin secretion and SW activity,[45] vhereas prolonged awakenings during the sleep period are associated with ecreases in prolactin levels.[45]

Thus, shallow and fragmented sleep is associated with a dampening of the noc- urnal elevation of prolactin levels. This is indeed the case in healthy elderly subjects, vho exhibit a nearly 50% reduction of the nocturnal prolactin rise observed in young ndividuals.[38,46] Mean prolactin profiles in young and old healthy men are illustrated in **ig. 3**. No data are available concerning the chronology of age-related alterations in rolactin secretion.

HYROTROPIN AND THYROID HORMONES

n healthy young adults, thyroid-stimulating hormone (TSH) levels are low and fairly table during daytime. In late afternoon or early evening, well before sleep onset, SH levels begin to rise and reach maximum levels around sleep onset.[47] During ne sleep period, TSH levels progressively decline, to return to daytime values shortly

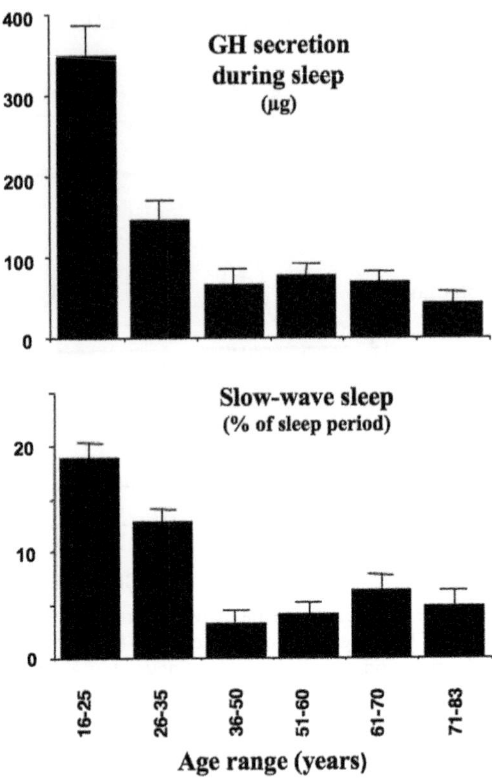

Fig. 4. Growth hormone secretion during sleep and slow-wave sleep (stages III and IV) as a function of age in 149 healthy men, aged 16 to 83 years. For each age group, values shown are mean (+SEM). Note the temporal concomitance between the decrease in GH secretion and the decline in SW sleep. (*Data from* Van Cauter E, Leproult R, Plat L. Age-related changes in slow wave sleep and REM sleep and relationship with growth hormone and cortisol levels in healthy men. JAMA 2000;284:861.)

after morning awakening.[47] While the evening increase is considered to reflect a circadian control, the nocturnal decrease throughout the sleep period seems to result from an inhibitory action of sleep on TSH secretion. Indeed, the nocturnal decrease is not observed in case of sleep deprivation.[47,48] This decrease is associated with SW sleep,[49,50] indicating that SW sleep is likely to be the primary determinant of the nocturnal TSH decline. Conversely, nocturnal awakenings are frequently associated with TSH peaks.[51]

TSH levels are reduced in healthy old subjects, in particular during the night (see **Fig. 3**).[38] In middle-aged subjects, this decrease is evidenced only after nocturnal sleep deprivation. Thus, TSH secretory capacity seems to progressively decline with aging. Because deep non-REM sleep inhibits TSH secretion, this decrease is clearly not dependent on age-related sleep alterations. It might result from an increased sensitivity of the pituitary thyrotropic cells to the negative feedback action of thyroid hormones, or from a diminished capacity of the hypothalamus to synthesize and release thyrotropin-releasing hormone.[52] Thyroid hormone secretion is diminished in the elderly, but circulating thyroxin levels remain fairly unchanged because the clearance of the hormone is also decreased.[52]

ADRENOCORTICOTROPIC HORMONE AND CORTISOL

In healthy young subjects, the 24-hour profile of adrenocorticotropic hormone and cortisol is characterized by an early morning peak; a progressive decline toward minimal levels centered around midnight (referred to as the quiescent period); followed during late sleep by an abrupt elevation (referred to as the circadian rise) toward the morning peak.[1] This pattern remains largely unchanged by sleep manipulations, such as sleep presence or absence at abnormal times.[1] Thus, this rhythm is primarily controlled by the circadian clock, presumably by the hypothalamic corticotropin-releasing hormone (CRH).

However, cortisol secretion is modulated by the sleep-wake homeostasis. Sleep onset is consistently followed by an immediate decrease in cortisol levels (which may not be detectable when sleep is initiated in early morning, at a peak of corticotropic activity).[53–56] This inhibitory effect of sleep has been shown to be related to SW sleep.[57–59] Conversely, final morning awakening and transient awakenings during the sleep period are consistently followed by pulses of cortisol secretion.[53,58,60,61] In an analysis of cortisol profiles recorded during nocturnal sleep, all transient awakenings that interrupted sleep for at least 10 minutes were followed, within the next 20 minutes, by significant cortisol pulses.[53]

Chronic insomnia, resulting in a reduction of total sleep time, is associated with an elevation of nocturnal cortisol levels.[62] In normal sleepers, total nocturnal wake time is positively associated with 24-hour circulating cortisol levels.[63] Moreover, during daytime wakefulness, a temporal coupling has been evidenced between cerebral alertness and cortisol secretion.[64] However, none of these studies allowed to determine whether the hyperactivity of the corticotropic axis resulted from the brain activity, or the opposite.

In rats and rabbits, intracerebral injections of CRH inhibit SW sleep.[65,66] Conversely, blockade of CRH receptors reduces wakefulness.[67] In humans, intravenous injections of CRH during the night were found either to inhibit sleep efficiency and SW sleep, or to have no significant effects on sleep, depending on the protocol used and the age of the subjects.[68–71] Conversely, cortisol administration was found to enhance SW sleep in young[72,73] and older subjects,[74] presumably by a negative feedback action on endogenous secretion of CRH.

In healthy subjects, the circadian rhythm of cortisol persists throughout the aging process, and is still present in very old individuals.[38,75,76] However, from 50 years of age onward, aging is associated with significant alterations of cortisol profiles: evening cortisol levels increase progressively and late evening levels are markedly higher in healthy subjects older than 70 years of age than in young adults.[75,76] In the elderly, the quiescent period starts later and ends earlier, is fragmented, and is markedly shortened. Alterations are more pronounced in women than in men: between 25 and 65 years of age, the reduction in the duration of the quiescent period is less than 3 hours in men but averages approximately 4.5 hours in women.[75,76] Elevated evening cortisol levels are likely to reflect a reduced resiliency of the hypothalamic-pituitary-adrenal axis, resulting from alterations of hippocampal neurons in the elderly.[77]

It is of interest to note that this age-related increase in evening cortisol concentrations and the age-related decline in REM sleep occur in a mirror image (**Fig. 5**).[17] Thus, age-related alterations of sleep quality could contribute to alterations of the corticotropic axis observed in the elderly. Indeed, in young subjects, acute total or partial (4 hours in bed) sleep deprivation results on the following day in elevated cortisol levels in late afternoon and evening.[78] Similar alterations are observed when partial sleep

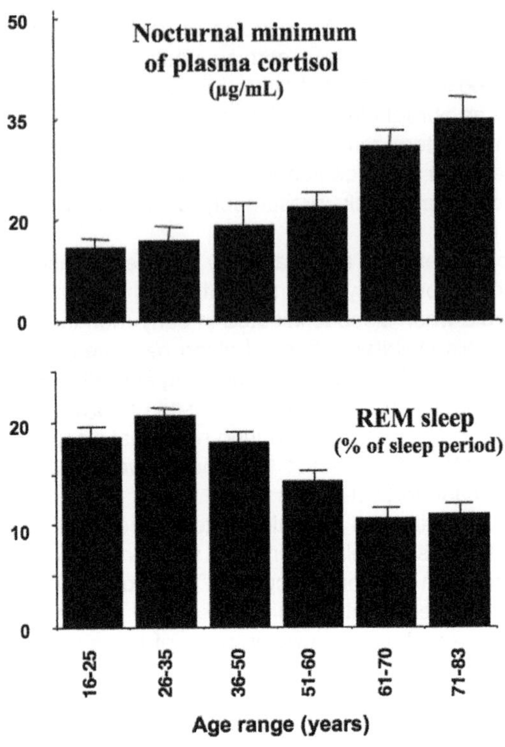

Fig. 5. Nocturnal minimum of plasma cortisol levels and REM sleep as a function of age in 149 healthy men, aged 16 to 83 years. For each age group, values shown are mean (+SEM). Note the temporal concomitance between the increase in nocturnal minimum cortisol levels and the decline in REM sleep. (*Data from* Van Cauter E, Leproult R, Plat L. Age-related changes in slow wave sleep and REM sleep and relationship with growth hormone and cortisol levels in healthy men. JAMA 2000;284:861.)

restriction (4 hours in bed per night) is enforced for 6 consecutive nights.[79] These alterations are strikingly similar to those observed in older healthy subjects with normal sleep schedules (**Fig. 6**). Thus, sleep curtailment seems to accelerate the senescence process of the hypothalamic-pituitary-adrenal axis. Both animal and human studies indicate that hyperactivity of the hypothalamic-pituitary-adrenal axis may have deleterious effects, especially at a time of the day when cortisol levels are normally low.[80,81] Thus, even modest elevations in evening cortisol levels could favor the development of central and peripheral disturbances associated with glucocorticoid excess, such as insulin resistance, osteoporosis, and memory deficits.[80–84]

GONADOTROPINS AND SEX STEROIDS

Women

An association between sleep and pulsatile gonadotropin secretion is already observed in prepubertal girls.[85] In pubertal girls, the pulse amplitude of the follicle-stimulating hormone (FSH) and of luteinizing hormone (LH) is increased during sleep.[85] In healthy adult cycling women, the amplitude and frequency of gonadotropin pulses appear to be modulated by circulating estrogen levels and vary markedly throughout the menstrual cycle. However, they are also modulated by sleep: in early follicular

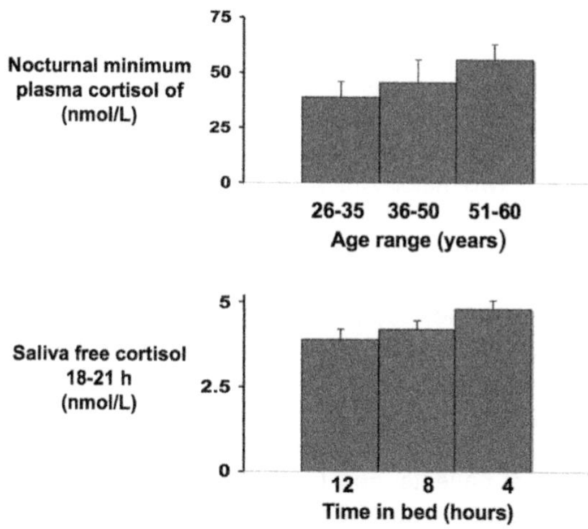

ig. 6. (*Upper panel*) Nocturnal minimum plasma cortisol levels in healthy men as a function of age. Values shown are mean (+SEM). (*Lower panel*) Evening saliva levels of free cortisol in healthy young men as a function of sleep schedule. Values shown are mean (+SEM). Note the similarity between the effects of aging and the effects of sleep curtailment. (*Data from* Van Cauter E, Leproult R, Plat L. Age-related changes in slow wave sleep and REM sleep and relationship with growth hormone and cortisol levels in healthy men. JAMA 2000;284:861; and Spiegel K, Leproult R, Van Cauter E. Impact of sleep debt on metabolic and endocrine function. Lancet 1999;354:1435.)

phase and in early luteal phase, pulse frequency is reduced during the night.[86,87] This slowing is specifically related to sleep and not to time of the day, because it is also observed during daytime sleep, but not during nighttime wakefulness.[88] Moreover, LH pulses during the sleep period occur preferentially in association with brief awakenings.[88] Sleep alterations (shorter and more fragmented sleep), rather common in night and shift workers, are likely to play a role in alterations of the menstrual function frequently observed in those individuals.

Few studies have investigated the potential confounding effects of the menstrual cycle on sleep architecture.[89] Awakenings are less frequent in the early luteal phase, presumably because estrogen and progesterone levels are rising. Conversely, awakenings are more frequent at the end of luteal phase, when both hormones levels are declining. Highest durations of light non-REM sleep (stage II) are found in late follicular phase and in early luteal phase, and a significant positive association was found between progesterone levels and the duration of stage III sleep.

A decrease in circulating levels of inhibin B seems to be the earliest hormonal marker of the onset of menopausal transition, resulting in increased FSH levels.[90] At menopause, ovarian steroid secretion falls markedly and in postmenopausal women, circulating levels of estradiol, progesterone, and androgens are very low, resulting in major elevations of gonadotropin levels, principally FSH. Sleep may be severely impaired, with increased sleep complaints and more nocturnal intermittent awakenings, especially in women with hot flushes.[89,91,92] Awakenings are not always associated with vasomotor symptoms (hot flushes), but nighttime flushes are consistently associated with transient awakenings. Major sleep disruptions and hot flushes occur mostly during the second half of the night, around 4 to 5 AM, at the time of the cortisol circadian rise, suggesting a possible involvement of the corticotropic axis. Hot flushes and low inhibin B levels have been shown to be independent predictors of poor sleep quality.[93]

Vasomotor symptoms were reported to be associated with higher body mass index, elevated blood pressure, increased cholesterol levels, reduced heart rate variability (a marker of increased cardiovascular risk), impaired endothelial function, increased aortic calcification and increased intima media thickness,[94–100] suggesting that women with hot flushes may be at greater risk for cardiovascular disease. Furthermore, careful analyses of two major clinical trials indicate that the increase in coronary heart disease associated with late hormone-replacement therapy was concentrated among women who reported clinically significant vasomotor symptoms.[101,102] However, an ongoing longitudinal population-based study conducted on more than 60,000 postmenopausal women found that the risk of cardiovascular disease was increased in women with late-onset vasomotor symptoms, but not in women with a history of perimenopausal vasomotor symptoms.[103]

The data concerning the effects of hormonal-replacement therapy on sleep architecture in postmenopausal women are largely inconsistent, probably because the protocol, the selection of patients, and the nature and the dose of the compounds used vary considerably across studies. A recent study indicates that oral administration of progesterone may improve sleep duration and quality in postmenopausal women when sleep is disturbed by environmental conditions.[104]

Men

In young adults, LH secretory pulses mainly reflect gonadotropin-releasing hormone pulsatility. During sleep, LH pulses appear to be temporally related to the REM–non-REM cycle: initiation of LH pulses was found to occur preferentially during non-REM stages, whereas REM sleep was generally associated with decreasing LH levels.[105] Diurnal variations over the 24-hour span are of low amplitude, or even undetectable. In contrast, circulating testosterone exhibits a major diurnal rhythm, superimposed on episodic pulses, with maximal levels in the early morning and minimal levels in the late evening.[106] This rhythm seems to be primarily driven by the sleep-wake cycle. Indeed, daytime sleep and nighttime sleep are associated with a robust rise in circulating testosterone levels.[107] However, albeit blunted compared with nocturnal sleep, a progressive increase in testosterone levels persists during nocturnal wakefulness,[107] indicating the existence of a circadian component that could reflect adrenal testosterone secretion.

From 30 years of age onward, aging is associated with a progressive decline in circulating testosterone levels by 1% to 2% per year,[75] together with an increase in sex hormone-binding globulin, so that the decrease in bioavailable testosterone is more pronounced than the decline in total testosterone.[108] Diurnal circadian variations are dampened.[109,110]

In contrast to the decline in testosterone levels, gonadotropin levels are increased in older men,[111,112] indicating that the decline in testosterone secretion is primarily caused by partial testicular failure. However, this decline seems to be modulated by age-related sleep alterations. Indeed, the duration of nighttime sleep has been shown to be an independent predictor of morning total and free testosterone in old men.[113] Consistent with this finding, a recent study conducted in young healthy men found that 1 week of sleep restriction (5 hours in bed per night) resulted in a significant decrease in 24-hour testosterone levels and in lower vigor scores.[114]

MELATONIN

The 24-hour profile of plasma melatonin by the pineal gland is primarily controlled by the circadian clock.[115] Under normal conditions, low and stable daytime levels are followed by a major circadian rise starting in the evening, between 9 and 11 PM and culminating around the middle of the sleep period. Thereafter, melatonin levels progressively return to low daytime values between 8 and 9 AM. Exposure to light during the night results in a dose-dependent suppression of circulating melatonin levels.[116,117] However, melatonin secretion is modulated by the sleep-wake cycle: in young healthy subjects, the amplitude of the circadian elevation was found to be mildly but significantly reduced when the subjects remain awake.[118]

Daytime melatonin levels are similar in old and young subjects. Most studies indicate that nocturnal melatonin elevations are dampened in the elderly.[38,118–120] This dampening might be caused by insufficient daytime environmental illumination frequently encountered by elderly individuals.[121] In contrast with young control subjects, the amplitude of the circadian melatonin rise was found to be enhanced, rather than reduced, in old subjects when they remain awake.[119] Thus, the effect of sleep on melatonin secretion seems to be age dependent. The mechanism of the relationship between sleep and melatonin secretion is unknown.

GLUCOSE AND INSULIN

Glucose homeostasis primarily depends on the balance between glucose production by the liver, and glucose use by insulin-dependent tissues (for instance, muscle and adipose tissue) and non–insulin dependent tissues (for instance, the brain). However, in normal humans, glucose utilization varies with the time of the day.[122] In healthy young subjects, glucose levels remain stable or decrease only minimally during nocturnal sleep, despite relatively prolonged fasting, whereas they clearly decline during daytime wakefulness. Moreover, glucose levels also remain stable during daytime sleep, but decrease in case of nighttime wakefulness.[54] This means that some sleep-associated mechanisms are operative to maintain stable glucose levels despite prolonged fasting. Experimental protocols involving constant enteral nutrition or intravenous glucose infusion have shown that during the first part of nocturnal sleep, glucose tolerance deteriorates to reach a minimum around mid-sleep, then improves to return to morning levels.[54,123,124] This decrease in glucose tolerance results from a reduction in cerebral[125] and peripheral glucose utilization. Indeed, positron emission tomography studies have evidenced that during SW sleep, which is a dominant sleep stage during the first half of the sleep period, cerebral glucose utilization (estimated to represent at least 20% of total body glucose utilization)[126,127] is markedly lower than during either wake or REM sleep.[128,129] On the other hand, the sleep onset–associated GH release is likely to inhibit glucose uptake by insulin-dependent tissues.[130] Thus, sleep-wake homeostasis appears to exert important modulatory effects on glucose regulation.

Well-controlled laboratory studies indicate that partial sleep restriction for 1 to 7 days may result in increased insulin resistance.[79,131–133] Prolonged voluntary sleep curtailment (at least 6 months) was also found to result in the development of insulin resistance.[134] These observations are consistent with data obtained in multiple epidemiologic studies, revealing an association between short sleep duration and the risk of developing diabetes.[135] Moreover, alterations in sleep quality are also important: using sound delivery to disturb normal sleep, an elegant study has evidenced that all-night selective suppression of SW sleep also resulted in reduced glucose tolerance, despite preservation of sleep duration and REM sleep.[136]

Aging is associated with a decrease in glucose tolerance, resulting from a decline in insulin secretion and insulin sensitivity.[137] Interestingly, the amplitude of the decrease in glucose clearance rate after intravenous glucose injection (intravenous glucose tolerance test) observed in elderly subjects older than 65 years as compared with

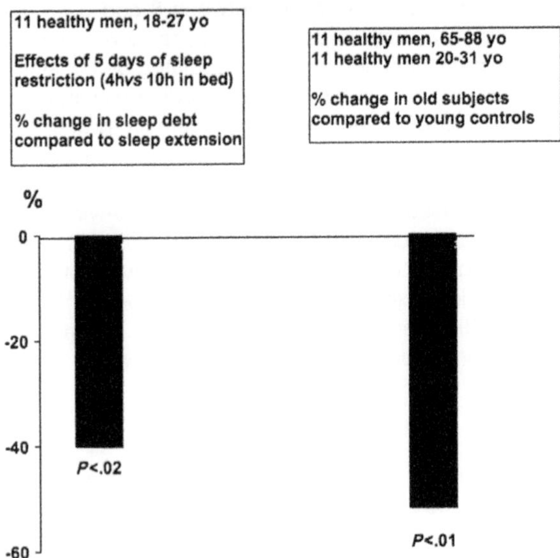

Fig. 7. Relative decrease in glucose tolerance after intravenous glucose injection (IVGTT) in healthy young subjects after partial sleep restriction compared with fully rested condition, and in old healthy subjects compared with young control subjects. Note the similarity between the effects of aging and the effects of sleep curtailment. (*Data from* Palmer JP, Ensinck JW. Acute-phase insulin secretion and glucose tolerance in young and aged normal men and diabetic patients. J Clin Endocrinol Metab 1975;41:498; and Spiegel K, Leproult R, Van Cauter E. Impact of sleep debt on metabolic and endocrine function. Lancet 1999;354:1435.)

young control subjects is fairly similar to the amplitude of the decrease observed in young healthy subjects submitted to partial sleep restriction as compared with fully rested condition (**Fig. 7**), so that glucose tolerance in young healthy subjects after partial sleep curtailment was found to fall in the range observed in elderly subjects with normal sleep schedule.[79,138,139] The similarity between the effects of aging and the effects of sleep curtailment suggests that sleep curtailment might accelerate the age-related deterioration of glucose metabolism.

SUMMARY

Age-related sleep and endocrinometabolic alterations frequently interact with each other. For many hormones, sleep curtailment in young healthy subjects results in alterations strikingly similar to those observed in healthy old subjects not submitted to sleep restriction. Thus, recurrent sleep restriction, which is currently experienced by a substantial and rapidly growing proportion of children and young adults, might contribute to accelerate the senescence of endocrine and metabolic function.

REFERENCES

1. Copinschi G, Turek FW, Van Cauter E. Endocrine rhythms, the sleep-wake cycle and biological clocks. In: Jameson LJ, DeGroot LJ, editors. Endocrinology, vol. 1, 6th edition. Philadelphia: Elsevier-Saunders; 2010. p. 199.

2. Rosenwasser AM, Turek FW. Physiology of the mammalian circadian system. Section 4-chronobiology. In: Kryger MH, Roth T, Dement WC, editors. Principles and practices of sleep medicine. New York: WB Saunders; 2005. p. 351.
3. Turek FW, Dugovic C, Laposky A. Master circadian clock, master circadian rhythm. Section 4-chronobiology. In: Kryger MH, Roth T, Dement WC, editors. Principles and practices of sleep medicine. 4 edition. New York: W B Saunders; 2005. p. 318.
4. Siegel JM. REM sleep: a biological and psychological paradox. Sleep Med Rev 2011;15:139.
5. Bliwise DL. Sleep in normal aging and dementia. Sleep 1993;16:40.
6. Prinz PN. Sleep and sleep disorders in older adults. J Clin Neurophysiol 1995; 12:139.
7. Prinz PN, Vitiello MV, Raskind MA, et al. Geriatrics: sleep disorders and aging. N Engl J Med 1990;323:520.
8. Buysse DJ, Browman KE, Monk TH, et al. Napping and 24-hour sleep/wake patterns in healthy elderly and young adults. J Am Geriatr Soc 1992;40:779.
9. Carrier J, Land S, Buysse DJ, et al. The effects of age and gender on sleep EEG power spectral density in the middle years of life (ages 20–60 years old). Psychophysiology 2001;38:232.
10. Ehlers CL, Kupfer DJ. Effects of age on delta and REM sleep parameters. Electroencephalogr Clin Neurophysiol 1989;72:118.
11. Feinberg I, Koresko RL, Heller N. EEG sleep patterns as a function of normal and pathological aging in man. J Psychiatr Res 1967;5:107.
12. Hayashi Y, Endo S. All-night sleep polygraphic recordings of healthy aged persons: REM and slow-wave sleep. Sleep 1982;5:277.
13. Kahn E, Fisher C. The sleep characteristics of the normal aged male. J Nerv Ment Dis 1969;148:477.
14. Landolt HP, Dijk DJ, Achermann P, et al. Effect of age on the sleep EEG: slow-wave activity and spindle frequency activity in young and middle-aged men. Brain Res 1996;738:205.
15. Miles LE, Dement WC. Sleep and aging. Sleep 1980;3:1.
16. Ohayon MM, Carskadon MA, Guilleminault C, et al. Meta-analysis of quantitative sleep parameters from childhood to old age in healthy individuals: developing normative sleep values across the human lifespan. Sleep 2004;27:1255.
17. Van Cauter E, Leproult R, Plat L. Age-related changes in slow wave sleep and REM sleep and relationship with growth hormone and cortisol levels in healthy men. JAMA 2000;284:861.
18. Groeger JA, Zijlstra FR, Dijk DJ. Sleep quantity, sleep difficulties and their perceived consequences in a representative sample of some 2000 British adults. J Sleep Res 2004;13:359.
19. Middelkoop HA, Smilde-van den Doel DA, Neven AK, et al. Subjective sleep characteristics of 1,485 males and females aged 50–93: effects of sex and age, and factors related to self-evaluated quality of sleep. J Gerontol A Biol Sci Med Sci 1996;51:M108.
20. Vitiello MV, Larsen LH, Moe KE. Age-related sleep change: gender and estrogen effects on the subjective-objective sleep quality relationships of healthy, noncomplaining older men and women. J Psychosom Res 2004;56:503.
21. Latta F, Leproult R, Tasali E, et al. Sex differences in delta and alpha EEG activities in healthy older adults. Sleep 2005;28:1525.
22. Van Cauter E, Plat L, Copinschi G. Interrelations between sleep and the somatotropic axis. Sleep 1998;21:553.

23. Ho KY, Evans WS, Blizzard RM, et al. Effects of sex and age on the 24-hour profile of growth hormone secretion in man: importance of endogenous estradiol concentrations. J Clin Endocrinol Metab 1987;64:51.
24. Caufriez A, Leproult R, L'Hermite-Baleriaux M, et al. A potential role of endogenous progesterone in modulation of GH, prolactin and thyrotrophin secretion during normal menstrual cycle. Clin Endocrinol (Oxf) 2009;71:535.
25. Van Cauter E, Spiegel K. Circadian and sleep control of endocrine secretions. In: Turek FW, Zee PC, editors. Regulation of sleep and circadian rhythms. New York: Marcel Dekker, Inc; 1999. p. 397.
26. Gronfier C, Luthringer R, Follenius M, et al. A quantitative evaluation of the relationships between growth hormone secretion and delta wave electroencephalographic activity during normal sleep and after enrichment in delta waves. Sleep 1996;19:817.
27. Holl RW, Hartman ML, Veldhuis JD, et al. Thirty-second sampling of plasma growth hormone in man: correlation with sleep stages. J Clin Endocrinol Metab 1991;72:854.
28. Van Cauter E, Kerkhofs M, Caufriez A, et al. A quantitative estimation of growth hormone secretion in normal man: reproducibility and relation to sleep and time of day. J Clin Endocrinol Metab 1992;74:1441.
29. Van Cauter E, Caufriez A, Kerkhofs M, et al. Sleep, awakenings, and insulin-like growth factor-I modulate the growth hormone (GH) secretory response to GH-releasing hormone. J Clin Endocrinol Metab 1992;74:1451.
30. Obal F Jr, Krueger JM. Biochemical regulation of non-rapid-eye-movement sleep. Front Biosci 2003;8:d520.
31. Ocampo-Lim B, Guo W, DeMott-Friberg R, et al. Nocturnal growth hormone (GH) secretion is eliminated by infusion of GH-releasing hormone antagonist. J Clin Endocrinol Metab 1996;81:4396.
32. Obal F Jr, Alfoldi P, Cady AB, et al. Growth hormone-releasing factor enhances sleep in rats and rabbits. Am J Physiol 1988;255:R310.
33. Obal F Jr, Floyd R, Kapas L, et al. Effects of systemic GHRH on sleep in intact and hypophysectomized rats. Am J Physiol 1996;270:E230.
34. Kerkhofs M, Van Cauter E, Van Onderbergen A, et al. Sleep-promoting effects of growth hormone-releasing hormone in normal men. Am J Physiol 1993;264:E594.
35. Marshall L, Molle M, Boschen G, et al. Greater efficacy of episodic than continuous growth hormone-releasing hormone (GHRH) administration in promoting slow-wave sleep (SWS). J Clin Endocrinol Metab 1996;81:1009.
36. Ziegenbein M, Held K, Kuenzel HE, et al. The somatostatin analogue octreotide impairs sleep and decreases EEG sigma power in young male subjects. Neuropsychopharmacology 2004;29:146.
37. Van Cauter E, Plat L, Scharf MB, et al. Simultaneous stimulation of slow-wave sleep and growth hormone secretion by gamma-hydroxybutyrate in normal young Men. J Clin Invest 1997;100:745.
38. Van Coevorden A, Mockel J, Laurent E, et al. Neuroendocrine rhythms and sleep in aging men. Am J Physiol 1991;260:E651.
39. Clemmons DR, Van Wyk JJ. Factors controlling blood concentration of somatomedin C. Clin Endocrinol Metab 1984;13:113.
40. Landin-Wilhelmsen K, Wilhelmsen L, Lappas G, et al. Serum insulin-like growth factor I in a random population sample of men and women: relation to age, sex, smoking habits, coffee consumption and physical activity, blood pressure and concentrations of plasma lipids, fibrinogen, parathyroid hormone and osteocalcin. Clin Endocrinol (Oxf) 1994;41:351.

41. Veldhuis JD, Liem AY, South S, et al. Differential impact of age, sex steroid hormones, and obesity on basal versus pulsatile growth hormone secretion in men as assessed in an ultrasensitive chemiluminescence assay. J Clin Endocrinol Metab 1995;80:3209.
42. Vermeulen A. Nyctohemeral growth hormone profiles in young and aged men: correlation with somatomedin-C levels. J Clin Endocrinol Metab 1987;64:884.
43. Spiegel K, Follenius M, Simon C, et al. Prolactin secretion and sleep. Sleep 1994;17:20.
44. Waldstreicher J, Duffy JF, Brown EN, et al. Gender differences in the temporal organization of proclactin (PRL) secretion: evidence for a sleep-independent circadian rhythm of circulating PRL levels- a clinical research center study. J Clin Endocrinol Metab 1996;81:1483.
45. Spiegel K, Luthringer R, Follenius M, et al. Temporal relationship between prolactin secretion and slow-wave electroencephalic activity during sleep. Sleep 1995;18:543.
46. Greenspan SL, Klibanski A, Rowe JW, et al. Age alters pulsatile prolactin release: influence of dopaminergic inhibition. Am J Physiol 1990;258:E799.
47. Brabant G, Prank K, Ranft U, et al. Physiological regulation of circadian and pulsatile thyrotropin secretion in normal man and woman. J Clin Endocrinol Metab 1990;70:403.
48. Parker DC, Pekary AE, Hershman JM. Effect of normal and reversed sleep-wake cycles upon nyctohemeral rhythmicity of plasma thyrotropin: evidence suggestive of an inhibitory influence in sleep. J Clin Endocrinol Metab 1976;43:318.
49. Goichot B, Brandenberger G, Saini J, et al. Nocturnal plasma thyrotropin variations are related to slow-wave sleep. J Sleep Res 1992;1:186.
50. Gronfier C, Luthringer R, Follenius M, et al. Temporal link between plasma thyrotropin levels and electroencephalographic activity in man. Neurosci Lett 1995; 200:97.
51. Hirschfeld U, Moreno-Reyes R, Akseki E, et al. Progressive elevation of plasma thyrotropin during adaptation to simulated jet lag: effects of treatment with bright light or zolpidem. J Clin Endocrinol Metab 1996;81:3270.
52. Mariotti S, Franceschi C, Cossarizza A, et al. The aging thyroid. Endocr Rev 1995;16:686.
53. Caufriez A, Moreno-Reyes R, Leproult R, et al. Immediate effects of an 8-h advance shift of the rest-activity cycle on 24-h profiles of cortisol. Am J Physiol Endocrinol Metab 2002;282:E1147.
54. Van Cauter E, Blackman JD, Roland D, et al. Modulation of glucose regulation and insulin secretion by circadian rhythmicity and sleep. J Clin Invest 1991;88:934.
55. Weibel L, Follenius M, Spiegel K, et al. Comparative effect of night and daytime sleep on the 24-hour cortisol secretory profile. Sleep 1995;18:549.
56. Weitzman ED, Zimmerman JC, Czeisler CA, et al. Cortisol secretion is inhibited during sleep in normal man. J Clin Endocrinol Metab 1983;56:352.
57. Bierwolf C, Struve K, Marshall L, et al. Slow wave sleep drives inhibition of pituitary-adrenal secretion in humans. J Neuroendocrinol 1997;9:479.
58. Follenius M, Brandenberger G, Bandesapt JJ, et al. Nocturnal cortisol release in relation to sleep structure. Sleep 1992;15:21.
59. Gronfier C, Luthringer R, Follenius M, et al. Temporal relationships between pulsatile cortisol secretion and electroencephalographic activity during sleep in man. Electroencephalogr Clin Neurophysiol 1997;103:405.
60. Spath-Schwalbe E, Gofferje M, Kern W, et al. Sleep disruption alters nocturnal ACTH and cortisol secretory patterns. Biol Psychiatry 1991;29:575.

61. Van Cauter E, van Coevorden A, Blackman JD. Modulation of neuroendocrine release by sleep and circadian rhythmicity. In: Yen S, Vale WV, editors. Advances in neuroendocrine regulation of reproduction. Norwell (MA): Serono symposium; 1990. p. 113.
62. Vgontzas AN, Bixler EO, Lin HM, et al. Chronic insomnia is associated with nyctohemeral activation of the hypothalamic-pituitary-adrenal axis: clinical implications. J Clin Endocrinol Metab 2001;86:3787.
63. Vgontzas AN, Zoumakis M, Bixler EO, et al. Impaired nighttime sleep in healthy old versus young adults is associated with elevated plasma interleukin-6 and cortisol levels: physiologic and therapeutic implications. J Clin Endocrinol Metab 2003;88:2087.
64. Chapotot F, Gronfier C, Jouny C, et al. Cortisol secretion is related to electroencephalographic alertness in human subjects during daytime wakefulness. J Clin Endocrinol Metab 1998;83:4263.
65. Ehlers CL, Reed TK, Henriksen SJ. Effects of corticotropin-releasing factor and growth hormone-releasing factor on sleep and activity in rats. Neuroendocrinology 1986;42:467.
66. Opp M, Obal F Jr, Krueger JM. Corticotropin-releasing factor attenuates interleukin 1-induced sleep and fever in rabbits. Am J Physiol 1989;257:R528.
67. Chang FC, Opp MR. Blockade of corticotropin-releasing hormone receptors reduces spontaneous waking in the rat. Am J Physiol 1998;275:R793.
68. Holsboer F, von Bardeleben U, Steiger A. Effects of intravenous corticotropin-releasing hormone upon sleep-related growth hormone surge and sleep EEG in man. Neuroendocrinology 1988;48:32.
69. Mann K, Roschke J, Benkert O, et al. Effects of corticotropin-releasing hormone on respiratory parameters during sleep in normal men. Exp Clin Endocrinol Diabetes 1995;103:233.
70. Tsuchiyama Y, Uchimura N, Sakamoto T, et al. Effects of hCRH on sleep and body temperature rhythms. Psychiatry Clin Neurosci 1995;49:299.
71. Vgontzas AN, Bixler EO, Wittman AM, et al. Middle-aged men show higher sensitivity of sleep to the arousing effects of corticotropin-releasing hormone than young men: clinical implications. J Clin Endocrinol Metab 2001;86:1489.
72. Born J, DeKloet ER, Wenz H, et al. Gluco- and antimineralocorticoid effects on human sleep: a role of central corticosteroid receptors. Am J Physiol 1991;260:E183.
73. Friess E, V Bardeleben U, Wiedemann K, et al. Effects of pulsatile cortisol infusion on sleep-EEG and nocturnal growth hormone release in healthy men. J Sleep Res 1994;3:73.
74. Bohlhalter S, Murck H, Holsboer F, et al. Cortisol enhances non-REM sleep and growth hormone secretion in elderly subjects. Neurobiol Aging 1997;18:423.
75. Harman SM, Metter EJ, Tobin JD, et al. Longitudinal effects of aging on serum total and free testosterone levels in healthy men. Baltimore Longitudinal Study of Aging. J Clin Endocrinol Metab 2001;86:724.
76. Van Cauter E, Leproult R, Kupfer DJ. Effects of gender and age on the levels and circadian rhythmicity of plasma cortisol. J Clin Endocrinol Metab 1996;81:2468.
77. McEwen BS. Stress, adaptation, and disease. Allostasis and allostatic load. Ann N Y Acad Sci 1998;840:33.
78. Leproult R, Copinschi G, Buxton O, et al. Sleep loss results in an elevation of cortisol levels the next evening. Sleep 1997;20:865.
79. Spiegel K, Leproult R, Van Cauter E. Impact of sleep debt on metabolic and endocrine function. Lancet 1999;354:1435.

80. Dallman MF, Strack AM, Akana SF, et al. Feast and famine: critical role of glucocorticoids with insulin in daily energy flow. Front Neuroendocrinol 1993;14:303.
81. Plat L, Leproult R, L'Hermite-Baleriaux M, et al. Metabolic effects of short-term elevations of plasma cortisol are more pronounced in the evening than in the morning. J Clin Endocrinol Metab 1999;84:3082.
82. Dennison E, Hindmarsh P, Fall C, et al. Profiles of endogenous circulating cortisol and bone mineral density in healthy elderly men. J Clin Endocrinol Metab 1999;84:3058.
83. McEwen BS. Protective and damaging effects of stress mediators. N Engl J Med 1998;338:171.
84. McEwen BS, Stellar E. Stress and the individual. Mechanisms leading to disease. Arch Intern Med 1993;153:2093.
85. Apter D, Butzow TL, Laughlin GA, et al. Gonadotropin-releasing hormone pulse generator activity during pubertal transition in girls: pulsatile and diurnal patterns of circulating gonadotropins. J Clin Endocrinol Metab 1993;76:940.
86. Filicori M, Santoro N, Merriam GR, et al. Characterization of the physiological pattern of episodic gonadotropin secretion throughout the human menstrual cycle. J Clin Endocrinol Metab 1986;62:1136.
87. Reame N, Sauder SE, Kelch RP, et al. Pulsatile gonadotropin secretion during the human menstrual cycle: evidence for altered frequency of gonadotropin-releasing hormone secretion. J Clin Endocrinol Metab 1984;59:328.
88. Hall JE, Sullivan JP, Richardson GS. Brief wake episodes modulate sleep-inhibited luteinizing hormone secretion in the early follicular phase. J Clin Endocrinol Metab 2005;90:2050.
89. Manber R, Armitage R. Sex, steroids, and sleep: a review. Sleep 1999;22:540.
90. Burger HG, Dudley EC, Robertson DM, et al. Hormonal changes in the menopause transition. Recent Prog Horm Res 2002;57:257.
91. Freedman RR. Biochemical, metabolic, and vascular mechanisms in menopausal hot flashes. Fertil Steril 1998;70:332.
92. Moe KE. Hot flashes and sleep in women. Sleep Med Rev 2004;8:487.
93. Pien GW, Sammel MD, Freeman EW, et al. Predictors of sleep quality in women in the menopausal transition. Sleep 2008;31:991.
94. Bechlioulis A, Kalantaridou SN, Naka KK, et al. Endothelial function, but not carotid intima-media thickness, is affected early in menopause and is associated with severity of hot flushes. J Clin Endocrinol Metab 2010;95:1199.
95. Brown DE, Sievert LL, Aki SL, et al. Effects of age, ethnicity and menopause on ambulatory blood pressure: Japanese-American and Caucasian school teachers in Hawaii. Am J Hum Biol 2001;13:486.
96. Gast GC, Grobbee DE, Pop VJ, et al. Menopausal complaints are associated with cardiovascular risk factors. Hypertension 2008;51:1492.
97. Gerber LM, Sievert LL, Warren K, et al. Hot flashes are associated with increased ambulatory systolic blood pressure. Menopause 2007;14:308.
98. Thurston RC, Christie IC, Matthews KA. Hot flashes and cardiac vagal control: a link to cardiovascular risk? Menopause 2010;17:456.
99. Thurston RC, Sutton-Tyrrell K, Everson-Rose SA, et al. Hot flashes and subclinical cardiovascular disease: findings from the Study of Women's Health Across the Nation Heart Study. Circulation 2008;118:1234.
100. Thurston RC, Sutton-Tyrrell K, Everson-Rose SA, et al. Hot flashes and carotid intima media thickness among midlife women. Menopause 2011;18:352.
101. Huang AJ, Sawaya GF, Vittinghoff E, et al. Hot flushes, coronary heart disease, and hormone therapy in postmenopausal women. Menopause 2009;16:639.

102. Rossouw JE, Prentice RL, Manson JE, et al. Postmenopausal hormone therapy and risk of cardiovascular disease by age and years since menopause. JAMA 2007;297:1465.
103. Szmuilowicz ED, Manson JE, Rossouw JE, et al. Vasomotor symptoms and cardiovascular events in postmenopausal women. Menopause 2011;18:603.
104. Caufriez A, Leproult R, L'Hermite-Baleriaux M, et al. Progesterone prevents sleep disturbances and modulates GH, TSH, and melatonin secretion in post-menopausal women. J Clin Endocrinol Metab 2011;96:E614.
105. Fehm HL, Clausing J, Kern W, et al. Sleep-associated augmentation and synchronization of luteinizing hormone pulses in adult men. Neuroendocrinology 1991;54:192.
106. Lejeune-Lenain C, Van Cauter E, Desir D, et al. Control of circadian and episodic variations of adrenal androgens secretion in man. J Endocrinol Invest 1987;10:267.
107. Axelsson J, Ingre M, Akerstedt T, et al. Effects of acutely displaced sleep on testosterone. J Clin Endocrinol Metab 2005;90:4530.
108. Lejeune H, Dechaud H, Pugeat M. Contribution of bioavailable testosterone assay for the diagnosis of androgen deficiency in elderly men. Ann Endocrinol (Paris) 2003;64:117 [in French].
109. Bremner WJ, Vitiello MV, Prinz PN. Loss of circadian rhythmicity in blood testosterone levels with aging in normal men. J Clin Endocrinol Metab 1983; 56:1278.
110. Tenover JS, Matsumoto AM, Clifton DK, et al. Age-related alterations in the circadian rhythms of pulsatile luteinizing hormone and testosterone secretion in healthy men. J Gerontol 1988;43:M163.
111. Morley JE, Kaiser FE, Perry HM III, et al. Longitudinal changes in testosterone, luteinizing hormone, and follicle-stimulating hormone in healthy older men Metabolism 1997;46:410.
112. Veldhuis JD, Iranmanesh A, Demers LM, et al. Joint basal and pulsatile hyper-secretory mechanisms drive the monotropic follicle-stimulating hormone (FSH) elevation in healthy older men: concurrent preservation of the orderliness of the FSH release process: a general clinical research center study. J Clin Endocrinol Metab 1999;84:3506.
113. Penev PD. Association between sleep and morning testosterone levels in older men. Sleep 2007;30:427.
114. Leproult R, Van Cauter E. Effect of 1 week of sleep restriction on testosterone levels in young healthy men. JAMA 2011;305:2173.
115. Rosenthal NE. Plasma melatonin as a measure of the human clock. J Clin Endocrinol Metab 1991;73:225.
116. Lewy AJ, Wehr TA, Goodwin FK, et al. Light suppresses melatonin secretion in humans. Science 1980;210:1267.
117. Zeitzer JM, Dijk DJ, Kronauer R, et al. Sensitivity of the human circadian pacemaker to nocturnal light: melatonin phase resetting and suppression. J Physio 2000;526(Pt 3):695.
118. Zeitzer JM, Duffy JF, Lockley SW, et al. Plasma melatonin rhythms in young and older humans during sleep, sleep deprivation, and wake. Sleep 2007;30:1437
119. Sharma M, Palacios-Bois J, Schwartz G, et al. Circadian rhythms of melatonin and cortisol in aging. Biol Psychiatry 1989;25:305.
120. Waldhauser F, Weiszenbacher G, Tatzer E, et al. Alterations in nocturnal serum melatonin levels in humans with growth and aging. J Clin Endocrinol Metab 1988;66:648.

121. Mishima K, Okawa M, Shimizu T, et al. Diminished melatonin secretion in the elderly caused by insufficient environmental illumination. J Clin Endocrinol Metab 2001;86:129.
122. Van Cauter E, Polonsky KS, Scheen AJ. Roles of circadian rhythmicity and sleep in human glucose regulation. Endocr Rev 1997;18:716.
123. Scheen AJ, Byrne MM, Plat L, et al. Relationships between sleep quality and glucose regulation in normal humans. Am J Physiol 1996;271:E261.
124. Simon C, Gronfier C, Schlienger JL, et al. Circadian and ultradian variations of leptin in normal man under continuous enteral nutrition: relationship to sleep and body temperature. J Clin Endocrinol Metab 1998;83:1893.
125. Boyle PJ, Scott JC, Krentz AJ, et al. Diminished brain glucose metabolism is a significant determinant for falling rates of systemic glucose utilization during sleep in normal humans. J Clin Invest 1994;93:529.
126. DeFronzo RA. Pathogenesis of type 2 diabetes mellitus. Med Clin North Am 2004;88:787.
127. Magistretti PJ. Neuron-glia metabolic coupling and plasticity. J Exp Biol 2006; 209:2304.
128. Maquet P. Functional neuroimaging of normal human sleep by positron emission tomography. J Sleep Res 2000;9:207.
129. Maquet P. Positron emission tomography studies of sleep and sleep disorders. J Neurol 1997;244:S23.
130. Moller N, Jorgensen JO, Schmitz O, et al. Effects of a growth hormone pulse on total and forearm substrate fluxes in humans. Am J Physiol 1990;258:E86.
131. Buxton OM, Pavlova M, Reid EW, et al. Sleep restriction for 1 week reduces insulin sensitivity in healthy men. Diabetes 2010;59:2126.
132. Spiegel K, Knutson K, Leproult R, et al. Sleep loss: a novel risk factor for insulin resistance and Type 2 diabetes. J Appl Physiol 2005;99:2008.
133. Spiegel K, Leproult R, L'Hermite-Baleriaux M, et al. Leptin levels are dependent on sleep duration: relationships with sympathovagal balance, carbohydrate regulation, cortisol, and thyrotropin. J Clin Endocrinol Metab 2004;89:5762.
134. Mander B, Colecchia E, Spiegel K, et al. Short sleep: a risk factor for insulin resistance and obesity. Diabetes 2001;50:A45.
135. Knutson KL, Van Cauter E. Associations between sleep loss and increased risk of obesity and diabetes. Ann N Y Acad Sci 2008;1129:287.
136. Tasali E, Leproult R, Ehrmann DA, et al. Slow-wave sleep and the risk of type 2 diabetes in humans. Proc Natl Acad Sci U S A 2008;105:1044.
137. Chen M, Bergman RN, Pacini G, et al. Pathogenesis of age-related glucose intolerance in man: insulin resistance and decreased beta-cell function. J Clin Endocrinol Metab 1985;60:13.
138. Garcia GV, Freeman RV, Supiano MA, et al. Glucose metabolism in older adults: a study including subjects more than 80 years of age. J Am Geriatr Soc 1997; 45:813.
139. Palmer JP, Ensinck JW. Acute-phase insulin secretion and glucose tolerance in young and aged normal men and diabetic patients. J Clin Endocrinol Metab 1975;41:498.

Frailty, Sarcopenia, and Hormones

ohn E. Morley, MB, BCh[a,*], Theodore K. Malmstrom, PhD[a,b]

KEYWORDS

• Frailty • Sarcopenia • Hormones • Exercise

KEY POINTS

- Age-related changes in hormones play a major role in the development of frailty by reducing muscle mass and strength (sarcopenia).
- Selective Androgen Receptor Molecules and ghrelin agonists are being developed to treat sarcopenia.
- Exercise (resistance and aerobic), vitamin D and protein supplementation, and reduction of polypharmacy are keys to the treatment of frailty.

railty is now a definable clinical syndrome with a simple screening test. Age-related hanges in hormones play a major role in the development of frailty by reducing nuscle mass and strength (sarcopenia). Selective Androgen Receptor Molecules nd ghrelin agonists are being developed to treat sarcopenia. The role of Activin ype IIB soluble receptors and Follistatinlike 3 mimetics is less certain because of ide effects. Exercise (resistance and aerobic), vitamin D and protein supplementa-ion, and reduction of polypharmacy are keys to the treatment of frailty.

NTRODUCTION

he recognition that frailty is an important clinical syndrome in older persons is now well stablished.[1–3] Both physical and psychosocial forms of frailty have been identified. he understanding of physical frailty and its interaction with hormones is much better stablished, and is the focus of this review. Two models of physical frailty have been roposed. The deficit model of Rockwood and colleagues[4] is a comorbidity model nd, in general, does not easily allow itself to be analyzed with regard to specific auses. The Cardiovascular Health Model (CHS) of Fried and colleagues[5] allows an asier analysis of its causes, and the role of hormones in this physical model has een established. The frailty model of the Study of Osteoporotic Fractures (SOF) is imilar to the CHS Model.[6] The FRAIL model is a simple questionnaire modeled on

[a] Division of Geriatric Medicine, Saint Louis University School of Medicine, 1402 South Grand Boulevard, M238, St Louis, MO 63104, USA; [b] Department of Neurology and Psychiatry, Saint Louis University School of Medicine, 1438 South Grand Boulevard, St Louis, MO 63104, USA
* Corresponding author.
E-mail address: morley@slu.edu

Endocrinol Metab Clin N Am 42 (2013) 391–405
http://dx.doi.org/10.1016/j.ecl.2013.02.006
endo.theclinics.com
0889-8529/13/$ – see front matter

the CHS model, takes less than 30 seconds to complete, and has been validated.[7–11] This questionnaire is ideal for rapid screening in the primary care physician's or endocrinologist's office practice. The components of the FRAIL questionnaire are as follows:

F: Are you *F*atigued?
R: *R*esistance: Can you walk up a flight of stairs?
A: *A*erobic: Can you walk a block?
I: Do you have more than 5 *I*llnesses?
L: Have you *L*ost 5% of weight in the past 6 months?

A positive answer to 1 or 2 questions is considered prefrail and 3 or more is frail. A variety of other models exist that are a mixture of physical and psychosocial frailty.[12–16]

The term sarcopenia was originally created to refer to age-related muscle mass.[17] There are now 4 international definitions of sarcopenia.[18–21] In essence they all agree, requiring a measure of walking capability (either low gait speed or a limited endurance [distance] in a 6-minute walk), together with an appendicular lean mass of less than 2 SDs of a sex and ethnically corrected normal level for individuals 20 to 30 years old. Sarcopenia needs to be differentiated from cachexia, which is a combination of both muscle and fat loss and is usually attributable to an excess of catabolic cytokines associated with a disease process.[22–24] It is important to recognize that muscle mass measurements are often poorly associated with muscle strength or power. Sarcopenia is a prime component of the frailty syndrome, and both sarcopenia and frailty are associated with increased disability, falls, hospitalization, nursing home admission, and mortality.[25–28]

Recently there has been increased evidence that osteoporosis and risk of fracture can be identified in many persons without direct measurement of bone mineral density by using the questions used in the Fracture Risk Assessment Tool (FRAX).[29,30] It has been suggested that it should be easier to identify sarcopenia using simple questions than it is to identify persons with osteoporosis. One measure has been proposed to identify sarcopenia by a set of questions, the SARC-F[31]:

*S*trength: Difficulty in lifting or carrying 10 lb
*A*ssistance in walking
*R*ise from chair
*C*limb stairs
*F*alls: 2 or more

ENDOCRINE DISEASE AND FRAILTY

Endocrine disorders are recognized as having early presentations that are nonspecific and often missed until the disorder has been present for a long time. In this way, they are similar to frailty. In fact, the presentation of many endocrine disorders is the same as frailty, ie, fatigue, weakness, and weight loss. Thus, in older persons, one of the few times frailty is caused by a single condition is when an endocrine disorder, such as hypothyroidism, apathetic thyrotoxicosis, hypercalcemia, Addison disease, hypopituitarism, or uncontrolled diabetes mellitus, has not been diagnosed! Polyglandular insufficiency syndromes, when one or more endocrine disorders coexist with vitamin B12 deficiency and/or celiac disease, is another cause of frailty.[32]

TESTOSTERONE

Testosterone levels decline in men at the rate of 1% per year from the age of 30 years paralleling declines in muscle mass and strength.[33] Epidemiologic studies support the relationship of low testosterone to the loss of muscle mass and strength with aging.[34–36] When testosterone is lowered in a healthy older man by administration of a gonadotropin-releasing hormone agonist, muscle mass, strength, and power decline, returning to normal with testosterone replacement.[37] Many studies in older men who have low testosterone levels (<300 ng/mL) have shown that testosterone increases muscle mass and strength[38,39]; however, in general, relatively high doses of testosterone are necessary to increase muscle strength compared with the lower doses necessary to increase muscle mass.[40] Testosterone increases muscle strength by bypassing the *Wnt* pathway and directly stimulating beta-catenin (**Fig. 1**).[41] High doses of testosterone activate satellite cells. The available data support the concept that the loss of muscle mass with aging is partly related to the age-related decline in testosterone.

Similarly, epidemiologic studies have found a relationship between low testosterone and frailty.[8,42,43] Three studies have specifically looked at the role of testosterone replacement in frailty. One study, using a low dose of testosterone, found no effect.[44] The other 2 studies found improvements in muscle mass and strength, and in 1 study, a strong tendency to improve function.[45,46] Two of the studies found no major side effects, but the third was stopped early because of increased cardiovascular disease; however, much of the cardiovascular disease was driven by an increase in edema. Older persons with heart failure have been shown to have an improvement in gait speed when given testosterone, without a worsening of heart failure,[47–49] although testosterone does increase fluid retention, which could increase peripheral edema.[50] In our pilot study in older persons residing in assisted living, we found a marked decrease in hospitalization in those receiving a combination of testosterone and a caloric supplement, but not in those receiving either testosterone or

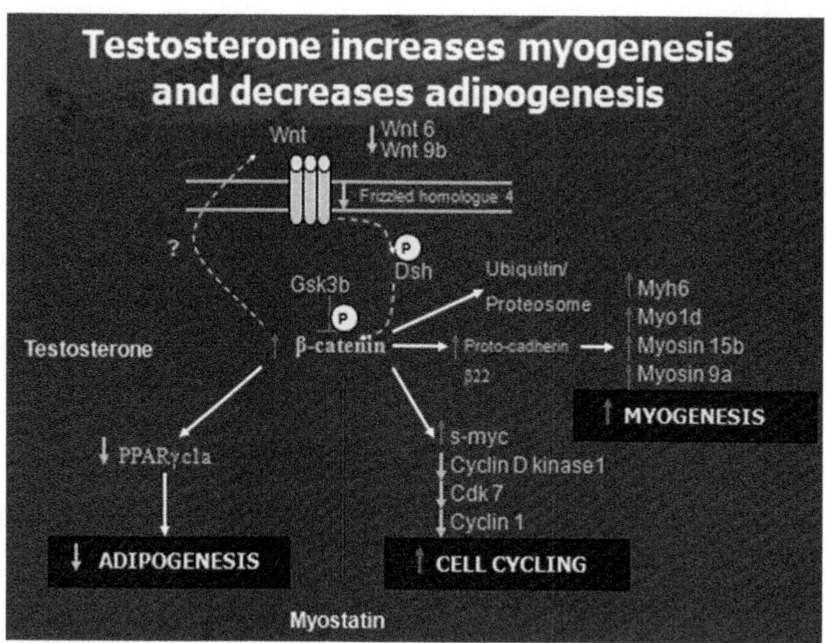

Fig. 1. Testosterone increases muscle strength by bypassing the *Wnt* pathway and directly stimulating beta-catenin.

extra calories alone.[51] Data for women are similar to those for men, but there are much fewer data.[52,53]

Selective Androgen Receptor Molecules (SARMs) have been developed to produce the positive effects of testosterone without the negative effects. Nandrolone, which was used for many years as an injectable SARM, has been shown to produce a variety of positive effects on muscle in older persons.[54,55] Enabosarm (ostarine) is a SARM developed by GTx (Memphis, TN). In healthy older persons (men and women), this SARM increases both muscle mass and stair-climbing power.[56] It has also been used in persons with lung cancer cachexia. A SARM developed by Merck (Whitehouse Station, NJ) has also shown small effects in frail older persons.[57]

Overall, testosterone and SARMs show promise in treating sarcopenia and frailty; however, larger more definitive trials are needed before they can be recommended for this purpose. In addition, whether their therapeutic benefit will be seen only in men with hypogonadism needs to be determined.

VITAMIN D

Levels of 25(OH) vitamin D decline over the life span.[58] Low 25(OH) vitamin D levels are common in older persons.[59–62] Many, but not all, epidemiologic studies have suggested that 25(OH) vitamin D is related to muscle strength and frailty.[63–66] It would appear that there is a threshold level below which 25(OH) vitamin D has an effect on muscle function. This may be at the level when low vitamin D triggers an increase in parathyroid hormone.[67] Replacement with 25(OH) vitamin D reduces falls in persons with low levels.[68,69] Similarly, it appears to improve muscle function in persons with low levels.[70]

Agrin is a proteoglycan that plays a role in maintaining neuromuscular function. Much of age-related loss of muscle mass is because of a loss of neuromuscular units.[71] C-terminal agrin levels are elevated in older persons with sarcopenia, as well as in renal failure.[72] Vitamin D replacement lowers agrin levels.

Overall, it would appear that low levels of vitamin D play a role in sarcopenia and frailty. It is possible that this effect is predominantly attributable to its effect on neuromuscular function rather than directly on muscle.

DEHYDROEPIANDROSTERONE

Dehydroepiandrosterone (DHEA) and its sulfate are anabolic hormones produced from the adrenal cortex. Levels decline rapidly with aging and this decline is correlated with loss of muscle mass.[73,74] DHEA replacement failed to increase muscle mass or strength in older persons,[75,76] although, in a recent study when given with vitamin D, it improved the short physical performance battery (SPPB).[77] There is some evidence that low DHEA levels may cause fatigue. At present, no clear role exists for DHEA in sarcopenia or frailty.

GROWTH HORMONE, INSULINLIKE GROWTH FACTOR-1, AND GHRELIN

Both growth hormone and insulinlike growth factor-1 (IGF-1) levels decline with aging. IGF-1 can be produced in either the liver or in muscle. Different isoforms of IGF-1 have differing effects. Liver-derived IGF-1 appears to predominantly increase muscle mass, whereas muscle-derived IGF-1 has effects on the development of satellite cells and on maintenance of neuromuscular function.[78] IGF-1 has been associated with frailty.[79]

The concept that growth hormone would decrease frailty with aging was first proposed by Dan Rudman.[80] Unfortunately, most growth hormone studies have hown that it can increase muscle mass and nitrogen retention but has little effect on nuscle strength, unless coupled with exercise or testosterone.[81] Growth hormone ends to increase type II muscle fibers. In addition, it has been shown to have a variety f unacceptable side effects.

In mice, introduction of stem cells to muscles that express IGF-1 or overexpression f IGF-1 both lead to increased muscle mass and strength.[82,83] A major effect of IGF-1 ppears to be on the phosphatidylinositol 3'-kinase (PI_3K)-AKT system, increasing rotein synthesis through mammalian target of rapamycin (mTOR) and reducing nuscle degradation through the ubiquitin ligase system. In humans, recombinant uman (*rh*)IGF-1 trials in motor neuron disease have suggested some clinical improvenent but no improvement in manual muscle strength testing.[84] In myotonia dystrophy, hIGF-1 increased muscle mass but not strength.[85] In patients with AIDS, *rh*IGF-1 ncreased muscle mass only.[86] These data do not support the use of *rh*IGF-1 for arcopenia.

Ghrelin is a hormone that is produced in the fundus of the stomach and enhances ood intake and activates growth release by increasing nitric oxide in the hypothalmus.[87] Ghrelin has been shown to increase food intake and prevent muscle loss in atients with cancer.[88] A ghrelin agonist, anamorelin, increased body weight in atients with cancer.[89] MK-0677 (ibutamoren mesylate), a ghrelin mimetic given to ealthy elderly persons for a year, increased fat-free mass and total and abdominal ubcutaneous fat.[90] It improved repeated chair rise but not the 6-minute walk r upper extremity strength. In one hip fracture study, it had no effect,[91] but in the other improved SPPB and halved fall rate.[92] Capromorelin, another ghrelin mimetic, given or 12 months, increased lean body mass, and improved power stair climb, 6-minute valk (only in 1 dose), and tandem walk.[93] Overall, these data provide some support for hrelin mimetics in the treatment of sarcopenia and frailty. However, research on the ast 2 ghrelin mimetics has not been continued by the pharmaceutical companies.

YOSTATIN AND ACTIVIN RECEPTORS

lyostatin is a compound found in muscle that inhibits muscle growth through the MAD pathway. Myostatin deletions lead to overmuscularization in Belgian Blue ows and in whippets. There is also a human with a homozygous myostatin deletion ading to excess musculature.[94] Myostatin levels are higher in young compared with lder men and increase in men receiving testosterone.[95] Numerous studies in mice ave demonstrated that myostatin antibodies increase muscle strength.[96] The first est in humans with muscular dystrophy found minimal effects of a myostatin antiody.[97] Eli Lilly and Company (Indianapolis, IN) have reported in abstract form that n antimyostatin compound (LY2495655) tends to increase thigh muscle volume nd, in advanced cancer, muscle volume and handgrip.

The activin receptor Type IIB is the receptor for myostatin. A soluble form of the actiin receptor type IIB promotes muscle growth by binding to myostatin. The activin eceptor type II B receptor inhibitor ACE-031 increased muscle mass and muscle thigh olume.[98] This compound also increased lumbar spine bone mineral density, ecreased total body fat mass, decreased leptin, and increased adiponectin. Unfortuately, in long-term use it may increase bleeding. Follistatinlike 3 is a potent inhibitor of ctivin signaling and may prove to be less toxic.

NGIOTENSIN-CONVERTING ENZYME INHIBITORS

pidemiologic studies have suggested that persons with the type II angiotensinonverting enzyme (ACE) genotype have greater endurance and, in some studies, persons taking ACE inhibitors have larger muscles and better walking speed.[99,100] Perindopril, an ACE inhibitor, given to persons without heart failure and hypertension, increased walking distance over 20 weeks.[101] In the Hypertension in the Very Elderly Trial (HYVET), perindopril reduced hip fracture, whereas in most studies, treatment of hypertension leads to an increase in hip fracture.[102]

Another cardiovascular drug that is being developed for treating sarcopenia is MT-102, a nonselective beta-blocker with 5HTla-blocking activity that upregulates pAKT and downregulates FOXO3a expression.

CORTISOL

It is well recognized that glucocorticoids cause myopathy. Frailty is significantly associated with increased 24-hour urinary cortisol.[103] Circulating cortisol levels with a blunted diurnal rhythm are elevated in frail persons.[104] Frail persons in nursing homes have higher levels of morning and afternoon cortisol levels.[105] A high cortisol:DHEA sulfate ratio was associated with increased frailty after 10 years of follow-up in the Hertfordshire Aging study.[106]

DIABETES AND INSULIN RESISTANCE

Individuals with diabetes are more likely than age-matched other persons to lose muscle mass.[107] Individuals with diabetes have decreased strength and are more likely to have injurious falls.[108] The metabolic syndrome is associated with loss of muscle and also a decrease in grip strength.[109] Through stimulation of protein synthesis, insulin plays a key role in maintaining muscle mass. Persons with sarcopenia, particularly those with sarcopenic obesity, are very likely to develop insulin resistance.[110] Frail persons with increased abdominal fat have been shown to be insulin resistant.[111–113]

CYTOKINES

Numerous studies have demonstrated that catabolic cytokines, eg, interleukin-6 and tumor necrosis factor-alpha, lead to a reduction in muscle mass, strength, and frailty.[114–117] This has been termed the cytokine-related aging process.[118]

NUTRITION

Besides low 25(OH) vitamin D, poor protein intake has also been identified as a risk factor for frailty.[119–123] There are increasing data showing that protein supplementation, perhaps optimally as a leucine-enriched essential amino acid mixture, will improve muscle mass and perhaps decrease frailty.[124–126] Protein supplementation acts synergistically with exercise.[127] It has been suggested that to prevent or treat sarcopenia, at least 1.2 g/kg of protein daily is necessary.[124]

WEIGHT LOSS

Although being overweight and obese is common in older persons, weight loss is a 2-edged sword. Most data suggest that weight loss in older persons is associated with increased mortality.[128–130] This is predominately because although 75% of weight loss is fat, the rest is muscle and bone.[131] Voluntary weight loss leads to an increase in hip fracture.[132] Thus, weight loss is an important component in the pathophysiology of sarcopenia and frailty. Studies by Villareal and colleagues[133] have suggested that caloric restriction together with exercise may be a reasonable option.

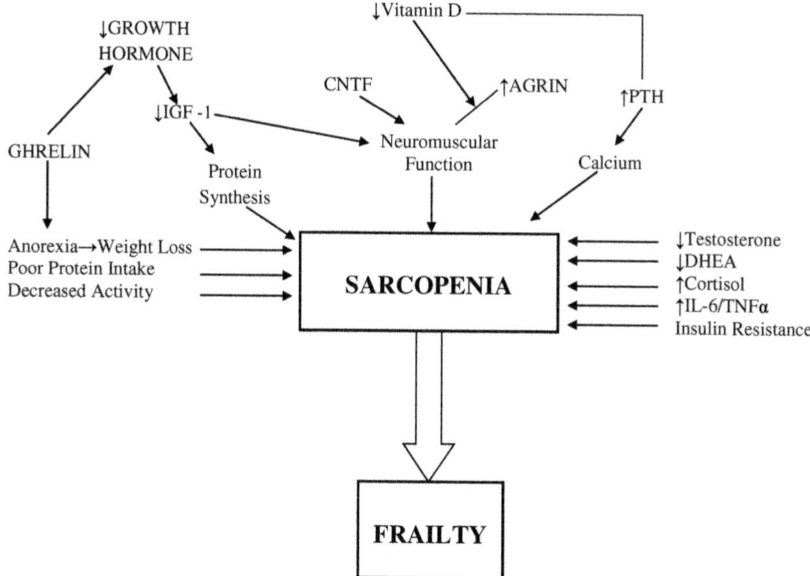

Fig. 2. The pathophysiology of sarcopenia and frailty. CNTF, ciliary neurotophic factor; IL-6, interleukin 6; TNFα, tumor necrosis factor alpha; DHEA, dehydroepiandrosterone; PTH, parathyroid hormone; IGF-1, Insulinlike growth factor-1.

EXERCISE

Overwhelmingly, resistance and aerobic exercise have been shown to increase muscle function.[134–139] An Australian study of persons with hip fracture showed that resistance exercise twice weekly for 12 months decreased nursing home admission, improved activities of daily living, and decreased mortality.[140] Exercise in frail elderly persons improved functional performance, increased walking speed, increased chair stand, increased stair climbing, increased balance, decreased depression, and decreased fear of falling.[141,142] In the Lifestyle Interventions and Independence for Elders (LIFE) pilot study, exercise improved functional status as measured by the SPPB.[143]

SUMMARY

There is now a large body of evidence that both sarcopenia and frailty are closely related to the decline in hormones that occurs with aging. As demonstrated in **Fig. 2**, these hormones appear to play an important role in the pathophysiology of sarcopenia and frailty. Based on the available data, it would appear that a low-dose hormonal cocktail that can return the hormonal milieu of a younger person may prove to be a more effective and safer method to treat these conditions. Hormonal treatment will need to be balanced with a sensible exercise and nutritional program.

REFERENCES

1. Abellan van Kan G, Rolland YM, Morley JE, et al. Frailty: toward a clinical definition. J Am Med Dir Assoc 2008;9:71–2.
2. Morley JE. Developing novel therapeutic approaches to frailty. Curr Pharm Des 2009;15:3384–95.

3. Morley JE, Perry HM 3rd, Miller DK. Editorial: something about frailty. J Gerontol A Biol Sci Med Sci 2002;57:M698–704.
4. Rockwood K, Abeysundera MJ, Mitnitski A. How should we grade frailty in nursing home patients? J Am Med Dir Assoc 2007;8:595–603.
5. Fried LP, Tangen CM, Walston J, et al. Frailty in older adults: evidence for a phenotype. J Gerontol A Biol Sci Med Sci 2001;56:M146–56.
6. Ensrud KE, Ewing SK, Taylor BC, et al. Comparison of 2 frailty indexes for prediction of falls, disability, fractures, and death in older women. Arch Intern Med 2008;168:382–9.
7. Abellan van Kan G, Rolland Y, Bergman H, et al. The I.A.N.A. task force on frailty assessment of older people in clinical practice. J Nutr Health Aging 2008;12: 29–37.
8. Hyde Z, Flicker L, Almeida OP, et al. Low free testosterone predicts frailty in older men: the Health in Men study. J Clin Endocrinol Metab 2010;95: 3165–72.
9. Lopez D, Flicker L, Dobson A. Validation of the frail scale in a cohort of older Australian women. J Am Geriatr Soc 2012;60:171–3.
10. Woo J, Leung J, Morley JE. Comparison of frailty indicators based on clinical phenotype and the multiple deficit approach in predicting mortality and physical limitation. J Am Geriatr Soc 2012;60:1478–86.
11. Morley JE, Malmstrom TK, Miller DK. A simple frailty questionnaire (FRAIL) predicts outcomes in middle aged African Americans. J Nutr Health Aging 2012;16:601–8.
12. Hoogendijk EO, van Hout HP. Investigating measurement properties of the Groningen Frailty Indicator: a more systematic approach is needed. J Am Med Dir Assoc 2012;13:757 [author reply: 757–8].
13. Gobbens RJ, van Assen MA, Luijkx KG, et al. The Tilburg Frailty Indicator: psychometric properties. J Am Med Dir Assoc 2010;11:344–55.
14. Gobbens RJ, Luijkx KG, Wijenen-Sponselee MT, et al. In search of an integral conceptual definition of frailty: opinions of experts. J Am Med Dir Assoc 2010; 11:338–43.
15. Andrew MK, Mitnitski A, Kirkland SA, et al. The impact of social vulnerability on the survival of the fittest older adults. Age Ageing 2012;41:161–5.
16. Gobbens RJ, Lujkx KG, Wijnen-Sponselee MT, et al. Toward a conceptual definition of frail community dwelling older people. Nurs Outlook 2010;58:76–86.
17. Morley JE, Baumgartner RN, Roubenoff R, et al. Sarcopenia. J Lab Clin Med 2001;137:231–43.
18. Cruz-Jentoft AJ, Baeyens JP, Bauer JM, et al. Sarcopenia: European consensus on definition and diagnosis: report of the European Working Group on Sarcopenia in Older People. Age Ageing 2010;39:412–23.
19. Morley JE, Abbatecola AM, Argiles JM, et al, Society on Sarcopenia, Cachexia and Wasting Disorders Trialist Workshop. Sarcopenia with limited mobility: an international consensus. J Am Med Dir Assoc 2011;12:403–9.
20. Fielding RA, Vellas B, Evans WJ, et al. Sarcopenia: an undiagnosed condition in older adults. Current consensus definition: prevalence, etiology and consequences. International Working Group on Sarcopenia. J Am Med Dir Assoc 2011;12:249–56.
21. Muscaritoli M, Anker SD, Argiles J, et al. Consensus definition of sarcopenia, cachexia and pre-cachexia: joint document elaborated by Special Interest Groups (SIG) "cachexia-anorexia in chronic wasting disease" and "nutrition in geriatrics." Clin Nutr 2010;29:154–9.

22. Argiles JM, Anker SD, Evans WJ, et al. Consensus on cachexia definitions. J Am Med Dir Assoc 2010;11:229–30.
23. Yeh SS, Lovitt S, Schuster MW. Pharmacological treatment of geriatric cachexia: evidence and safety in perspective. J Am Med Dir Assoc 2007;8:363–77.
24. Evans WJ, Morley JE, Argiles J, et al. Cachexia: a new definition. Clin Nutr 2008; 27:793–9.
25. Landi F, Liperoti R, Fusco D, et al. Sarcopenia and mortality among older nursing home residents. J Am Med Dir Assoc 2012;13:121–6.
26. Cesari M, Vellas B. Sarcopenia: a novel clinical condition or still a matter for research? J Am Med Dir Assoc 2012;13:766–7.
27. von Haehling S, Morley JE, Anker SD. From muscle wasting to sarcopenia and myopenia: update 2012. J Cachexia Sarcopenia Muscle 2012;3:213–7.
28. Rolland Y, Czerwinski S, Abellan van Kan G, et al. Sarcopenia: its assessment, etiology, and pathogenesis, consequences and future perspectives. J Nutr Health Aging 2008;12:433–50.
29. Leslie WD, Majumdar SR, Lix LM, et al, Manitoba Bone Density Program. High fracture probability with FRAX usually indicates densitometric osteoporosis: implications for clinical practice. Osteoporos Int 2012;23:391–7.
30. Leslie WD, Morin S, Lix LM, et al, Manitoba Bone Density Program. Fracture risk assessment without bone density measurement in routine clinical practice. Osteoporos Int 2012;23:75–85.
31. Malmstrom TK, Morley JE. Sarcopenia: the target population. J Frailty Aging 2013;2:55–6.
32. Trence DL, Morley JE, Handwerger BS. Polyglandular autoimmune syndromes. Am J Med 1984;77:107–16.
33. Wang C, Nieschlag E, Swerdloff R, et al. Investigation, treatment and monitoring of late-onset hypogonadism in males: ISA, ISSAM, EAU, EAA and ASA recommendations. Eur J Endocrinol 2008;159:507–14.
34. Baumgartner RN, Waters DL, Gallagher D, et al. Predictors of skeletal muscle mass in elderly men and women. Mech Ageing Dev 1999;107:123–36.
35. Maggio M, Ceda GP, Lauretani F, et al. Gonadal status and physical performance in older men. Aging Male 2011;14:42–7.
36. Perry HM 3rd, Miller DK, Patrick P, et al. Testosterone and leptin in older African-American men: relationship to age, strength, function, and season. Metabolism 2000;49:1085–91.
37. Bhasin S, Woodhouse L, Casaburi R, et al. Older men are as responsive as young men to the anabolic effects of graded doses of testosterone on the skeletal muscle. J Clin Endocrinol Metab 2005;90:678–88.
38. Morley JE, Perry HM 3rd, Kaiser FE, et al. Effects of testosterone replacement therapy in old hypogonadal males: a preliminary study. J Am Geriatr Soc 1993;41:149–52.
39. Isidori AM, Giannetta E, Greco EA, et al. Effects of testosterone on body composition, bone metabolism and serum lipid profile in middle-aged men: a meta-analysis. Clin Endocrinol (Oxf) 2005;63:280–93.
40. Wittert GA, Chapman IM, Haren MT, et al. Oral testosterone supplementation increases muscle and decreases fat mass in healthy elderly males with low-normal gonadal status. J Gerontol A Biol Sci Med Sci 2003;58:618–25.
41. Haren MT, Siddiqui AM, Armbrecht HJ, et al. Testosterone modulates gene expression pathways regulating nutrient accumulation, glucose metabolism and protein turnover in mouse skeletal muscle. Int J Androl 2011;34: 55–68.

42. Cawthon PM, Ensrud KE, Laughlin GA, et al. Sex hormones and frailty in older men: the osteoporotic fractures in men (MrOS) study. J Clin Endocrinol Metab 2009;94:3806–15.
43. Eichholzer M, Barbir A, Basaria S, et al. Serum sex steroid hormones and frailty in older American men of the Third National Health and Nutrition Examination Survey (NHANES III). Aging Male 2012;15:208–15.
44. Kenny AM, Kleppinger A, Annis K, et al. Effects of transdermal testosterone on bone and muscle in older men with low bioavailable testosterone levels, low bone mass, and physical frailty. J Am Geriatr Soc 2010;58:1134–43.
45. Srinivas-Shankar U, Roberts SA, Connolly MJ, et al. Effects of testosterone on muscle strength, physical function, body composition, and quality of life in intermediate-frail and frail elderly men: a randomized, double-blind, placebo-controlled study. J Clin Endocrinol Metab 2010;95:639–50.
46. Travison TG, Basaria S, Storer TW, et al. Clinical meaningfulness of the changes in muscle performance and physical function associated with testosterone administration in older men with mobility limitation. J Gerontol A Biol Sci Med Sci 2011;66:1090–9.
47. Stout M, Tew GA, Doll H, et al. Testosterone therapy during exercise rehabilitation in male patients with chronic heart failure who have low testosterone status: a double-blind randomized controlled feasibility study. Am Heart J 2012;164:893–901.
48. Caminiti G, Volterrani M, Iellamo F, et al. Effect of long-acting testosterone treatment on functional exercise capacity, skeletal muscle performance, insulin resistance, and baroreflex sensitivity in elderly patients with chronic heart failure: a double-blind, placebo-controlled, randomized study. J Am Coll Cardiol 2009;54:919–27.
49. Malkin CJ, Pugh PJ, West JN, et al. Testosterone therapy in men with moderate severity heart failure: a double-blind randomized placebo controlled trial. Eur Heart J 2006;27:57–64.
50. Chahla EJ, Hayek ME, Morley JE. Testosterone replacement therapy and cardiovascular risk factors modification. Aging Male 2011;14:83–90.
51. Chapman IM, Visvanathan R, Hammond AJ, et al. Effect of testosterone and a nutritional supplement, alone and in combination, on hospital admissions in undernourished older men and women. Am J Clin Nutr 2009;89:880–9.
52. Morley JE, Perry HM 3rd. Androgens and women at the menopause and beyond. J Gerontol A Biol Sci Med Sci 2003;58:M409–16.
53. Iellamo F, Volterrani M, Caminiti G, et al. Testosterone therapy in women with chronic heart failure: a pilot double-blind, randomized, placebo-controlled study. J Am Coll Cardiol 2010;56:1310–6.
54. Johansen KL, Patiner PL, Sakkas GK, et al. Effects of resistance exercise training and nandrolone decanoate on body composition and muscle function among patients who receive hemodialysis: a randomized, controlled trial. J Am Soc Nephrol 2006;17:2307–14.
55. Frisoli A Jr, Chaves PH, Pinheiro MM, et al. The effect of nandrolone decanoate on bone mineral density, muscle mass, and hemoglobin levels in elderly women with osteoporosis: a double-blind, randomized, placebo-controlled clinical trial. J Gerontol A Biol Sci Med Sci 2005;60:648–53.
56. Dalton JT, Barnette KG, Bohl CE, et al. The selective androgen receptor modulator GTx-024 (enobosarm) improves lean body mass and physical function in healthy elderly men and postmenopausal women: results of a double-blind, placebo-controlled phase II trial. J Cachexia Sarcopenia Muscle 2011;2:153–61

57. A study to evaluate the safety, tolerability, and efficacy of MK-0773 in women with sarcopenia (loss of muscle mass) (MK-0773-005). Available at: www.clinicaltrials.gov. Accessed December 12, 2012.
58. Perry HM 3rd, Horowitz M, Morley JE, et al. Longitudinal changes in serum 25-hydroxyvitamin D in older people. Metabolism 1999;48:1028–32.
59. Islam T, Peiris P, Copeland RJ, et al. Vitamin D: lessons from the veterans population. J Am Med Dir Assoc 2011;12:257–62.
60. McKinny JD, Bailey BA, Garrett LH, et al. Relationship between vitamin D status and ICU outcomes in veterans. J Am Med Dir Assoc 2011;12:208–11.
61. Braddy KK, Imam SN, Palla KR, et al. Vitamin D deficiency/insufficiency practice patterns in a Veterans Health Administration long-term care population: a retrospective analysis. J Am Med Dir Assoc 2009;10:653–7.
62. Demontiero O, Herrmann M, Duque G. Supplementation with vitamin D and calcium in long-term care residents. J Am Med Dir Assoc 2011;12:190–4.
63. Ensrud KE, Ewing SK, Fredman L, et al, Study of Osteoporotic Fractures Research Group. Circulating 25-hydroxyvitamin D levels and frailty status in older women. J Clin Endocrinol Metab 2010;95:5266–73.
64. Ensrud KE, Blackwell TL, Cauley JA, et al, Osteoporotic Fractures in Men Study Group. Circulating 25-hydroxyvitamin D levels and frailty in older men: the Osteoporotic Fractures in Men study. J Am Geriatr Soc 2011;59:101–6.
65. Morley JE. Should all long-term care residents receive vitamin D? J Am Med Dir Assoc 2007;8:69–70.
66. Tajar A, Lee DM, Pye SR, et al. The association of frailty with serum 25-hydroxyvitamin D and parathyroid hormone levels in older European men. Age Ageing 2012. [Epub ahead of print].
67. Morley JE. Hip fractures. J Am Med Dir Assoc 2010;11:81–3.
68. Murad MH, Elamin KB, Abu Elnour NO, et al. Clinical review: the effect of vitamin D on falls: a systematic review and meta-analysis. J Clin Endocrinol Metab 2011; 96:2997–3006.
69. Kalyani RR, Stein B, Valiyil R, et al. Vitamin D treatment for the prevention of falls in older adults: systematic review and meta-analysis. J Am Geriatr Soc 2010;58: 1299–310.
70. Daly RM. Independent and combined effects of exercise and vitamin D on muscle morphology, function and falls in the elderly. Nutrients 2010;2:1005–17.
71. Ryall JG, Schertzer JD, Lynch GS. Cellular and molecular mechanisms underlying age-related skeletal muscle wasting and weakness. Biogerontology 2008;9:213–28.
72. Drey M, Sieber CC, Bauer JM, et al. C-terminal Agrin Fragment as a potential marker for sarcopenia caused by degeneration of the neuromuscular junction. Exp Gerontol 2012;48(1):76–80.
73. Haren MT, Malmstrom TK, Banks WA, et al. Lower serum DHEAS levels are associated with a higher degree of physical disability and depressive symptoms in middle-aged to older African American women. Maturitas 2007;57: 347–60.
74. Voznesensky M, Walsh S, Dauser D, et al. The association between dehydroepiandrosterone and frailty in older men and women. Age Ageing 2009;38: 401–6.
75. Percheron G, Hogrel JY, Denot-Ledunois S, et al. Effect of 1-year oral administration of dehydroepiandrosterone to 60- to 80-year-old individuals on muscle function and cross-sectional area: a double-blind placebo-controlled trial. Arch Intern Med 2003;163:720–7.

76. Kim MJ, Morley JE. The hormonal fountains of youth: myth or reality? J Endocrinol Invest 2005;28(Suppl 11):5–14.
77. Kenny AM, Boxer RS, Kleppinger A, et al. Dehydroepiandrosterone combined with exercise improves muscle strength and physical function in frail older women. J Am Geriatr Soc 2010;58:1707–14.
78. Perrini S, Laviola L, Carreira MC, et al. The GH/IGF1 axis and signaling pathways in the muscle and bone: mechanisms underlying age-related skeletal muscle wasting and osteoporosis. J Endocrinol 2010;205:201–10.
79. Yeap BB, Paul Chubb SA, Lopez D, et al. Associations of insulin-like growth factor-1 and its binding proteins, and testosterone, with frailty in older men. Clin Endocrinol (Oxf) 2012. [Epub ahead of print]. http://dx.doi.org/10.1111/cen.12052.
80. Rudman D, Feller AG, Nagraj HS, et al. Effects of human growth hormone in men over 60 years old. N Engl J Med 1990;323:1–6.
81. Lissett CA, Shalet SM. Effects of growth hormone on bone and muscle. Growth Horm IGF Res 2000;10(Suppl B):S95–101.
82. Palazzolo I, Stack C, Kong L, et al. Overexpression of IGF-1 in muscle attenuates disease in a mouse model of spinal and bulbar muscular atrophy. Neuron 2009;63:316–28.
83. Muscarò A, Giacinti C, Borsellino G, et al. Stem cell-mediated muscle regeneration is enhanced by local isoform of insulin-like growth factor 1. Proc Natl Acad Sci U S A 2004;101:1206–10.
84. Beauverd M, Mitchell JD, Wokke JH, et al. Recombinant human insulin-like growth factor 1 (rhIGF-1) for the treatment of amyotrophic lateral sclerosis/motor neuron disease. Cochrane Database Syst Rev 2012;(11):CD002064.
85. Heatwole CR, Eichinger KJ, Friedman DI, et al. Open-label trial of recombinant human insulin-like growth factor 1/recombinant human insulin-like growth factor binding protein 3 in myotonic dystrophy type 1. Arch Neurol 2011;68:37–44.
86. Waters D, Danska J, Hardy K, et al. Recombinant human growth hormone, insulin-like growth factor 1, and combination therapy in AIDS-associated wasting. A randomized, double-blind, placebo-controlled trial. Ann Intern Med 1996;125:865–72.
87. Gaskin FS, Farr SA, Banks WA, et al. Ghrelin-induced feeding is dependent on nitric oxide. Peptides 2003;24:913–8.
88. Fouladuin M, Körner U, Bosaeus I, et al. Body composition and time course changes in regional distribution of fat and lean tissue in unselected cancer patients on palliative care—correlations with food intake, metabolism, exercise capacity, and hormones. Cancer 2005;103:2189–98.
89. Garcia JM, Friend J, Allen S. Therapeutic potential of anamorelin, a novel, oral ghrelin mimetic, in patients with cancer-related cachexia: a multicenter, randomized, double-blind, crossover, pilot study. Support Care Cancer 2013;21:129–37.
90. Nass R, Pezzoli SS, Oliveri MC, et al. Effects of an oral ghrelin mimetic on body composition and clinical outcomes in healthy older adults: a randomized trial. Ann Intern Med 2008;149:610–1.
91. Bach MA, Rockwood K, Zetterberg C, et al, MK 0677 Hip Fracture Study Group. The effects of MK-0677, an oral growth hormone secretagogue, in patients with hip fracture. J Am Geriatr Soc 2004;52:516–23.
92. Adunsky A, Chandler J, Heyden N, et al. MK-0677 (ibutamoren mesylate) for the treatment of patients recovering from hip fracture: a multicenter, randomized, placebo-controlled phase IIb study. Arch Gerontol Geriatr 2011;53:183–9.

93. White HK, Petrie CD, Landschulz W, et al. Effects of an oral growth hormone secretagogue in older adults. J Clin Endocrinol Metab 2009;94:1198–206.
94. Schuelke M, Wagner KR, Stolz LE, et al. Myostatin mutation associated with gross muscle hypertrophy in a child. N Engl J Med 2004;350:2682–8.
95. Lakshman KM, Bhasin S, Corcoran C, et al. Measurement of myostatin concentrations in human serum: circulating concentrations in young and older men and effects on testosterone administration. Mol Cell Endocrinol 2009;302:26–32.
96. Han HQ, Mitch WE. Targeting the myostatin signaling pathway to treat muscle wasting diseases. Curr Opin Support Palliat Care 2011;5:334–41.
97. Wagner KR, Fleckenstein JL, Amato AA, et al. A phase I/II trial of MYO-029 in adult subjects with muscular dystrophy. Ann Neurol 2008;63:561–71.
98. Attie KM, Brogstein NG, Yang Y, et al. A single ascending-dose study of muscle regulator ACE-031 in healthy volunteers. Muscle Nerve 2012. [Epub ahead of print]. http://dx.doi.org/10.1002/mus.23539.
99. Sumukadas D, Witham MD, Struthers AD, et al. Ace inhibitors as a therapy for sarcopenia—evidence and possible mechanisms. J Nutr Health Aging 2008; 12:480–5.
100. Witham MD, Sumukadas D, McMurdo ME. ACE inhibitors for sarcopenia—as good as exercise training? Age Ageing 2008;37:363–5.
101. Sumukadas D, Witham MD, Struthers AD, et al. Effect of perindopril on physical function in elderly people with functional impairment: a randomized controlled trial. CMAJ 2007;177:867–74.
102. Peters R, Beckett N, Burch L, et al. The effect of treatment based on a diuretic (indapamide) +/- ACE inhibitor (perindopril) on fractures in the Hypertension in the Very Elderly Trial (HYVET). Age Ageing 2010;39:609–16.
103. Carvalhaes-Neto N, Ramos LR, Vieira JG, et al. Urinary free cortisol is similar in older and younger women. Exp Aging Res 2002;28:163–8.
104. Varadhan R, Walston J, Cappola AR, et al. Higher levels and blunted diurnal variation of cortisol in frail older women. J Gerontol A Biol Sci Med Sci 2008; 63:190–5.
105. Holanda CM, Guerra RO, Nóbrega PV, et al. Salivary cortisol and frailty syndrome in elderly residents of long-stay institutions: a cross-sectional study. Arch Gerontol Geriatr 2012;54:e146–51.
106. Baylis D, Bartlett DB, Syddall HE, et al. Immune-endocrine biomarkers as predictors of frailty and mortality: a 10-year longitudinal study in community-dwelling older people. Age (Dordr) 2012. [Epub ahead of print].
107. Sinclair A, Morley JE, Rodriguez-Manas L, et al. Diabetes mellitus in older people: position statement on behalf of the International Association of Gerontology and Geriatrics (IAGG), the European Diabetes Working Party for Older People (EDWPOP), and the International Task Force of Experts in Diabetes. J Am Med Dir Assoc 2012;13:497–502.
108. Miller DK, Lui LY, Perry HM 3rd, et al. Reported and measured physical functioning in older inner-city diabetic African Americans. J Gerontol A Biol Sci Med Sci 1999;54:M230–6.
109. Morley JE. Diabetes mellitus: "The times they are a-changin". J Am Med Dir Assoc 2012;13:574–5.
110. Bauer JM, Kaiser MJ, Sieber CC. Sarcopenia in nursing home residents. J Am Med Dir Assoc 2008;9:545–51.
111. Goulet ED, Hassaine A, Dionne IJ, et al. Frailty in the elderly is associated with insulin resistance of glucose metabolism in the postabsorptive state only in the presence of increased abdominal fat. Exp Gerontol 2009;44:740–4.

112. Kalyani RR, Varadhan R, Weiss CO, et al. Frailty status and altered glucose-insulin dynamics. J Gerontol A Biol Sci Med Sci 2012;67:1300–6.
113. Kalyani RR, Tian J, Xue WL, et al. Hyperglycemia and incidence of frailty and lower extremity mobility limitations in older women. J Am Geriatr Soc 2012;60:1701–7.
114. Leng SX, Xue QL, Tian J, et al. Inflammation and frailty in older women. J Am Geriatr Soc 2007;55:864–71.
115. Haren MT, Malmstrom TK, Miller DK, et al. Higher C-reactive protein and soluble tumor necrosis factor receptor levels are associated with poor physical function and disability: a cross-sectional analysis of a cohort of late middle-aged African Americans. J Gerontol A Biol Sci Med Sci 2010;65:274–81.
116. Kuikka LK, Salminen S, Ouwehand A, et al. Inflammation markers and malnutrition as risk factors for infections and impaired health-related quality of life among older nursing home residents. J Am Med Dir Assoc 2009;10:348–53.
117. Sullivan DH, Roberson PK, Johnson LE, et al. Association between inflammation-associated cytokines, serum albumins, and mortality in the elderly. J Am Med Dir Assoc 2007;8:458–63.
118. Morley JE, Baumgartner RN. Cytokine-related aging process. J Gerontol A Biol Sci Med Sci 2004;59:M924–9.
119. Bartali B, Frongillo EA, Bandinelli S, et al. Low nutrient intake is an essential component of frailty in older persons. J Gerontol A Biol Sci Med Sci 2006;61: 589–93.
120. Malafarina V, Uriz-Otano F, Iniesta R, et al. Effectiveness of nutritional supplementation on muscle mass in treatment of sarcopenia in old age: a systematic review. J Am Med Dir Assoc 2013;14(1):10–7. http://dx.doi.org/10.1016/j.jamda.2012.08.001 pii:S1525-8610(12)00245-9.
121. Morley JE. Undernutrition: a major problem in nursing homes. J Am Med Dir Assoc 2011;12:243–6.
122. van Wetering CR, Hoogendoorn M, Broekhuizen R, et al. Efficacy and costs of nutritional rehabilitation in muscle-wasted patients with chronic obstructive pulmonary disease in a community-based setting: a prespecified subgroup analysis of the INTERCOM trial. J Am Med Dir Assoc 2010;11:179–87.
123. Neelemaat F, Bosmans JE, Thijs A, et al. Post-discharge nutritional support in malnourished elderly individuals improves functional limitations. J Am Med Dir Assoc 2011;12:295–301.
124. Morley JE, Argiles JM, Evans WJ, et al. Society for Sarcopenia, Cachexia, and Wasting Disease. Nutritional recommendations for the management of sarcopenia. J Am Med Dir Assoc 2010;11:391–6.
125. Tieland M, van de Rest O, Dirks ML, et al. Protein supplementation improves physical performance in frail elderly people: a randomized, double-blind, placebo-controlled trial. J Am Med Dir Assoc 2012;13:720–6.
126. Morley JE. Do frail older persons need more protein? J Am Med Dir Assoc 2012; 13:667–8.
127. Tieland M, Dirks ML, van der Zwaluw N, et al. Protein supplementation increases muscle mass gain during prolonged resistance-type exercise training in frail elderly people: a randomized, double-blind, placebo-controlled trial. J Am Med Dir Assoc 2012;13:713–9.
128. Morley JE. Weight loss in the nursing home. J Am Med Dir Assoc 2007;8:201–4.
129. Rolland Y, Perrin A, Gardette V, et al. Screening older people at risk of malnutrition or malnourished using the Simplified Nutritional Appetite Questionnaire (SNAQ): a comparison with the Mini-Nutritional Assessment (MNA) tool. J Am Med Dir Assoc 2012;13:31–4.

130. Morley JE. Anorexia, weight loss, and frailty. J Am Med Dir Assoc 2010;11:225–8.
131. Morley JE. Weight loss in older persons: new therapeutic approaches. Curr Pharm Des 2007;13:3637–47.
132. Ensrud KE, Ewing SK, Stone KL, et al, Study of Osteoporotic Fractures Research Group. Intentional and unintentional weight loss increase bone loss and hip fracture risk in older women. J Am Geriatr Soc 2003;51:1740–7.
133. Villareal DT, Chode S, Parimi N, et al. Weight loss, exercise, or both and physical function in obese older adults. N Engl J Med 2011;364:1218–29.
134. Valenzuela T. Efficacy of progressive resistance training interventions in older adults in nursing homes: a systematic review. J Am Med Dir Assoc 2012;13:418–28.
135. Yamada M, Arai H, Sonoda T, et al. Community-based exercise program is cost-effective by preventing care and disability in Japanese frail older adults. J Am Med Dir Assoc 2012;13:507–11.
136. Marzolini S, Oh PI, Brooks D. Effect of combined aerobic resistance training versus aerobic training alone in individuals with coronary artery disease: a meta-analysis. Eur J Prev Cardiol 2012;19:81–94.
137. Tschopp M, Sattelmayer MK, Hilfiker R. Is power training or conventional resistance training better for function in elderly persons? A meta-analysis. Age Ageing 2011;40:549–56.
138. Peterson MD, Gordon PM. Resistance exercise for the aging adult: clinical implications and prescription guidelines. Am J Med 2011;124:194–8.
139. Nicola F, Catherine S. Dose-response relationship of resistance training in older adults: a meta-analysis. Br J Sports Med 2011;45:233–4.
140. Singh NA, Quine S, Clemson LM, et al. Effects of high-intensity progressive resistance training and targeted multidisciplinary treatment of frailty on mortality and nursing home admissions after hip fracture: a randomized controlled trial. J Am Med Dir Assoc 2012;13:24–30.
141. Chou CH, Hwang CL, Wu YT. Effect of exercise on physical function, daily living activities, and quality of life in the frail older adults: a meta-analysis. Arch Phys Med Rehabil 2012;93:237–44.
142. Theou O, Stathokostas L, Roland KP, et al. The effectiveness of exercise interventions for the management of frailty: a systematic review. J Aging Res 2011;2011:569194. http://dx.doi.org/10.4061/2011/569194.
143. Rejeski WJ, Marsh AP, Chmelo E, et al. The Lifestyle Interventions and Independence for Elders Pilot (LIFE-P): 2-year followup. J Gerontol A Biol Sci Med Sci 2009;64:462–7.

ndex

ote: Page numbers of article titles are in **boldface** type.

A

Endocrinol Metab Clin N Am 42 (2013) 407–433
http://dx.doi.org/10.1016/S0889-8529(13)00032-7

C

D

E

G

H

I

K

L

M

N

O

S

U

V

Moving?

Make sure your subscription moves with you!

To notify us of your new address, find your **Clinics Account Number** (located on your mailing label above your name), and contact customer service at:

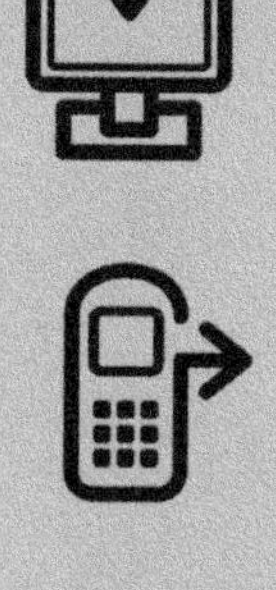

Email: journalscustomerservice-usa@elsevier.com

800-654-2452 (subscribers in the U.S. & Canada)
314-447-8871 (subscribers outside of the U.S. & Canada)

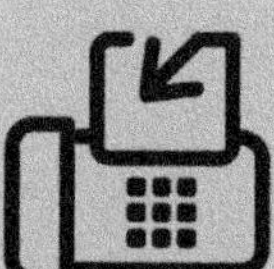

Fax number: 314-447-8029

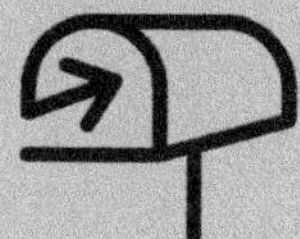

Elsevier Health Sciences Division
Subscription Customer Service
3251 Riverport Lane
Maryland Heights, MO 63043

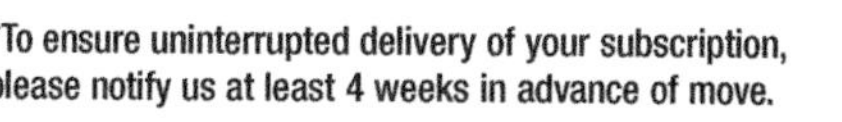

*To ensure uninterrupted delivery of your subscription, please notify us at least 4 weeks in advance of move.

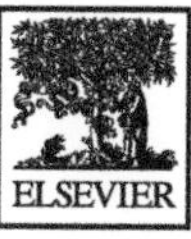

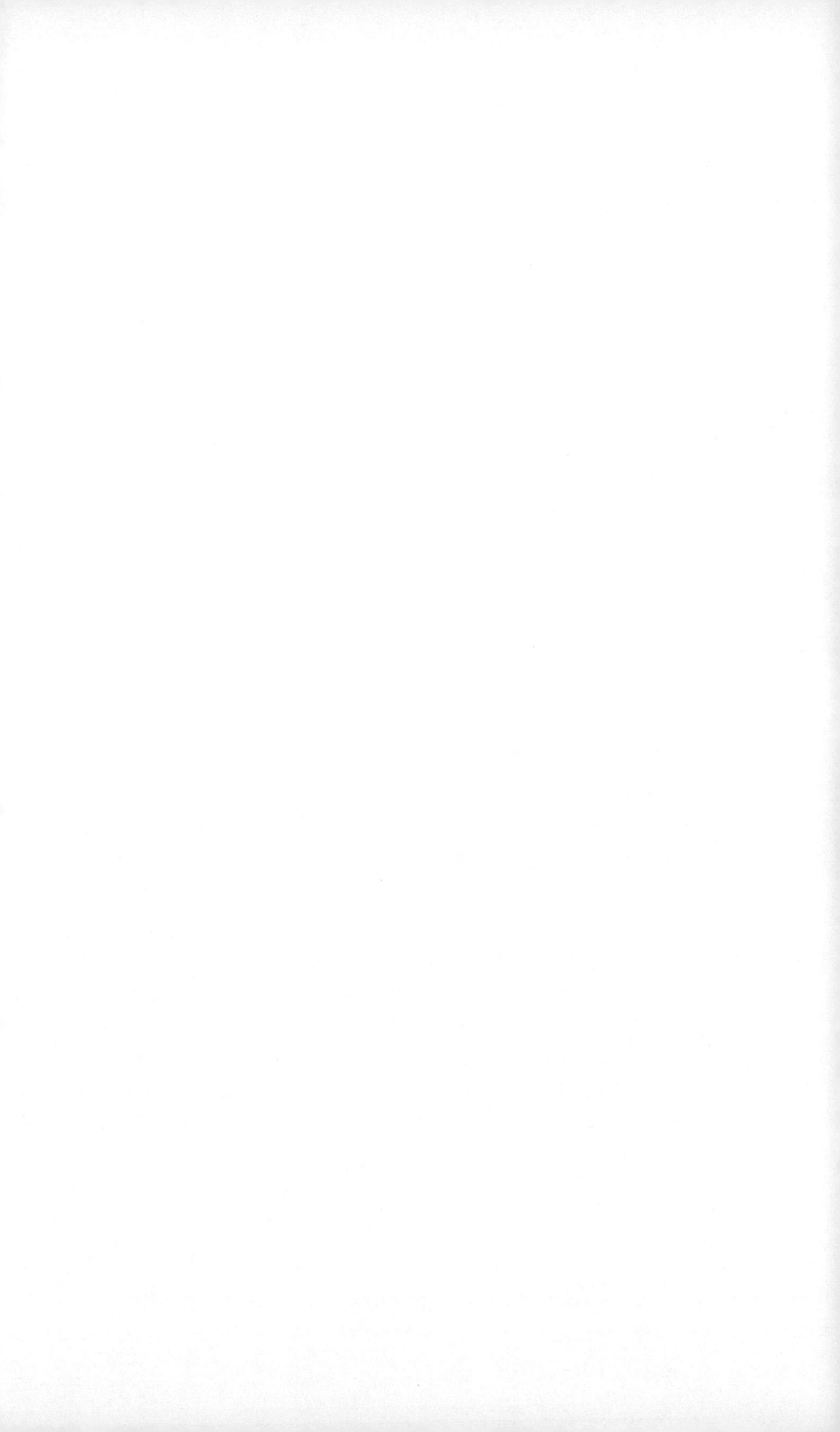

Printed and bound by CPI Group (UK) Ltd, Croydon, CR0 4YY

03/10/2024

01040440-0008